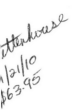

Essentials of
Nursing Law and Ethics

Susan J. Westrick, JD, MS, RN, CNE
Professor
Department of Nursing
Southern Connecticut State University
New Haven, Connecticut

Attorney at Law
Branford, Connecticut

Katherine Dempski, JD, BSN, RN
Director of Risk Management
Maine Medical Center
Portland, Maine

JONES AND BARTLETT PUBLISHERS
Sudbury, Massachusetts
BOSTON   TORONTO   LONDON   SINGAPORE

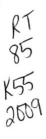

World Headquarters

Jones and Bartlett Publishers
40 Tall Pine Drive
Sudbury, MA 01776
978-443-5000
info@jbpub.com
www.jbpub.com

Jones and Bartlett Publishers
Canada
6339 Ormindale Way
Mississauga, Ontario L5V 1J2
Canada

Jones and Bartlett Publishers
International
Barb House, Barb Mews
London W6 7PA
United Kingdom

Jones and Bartlett's books and products are available through most bookstores and online booksellers. To contact Jones and Bartlett Publishers directly, call 800-832-0034, fax 978-443-8000, or visit our website www.jbpub.com.

Substantial discounts on bulk quantities of Jones and Bartlett's publications are available to corporations, professional associations, and other qualified organizations. For details and specific discount information, contact the special sales department at Jones and Bartlett via the above contact information or send an email to specialsales@jbpub.com.

The authors, editor, and publisher have made every effort to provide accurate information. However, they are not responsible for errors, omissions, or for any outcomes related to the use of the contents of this book and take no responsibility for the use of the products and procedures described. Treatments and side effects described in this book may not be applicable to all people; likewise, some people may require a dose or experience a side effect that is not described herein. Drugs and medical devices are discussed that may have limited availability controlled by the Food and Drug Administration (FDA) for use only in a research study or clinical trial. Research, clinical practice, and government regulations often change the accepted standard in this field. When consideration is being given to use of any drug in the clinical setting, the health care provider or reader is responsible for determining FDA status of the drug, reading the package insert, and reviewing prescribing information for the most up-to-date recommendations on dose, precautions, and contraindications, and determining the appropriate usage for the product. This is especially important in the case of drugs that are new or seldom used.

Production Credits
Publisher: Kevin Sullivan
Acquisitions Editor: Emily Ekle
Acquisitions Editor: Amy Sibley
Associate Editor: Patricia Donnelly
Editorial Assistant: Rachel Shuster
Supervising Production Editor: Carolyn F. Rogers
Associate Marketing Manager: Ilana Goddess
V.P., Manufacturing and Inventory Control: Therese Connell
Composition: Auburn Associates, Inc.
Cover Design: Kate Ternullo
Cover Image: A detail of the columns and entrance engravings of the US Supreme Court in Washington, DC.
    © Stephen Finn/ShutterStock, Inc.
Printing and Binding: Malloy, Inc.
Cover Printing: Malloy, Inc.

Library of Congress Cataloging-in-Publication Data
Killion, Susan Westrick.
    Essentials of nursing law and ethics / Susan J. Westrick, Katherine Dempski.
        p. ; cm.
    Includes bibliographical references and index.
    ISBN-13: 978-0-7637-5302-3 (pbk.)
    ISBN-10: 0-7637-5302-5 (pbk.)
    1. Nursing ethics. 2. Nursing—Law and legislation—United States. I. Dempski, Katherine. II. Title.
    [DNLM: 1. Legislation, Nursing—United States. 2. Ethics, Nursing—United States. WY 33 AA1 K48e 2009]
    RT85.K55 2009
    174.2--dc22

                                                                            2008043627

6048
Printed in the United States of America
12 11 10 09 08   10 9 8 7 6 5 4 3 2 1

Contents

Preface

The authors' first book on legal and ethical issues in the *Quick Look Nursing* series (2000) has been transformed into a second book that is extensively updated and documented. This new book has an in-depth and scholarly focus that provides a foundation for evidence-based accountability in nursing practice. The basic organization and structure of the new book remains the same with five major parts: The Law and Nursing Practice, Liability in Patient Care, Documentation Issues, Employment and the Workplace, and Ethics.

Essentials of Nursing Law and Ethics retains the same central purpose of offering the reader concise yet scholarly chapters that cover discrete topics of critical importance to nursing students and practicing nurses. In addition to updates, new content has been added that doubles the length of the previous book. Of most importance is that every chapter reviews current court cases involving nurses, in addition to core content that is essential to every nursing curriculum. These cases are the result of extensive legal research conducted by the authors and represent the most recent information. The legal issues and outcomes discussed in the case law, along with legislation, regulations, and statutes, guide nurses to ensure accountability in their practice.

Highlights of new or expanded legal and ethical content include:

- Focus on medication administration, including IV, patient controlled analgesia, criminalization of unintended medication errors, automated medication dispensing systems, high-alert drugs, and medication error reduction
- Error and event reporting, including CMS, Joint Commission, and state law requirements for mandatory disclosure of medical errors to patients and families
- Internal reporting for process improvement and mandatory reporting of adverse events under state statutes, accreditation, and regulatory agencies
- State board of nursing regulation and reporting to the National Practitioner Data Bank (NPDB) and Healthcare Integrity and Protection Data Bank (HIPDB)
- Staffing issues, short staffing, floating, and refusing assignments
- Working with unlicensed personnel, with student nurses, and as supervisors
- Accountability for patient advocacy, including refusal to implement unsafe orders
- Electronic documentation and record-keeping, electronic communication, and HIPAA privacy rules
- Workplace safety, including environmental health and safety and medical devices
- CMS and Joint Commission regulations in sentinel events, restraint use, patients' rights, and end-of-life issues
- Legal implications of passive euthanasia and terminal sedation
- A new and useful appendix guide to legal research, written by Susan Clerc, a reference librarian and attorney, includes how to search for cases, statutes and regulations; examples and explanations of case law components; identification of electronic databases; and search techniques for basic legal research

The target audience for the book is primarily nursing students in prelicensure educational programs, and for practicing nurses as an authoritative reference. Self-study questions for students with explicit rationales for correct and incorrect answers are included at the end of each section to enhance critical thinking and problem solving. In addition to scholarly legal and professional references and case law citations at the end of each chapter, many chapters cite additional bibliographic material and Web sites as supplements. The book is also useful as a text in selected graduate courses or as a resource for continuing education programs. Nursing faculty will find the book an invaluable tool to assist their teaching of these challenging but essential topics. The authors have prepared a secured TestBank to assist in evaluation of student learning which is available online at *http://nursing.jbpub.com*. Many of the questions incorporate the NCLEX® format and item structure.

Although this second book has been greatly expanded and changed in depth and focus, basic information from the first book has been retained. Therefore, the work of contributors to the first text is gratefully acknowledged as follows:

Diana C. Ballard, JD, MBA, RN
Doreen J. Bonadies, JD, RN

Regina M. Murphy, JD, BSN
Barbara Dunham, JD, RN
Roberta G. Geller, JD, BS, RN
Cynthia Keenan, JD, BA, RN
Melinda S. Monson, JD, MSN, RN
Lynda L. Nemeth, JD, RN
Susan B. Ramsey, JD, BSN
Joanne P. Sheehan, JD, RN
Maureen Townsend, JD, RN

As nurse attorneys with extensive experience in nursing practice and education, private law practice, and healthcare risk management, we have blended and integrated our unique perspectives into the content of the book. Our involvement with the American Association of Nurse Attorneys (TAANA) has further enriched our insights. In presenting this essential information we hope to broaden and deepen an understanding of many of the complex issues faced by nurses. This authoritative reference serves as a guide and framework for legally and ethically sound practice.

Susan J. Westrick and Katherine Dempski

Contributor

Susan J. Clerc, MLS, JD, PhD
Electronic Resource Coordinator/Reference Librarian
Southern Connecticut State University
New Haven, Connecticut

Acronyms

AAP	American Academy of Pediatrics
ADA	Americans with Disabilities Act
AHA	American Hospital Association
AHRQ	Agency for Healthcare Research and Quality
AIDS	acquired immunodeficiency syndrome
ANA	American Nurses Association
ANCC	American Nurses Credentialing Center
BSN	bachelor of science in nursing
CAPTA	Child Abuse Prevention and Treatment Act
CBA	collective bargaining agreement
CDC	Centers for Disease Control and Prevention
CMS	Centers for Medicare and Medicaid
CMV	cytomegalovirus
CPR	computerized patient record
EEOC	Equal Employment Opportunity Commission
EMTLA	Emergency Medical Treatment and Labor Act
ENA	Emergency Nurses Association
FCA	False Claims Act
FDA	Food and Drug Administration
FMLA	Family Medical Leave Act
FOIA	Freedom of Information Act
FTCA	Federal Tort Claims Act
HCFA	Health Care Financing Administration
HIPAA	Health Insurance Portability and Accountability Act
HIV	human immunodeficiency virus
HMO	health maintenance organization
HRSA	Health Resources and Services Administration
IOM	Institute of Medicine
IV	intravenous
IM	intramuscular
LMRA	Labor Management Relations Act
LPN	licensed practical nurse
NCSBN	National Council of State Boards of Nursing
NIOSH	National Institute for Occupational Safety and Health
NLRA	National Labor Relations Act
NLRB	National Labor Relations Board
NPA	nurse practice act
OBRA	Omnibus Reconciliation Act
OPO	organ procurement organization
OPTN	Organ Procurement and Transplantation Network

OSHA	Occupational and Safety Health Act
PCA	patient-controlled analgesia
Prn	as needed
PSDA	Patient Self-Determination Act
RN	registered nurse
STD	sexually transmitted disease
TAANA	The American Association of Nurse Attorneys
UAP	unlicensed assistive personnel
UNOS	United Network for Organ Sharing

The Law and Nursing Practice

Chapter 1

The Legal Environment

Susan J. Westrick and Katherine Dempski

Civil and Criminal Court System

Federal

U.S. Supreme Court
- Appeals from U.S. Court of Appeals
- Appeals from State Supreme Courts
  (involving federal or constitutional law)
  - Lawsuits between states

U.S. courts of appeals
- Appeals from lower district courts

U.S. district courts
- Civil lawsuits or criminal acts involving federal law
  or between litigants with diverse citizenship

State

State supreme court
- Appeals from state appellate courts
  final decision in that state
  (unless constitutional issue)

State appellate court
- Appeals from state trial courts

State district courts
- Criminal (divided by geographical area)
- Civil (divided in jurisdictions)

■ DEFINITION OF LAW

Law has been defined as the formalization of a body of rules of action or conduct prescribed that is enforced by binding legal authority or as the sum total of rules and regulations by which society is governed. Because law reflects society's values, it is by definition an ever-changing concept subject to modification. The law reflects the will of the people as represented by legislative or judicial bodies (almost all of whom are elected) that enact the law or interpret the law.

■ SOURCES AND TYPES OF LAW

Constitutional law is the organizational framework of a system of laws or principles that govern a nation, system, corporation, or other organization. It forms the basis of how that entity will be governed. The US Constitution (and its amendments) is the supreme law of the

United States and sets forth the general organization of the government and the powers and limitations of the federal government. The best-known limitations on the powers of the government are the first 10 amendments, known as the Bill of Rights. These incorporate such concepts as free speech, freedom of religion, and the right not to be deprived of life, liberty, or the pursuit of happiness without due process of law. Any rights not expressly granted to the federal government are reserved to the states.

Also established by the US Constitution are the three branches of government: executive, judicial, and legislative. These serve as a system of checks and balances, with powers distributed among them.

Individual states have constitutions as well and are an important source of legal rights. If there is a conflict between federal and state law, the federal law would take precedence as the supreme law. The Court can also declare that laws are invalid and unconstitutional when they are not consistent with the constitution (*Marbury v. Madison*, 1803).

Enactments by the legislative branches of government are known as *statutes,* the written laws that are "on the books" and codified or available in writing. Examples are the US code that contains federal statutes, state statutes (such as the Connecticut General Statutes), and ordinances passed by city or municipal government representatives. The nurse practice act (NPA) is an example of a statutory law that is available for review in the written statutes of each state.

Administrative agencies (e.g., National Labor Relations Board, state board of nursing) are empowered by legislative bodies to implement a certain area of law called *administrative law*. The administrative agency has delegated power to make administrative rules and regulations and to adjudicate disputes within the area of delegated power. Decisions by these agencies are subject to judicial review on a very limited basis, and the agency is considered to be the expert decision maker in its area of expertise.

Administrative rules, regulations, and decisions are subject to administrative procedure acts, which also govern their activities.

Attorney generals' opinions are another source of administrative law. An attorney general may be asked to render an opinion related to an important aspect of administrative law. This will stand as binding until it is overruled by a specific statute, regulation, or court order. These opinions serve as an important source of guidance in interpreting statutory or common law.

The *common law,* or *case law,* is the result of judicial decisions made from disputes that arise and are decided in courts of law. Case law is an important source of guidance for others who may be in similar circumstances because it serves as legal precedent in the jurisdiction where the decision was made. Even though case law is not precedent for other jurisdictions, courts often look to case law for guidance in similar situations. Important case law (usually that which has been appealed) is reported in case law books, which are available at law libraries.

■ THE COURT SYSTEM

Courts in the federal, state, and municipal systems are organized in a tierlike structure (see **Figure 1-1**). The lowest level is the trial court where cases are first heard. The second level is the intermediate court, or court of appeals, where the case is taken if one of the parties is not satisfied with the outcome in the trial court. The highest level in the system, the supreme court, often makes the final decision, but higher courts do not automatically take all cases that seek an appeal. The trial court for the federal system is called the *federal district court,* and the intermediate courts are divided into circuits that cover several states. It is important to know in which court a case is decided to determine if it is applicable as precedent in a subsequent case.

Many special branches of trial courts have a particular area of authority or jurisdiction (e.g., probate court often is the designated court for decisions related to competency of patients, family court may handle termination of parental rights).

■ PROCEDURAL AND SUBSTANTIVE RIGHTS

Procedural laws (e.g., evidence and jurisdictional laws) prescribe the manner in which rights and responsibilities are exercised and enforced in court. They provide the form and manner of conducting judicial business before the court. *Substantive laws* (contract, criminal, and civil laws) define and give rights that the court administers.

The due process clause in the 5th and 14th amendments provides citizens with *procedural* and *substantive due process*. *Procedural due process* applies when a citizen has been deprived of a life, liberty, or property interest. The person is entitled to be heard in a proceeding (hearing right) and must be notified of such a right before the deprivation (notice right). Substantive due process requires fair legislation that should be reasonable in context as well as application. No one should be unreasonably or arbitrarily deprived of life, liberty, or property.

■ LAWSUITS AND LEGAL PROCESSES

When parties disagree, or when someone wants to assert an individual right, a lawsuit may be filed to resolve the issues (see **Figure 1-2**). The purpose of bringing a lawsuit is to resolve the matter at hand in an orderly and fair manner. The person who brings the lawsuit, or *plaintiff*, files a *complaint* outlining allegations against one or more defendants. A *summons* is issued, and the complaint is served upon the defendants, who must answer the allegations set forth in the complaint. Failure to file and answer the complaint in a timely fashion may result in a default judgment in favor of the plaintiff. The defendant may answer the complaint with counterclaims of his own and may deny the allegations. Both the plaintiff and the defendant usually retain an attorney to represent them in the legal action.

Nurses are sometimes involved as defendants in lawsuits by a patient/plaintiff. The patient may allege malpractice or negligence by the nurse during a professional relationship. The hospital or agency that employs the nurse as well as other caregivers, such as physicians, are often named in the same lawsuit as party defendants. This results in multiple attorneys and insurance companies being involved in the same proceeding. Allegations against each of these parties must be proven for the plaintiff to prevail against that party. Plaintiffs are increasingly naming multiple defendants, including nurses, to improve their chances of a full recovery.

In other situations, the nurse may be the plaintiff party who is seeking reinstatement following an alleged wrongful discharge by the defendant employer. Although the nurse may have malpractice insurance to cover expenses related defending a malpractice claim, costs of litigation are most often the individual nurse's responsibility in other types of legal actions.

A period of *discovery* usually follows the defendant's answer during which the parties

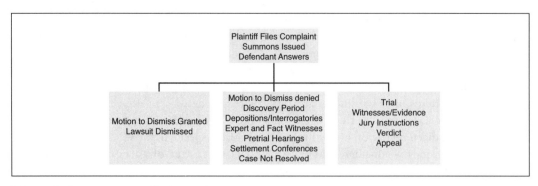

Figure 1-2 Anatomy of a lawsuit.

gather information and make official statements about the facts surrounding the incident in question. *Depositions*, or sworn statements, may be made in the presence of a court reporter, or written *interrogatories* may be answered, both of which preserve the evidence for later use at trial. During any of the discovery proceedings, either party may file a motion with the court for a *summary judgment* in their favor. If granted, the lawsuit is ended, unless the losing party seeks an appeal of that order.

One of the purposes of discovery is to reveal what facts the witnesses and parties know regarding the claim, thus "discovering" the facts that will be admitted at trial to resolve the case. By completing this less formal discovery process before the trial begins, the parties may reach a settlement, or a party may withdraw the lawsuit if it is anticipated that the case cannot be proven. Pretrial hearings and settlement conferences precede the actual trial.

If the case continues, there is a trial where either a judge or jury will hear the case and make a decision, depending on the nature of the proceedings. Various motions can be made by either party during the trial, including a *motion to dismiss* the action. Witnesses testify and are examined and cross examined by the opposing party's attorney, and other evidence is presented at the trial. The plaintiff presents his case first, and then the defendant presents his case, and either party may request a motion for dismissal or a *directed verdict* based on a lack of evidence presented by the opposing party.

The jury is instructed by the judge on the law related to the case, and then the jury deliberates and reviews the case. Finally a *verdict* or outcome of the case is reached, and the *judgment* is executed. The losing party may still make a motion for a *judgment notwithstanding the verdict* or take a later *appeal* of the judgment.

ALTERNATIVE DISPUTE RESOLUTION

Sometimes a lawsuit can be avoided if the parties agree to use other methods to settle a dispute or if this right arises, for example, from a contract. One process is to use a *mediator* or impartial party who meets with the parties and attempts to have each understand the other party's views. Thus a voluntary settlement or mediation of the matter may result, often at a considerable cost savings compared to having a lawsuit proceed.

Another method is an *arbitration* proceeding where an arbitrator is selected by the parties, and a legally binding decision is offered by the arbitrator. The arbitrator, a neutral party, who is sometimes an attorney, hears both sides of the dispute in a more informal proceeding where witnesses can be heard and questioned. There is no court reporter to make a formal recording of the proceeding. Both parties agree before the arbitration hearing that the arbitrator's judgment will be legally binding.

Increasingly, parties are using alternative dispute resolution processes to avoid both the costs and length of a lawsuit. There are attorneys and others who specialize in this area of practice.

The Appendix (p. 301) provides a comprehensive guide for basic legal research and explains how to read citations for case law, statutes, and regulations. Pointers for how to conduct legal research using electronic databases, search engines, library references, commercial law publishers, and public Web sites are discussed. Sample cases are illustrated to assist the reader in identifying components of opinions and to trace the path of a case through the legal system. This valuable resource provides guidance for nurses to find authoritative legal references and information when conducting a literature search.

REFERENCES

Marbury v. Madison, 5 U.S. (1 Cranch) 137 (1803).

Miller, R. (2006). Introduction to the American legal system. In *Problems in health care law* (9th ed.). Sudbury, MA: Jones and Bartlett.

Chapter 2

Regulation of Nursing Practice

Susan J. Westrick

A Licensure

Enables nurse to work as an RN and use this title

↓

Mandatory (all states):
Anyone performing nursing activities
and using title RN must be licensed

↓

Multistate licensure and mutual recognition
• Practice beyond state borders
• NCSBN created Nursing Licensure Compact (NLC)
• RN and LPN/VN Compact, APRN Compact
• Mutual recognition of license in participating NLC state

B Nurse Practice Acts

• Entry requirements	• License renewal	• Disciplinary actions
• Scope of practice	• Advanced practice	• Special provisions

C Credentialing

• Recognition of knowledge and skills exceeding basic practice
  (performance, knowledge, and preparation requirements)

• Recognition by specialty organization

• Can use initials with title RN, e.g., certified oncology nurse (CON)

■ LICENSURE

Licensure is the process by which a governmental agency (state health department through the board of nursing) entitles a person to practice a certain profession (see **Figure 2-1A**). Licensing laws derive their power from the police power of the state to protect the public. In addition to protecting the public, these statutes regulate the profession. Licensure of an individual as a nurse or a registered nurse (RN) assures the public that the person is qualified to assume the duties as specified for this professional practitioner. However, licensure only assures minimal safety and competence and does not specify a particular educational background or degree, unless required by the state statute or regulations.

All states have mandatory licensure—all persons who are compensated for nursing services and perform the duties of an RN must be licensed. Both the designation of "RN" and the actions of RNs are protected by the statute. Exceptions to this rule include student nurses who provide nursing services while enrolled in educational programs.

Violation of these statutes or practicing nursing without a license is a crime, as is aiding or assisting another to practice nursing without a license. Penalties may include fines or more severe sanctions, such as confinement. Those who harm patients may be liable for civil damages in suits that allege negligence.

■ MULTISTATE LICENSURE AND MUTUAL RECOGNITION

Regulation of nursing practice across state borders has become an increasing concern of professional nursing organizations. With the advent of telenursing, many issues have been raised concerning the "site" of practice and which state's NPA would prevail in questionable situations. In 1998, the National Council of State Boards of Nursing (NCSBN) approved the Nursing Licensure Compact (NLC) to address interstate licensure for registered nurses and licensed practical nurses or vocational nurses (RN and LVN/VN Compact). This allows an individual to have one license (in his or her state of residency) and to practice in other states (both physically and electronically), subject to that state's practice laws and regulations. This mutual recognition model of nurse licensure calls for recognition of persons licensed in another state, similar to the procedure used for drivers' licenses. In order to achieve mutual recognition, each state must enact legislation or regulations authorizing the Nurse Licensure Compact. States must also

adopt administrative rules and regulations for implementing the compact. To date, 23 states have entered into the NCL for RNs and LPN/VNs. In 2002 the NCSBN approved adoption of a licensure compact for advanced practice registered nurses (APRNs). Utah became the first state to pass the APRN Compact Law legislation in 2004, and to date Iowa and Texas have also passed these laws. Many specialty nursing organizations, other healthcare organizations, and state boards of nursing have endorsed the NLC. However, some professional nursing organizations, such as the American Nurses Association (ANA) and individual state boards of nursing, have expressed multiple concerns about multistate licensure and have not endorsed this plan. A few states have agreed to adopt the compact on a trial basis.

■ NURSE PRACTICE ACTS

NPAs are individual to each state. However, they typically follow model NPAs as defined by the NCSBN or the ANA. NPAs define entry requirements for the profession (such as graduation from an approved educational program for nursing), duties and composition of the state board of nursing, scope of practice, grounds for disciplinary action, license renewal and fees, and other regulatory rules (see Figure 2-1B).

State legislatures modify and update NPAs in what is often a long and challenging process. Changes are usually initiated by the state nurses association in response to a need identified by the professional community.

Provisions

Nurse practice acts contain the following:

- Scope of practice: These provisions are broad in nature and provide guidance for nursing actions. They provide the legal boundaries for practice. Most statutes incorporate language for nurses to "diagnose human responses to actual or potential health problems" and to "assess needs of patients." Many also specify "health counseling, referral, patient teaching, and prescribing nursing actions" as nursing activities. Nurses need to check the scope of their practice as related to the licensed practical nurse (LPN). Most often the LPN works under the supervision or direction of the RN. Independent nursing actions are identified along with those that are interdependent or dependent, such as administration of medications prescribed by other practitioners. These provisions are purposefully broad so that the practice act does not become outdated as nursing practice continues to evolve.

- Advanced practice: Many NPAs have separate sections for advanced practice nursing that often permit diagnosis of certain medical conditions, prescription of medications following practice protocols, and treatment of some conditions. Some specify that these nurses have written agreements with supervising physicians or work under the supervision of a physician. Some specialized advanced practice nurses, such as nurse midwives and nurse anesthetists, have separate statutes that regulate their practice.

- Special provisions: Some states have passed provisions for mandatory continuing education for license renewal to help ensure continued competency. Two states, North Dakota and Maine, have provisions or regulations specifying a bachelor of science in nursing (BSN) as the entry criterion for initial licensure of RNs. Each nurse needs to check the state NPA because the requirements for practice vary among states.

■ INTERACTION WITH RELATED HEALTHCARE PRACTITIONERS

Other healthcare practitioners (e.g., physicians, physician's assistants, social workers, etc.) have separate practice acts that can

potentially affect nursing practice. Practicing outside the scope of one's practice can have serious consequences, including successful malpractice claims if patient injury results. The person who acts outside the scope of practice usually is held to the standard of the other practitioner for purposes of malpractice. Thus, if an RN removed a patient's cast and this action was outside the scope of practice for an RN, the nurse would be held accountable to the standard required by the practitioner (herein an MD). Other actions may be sustained as well, including other tort actions for fraud, crimes, or disciplinary actions by the state board of nursing or other regulatory bodies.

■ CREDENTIALING

Another means to regulate practice is by credentialing (see Figure 2-1C). Credentialing usually involves endorsement or recognition by a specialized organization or specialty group that the nurse has certain qualifications that exceed basic competence. The nurse has met additional standards of performance and preparation and can then use initials appropriate to the credential or certification after the title RN. As an example, on behalf of the ANA, the American Nurses Credentialing Center (ANCC) certifies nurses in certain specialties, such as nursing administration or oncology nursing. Often educational, practice, and testing criteria have to be met. For advance practice nurses, the nurse practice act may require certification by a national certifying organization, such as ANCC. Certification is often for several years; thereafter, the nurse must become recertified. Many other specialty organizations, such as the Emergency Nurse Organization, certify nurses for specialty practice.

■ CHALLENGES TO NURSING PRACTICE

In *Sermchief v. Gonzales* (1983) the Missouri Board of Healing Arts, which regulated physicians, challenged the scope of practice for nurse practitioners working in a public clinic offering reproductive services. The nurses were supervised by physicians and performed gynecological exams, Papanicolaou (Pap) smears, and birth control counseling. Protocols were in place to guide their practice. In its declaratory ruling, the appeals court overruled the court below and found that the nurses were in fact practicing under the nurse practice act, not the statute that regulated physicians. The court looked to the historical development and broad language in the nursing statute that permitted nursing practice to evolve. Of particular relevance was the portion of the statute that permitted practice that "included but was not limited to" the nursing functions that were listed in the statute. The court also noted that there were no allegations that the nurses were not educated or trained to perform these tasks and that they were supervised and operating under protocols to support their practice. This case validated the legal foundation and support for the evolution of advanced practice nursing.

■ PRELICENSURE CONSIDERATIONS

Many states evaluate nursing licensure applicants for prior criminal convictions, especially felonies. Applicants or newly admitted nursing students should be informed that the question of licensure is a state board of nursing function, and criminal background will likely be considered in whether to initially license an individual or place restrictions on a nurse's license. In rare instances it could be possible for someone to graduate from a nursing program but later be denied licensure by the state board as a registered nurse. The justification for this is the mandate of the board of nursing to protect the public. The public places trust in nurses and other licensed healthcare practitioners, and they are expected to be of good moral and ethical character. In a recent study by Alison Chevette, Marla Erbin-Rosemann, and Charlene Kelly (2007), it was found that there was no correlation between prior criminal conviction and disciplinary action following licensure. These researchers compared records of 184 disciplined nurses in Nebraska who had prior criminal convictions to a control group of 184 nurses without any disciplinary actions on their licenses. Nevertheless, potential applicants to nursing education programs or for licensure should check with the state board of nursing in any state they expect to be working if they are concerned about prior criminal convictions.

■ REFERENCE

Chevette, A., Erbin-Rosemann, M., & Kelly, C. (2007). Nursing licensure: An examination of the relationship between criminal conviction and licensure. *Journal of Nursing Law, 11*(1), 5–11.

Sermchief v. Gonzales, 660 S.W.2d 683 (Mo., banc., 1983).

■ ADDITIONAL REFERENCE

National Council of State Boards of Nursing: www.ncsbn.org

Chapter 3

Nurses in Legal Actions

Katherine Dempski

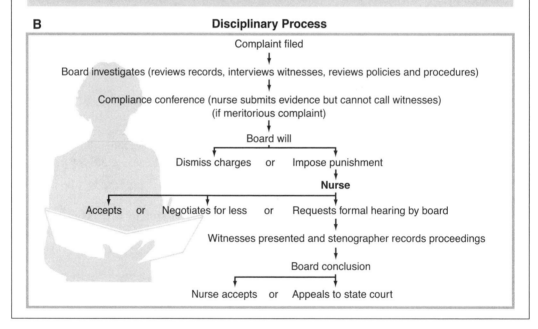

A

Most Common Grounds for Disciplinary Charges
- Fraud or deception in obtaining a nursing license, or falsifying insurance claim forms or patient hospital records.
- Physical or mental impairment such as loss of motor skill or mobility and mental illnesses such as schizophrenia. Having a physical or mental impairment doesn't necessarily mean that the nurse's license will be in jeopardy; however, the nurse must be able to perform the job. The board may request that the nurse undergo a physical or psychological examination to determine ability to practice nursing.
- Illegal conduct, incompetence, or negligence in carrying out a nursing function. A nurse can be disciplined even if the acts did not cause injury to the patient.
- Drug or alcohol abuse. Many state boards recognize the problems of chemical dependency and will require participation in a rehabilitation program.
- Abusive behavior, either physical or verbal.
- Conviction of a criminal offense.

B   **Disciplinary Process**

Complaint filed
↓
Board investigates (reviews records, interviews witnesses, reviews policies and procedures)
↓
Compliance conference (nurse submits evidence but cannot call witnesses)
(if meritorious complaint)
↓
Board will
┌──────────────┴──────────────┐
Dismiss charges   or   Impose punishment
↓
Nurse
┌──────────┬──────────────────┬──────────────┐
Accepts or Negotiates for less or Requests formal hearing by board
↓
Witnesses presented and stenographer records proceedings
↓
Board conclusion
┌──────────────┴──────────────┐
Nurse accepts   or   Appeals to state court

Nurses may become involved in different types of actions within the legal system, including criminal actions, administrative law actions, and civil actions. A nurse who makes an error administering medicine is susceptible to a civil malpractice action by the patient who is injured and a disciplinary proceeding by the licensing board. The same nurse may be subject to criminal charges if the error was so egregious that it constituted negligent homicide or manslaughter.

CRIMINAL ACTIONS

Criminal actions are brought by the state against a defendant accused of breaking a law. Nurses have been prosecuted for crimes such as negligent homicide, manslaughter, theft of narcotics, insurance fraud, and falsifying medical records. A nurse who attempts to conceal a negligent nursing action (civil action) by entering false information in a medical record commits fraud and falsification of a record and could face criminal charges for these crimes.

When a nurse's professional negligence rises to the level of "reckless disregard for human life" (a legal standard of conduct), the nurse may face criminal charges of negligent homicide or manslaughter. Each charge is defined in the state criminal statutes and requires certain elements the state must prove. Two well-known cases involving the initiation of criminal charges against nurses for clinical actions were the Colorado nurse who administered a lethal dose of penicillin and the New Jersey nurses who were accused of failing to notify the physician that the patient was lethargic and unresponsive. In those cases nurses either pleaded guilty, were acquitted, or took a pretrial intervention (in which no criminal charges are brought as long as the defendants meet certain criteria).

ADMINISTRATIVE LAW ACTIONS

Administrative law agencies are created by state statutes that define the agencies' purpose, functions, and powers. The state board of nursing is an administrative law agency. The governor of the state typically appoints members to the board of nursing, and most state statutes determine the number of board members, the professional requirements, and the length of appointment. The board of nursing is empowered by the NPA to administer and establish the rules and regulations of nursing practice, educational requirements, licensing for practice, licensure renewal requirements, and approval of schools of nursing. In addition, the board enforces the state's NPA and is responsible for disciplinary actions.

DISCIPLINARY ACTIONS

Each board of nursing is charged with the responsibility to maintain the standards of the nursing profession within the state and to protect the public. The board may conduct an investigation to determine whether a nurse has violated the NPA. This is a disciplinary procedure and differs from a civil action or criminal action. **Figure 3-1** lists the most common grounds for disciplinary charges.

A licensing action begins as a complaint and allegations by a patient, patient's family, or colleagues regarding a nurse's actions. Hospitals are required to report when disciplinary action was taken when the nurse's act puts a patient at a safety risk or is grounds for license suspension or revocation.

Administrative disciplinary actions can be against the nursing license or another denial of administrative privilege. Back-timing a morphine order was fraud and resulted in disciplinary action against the nurse's license by the board of nursing in *Nevada State Board of Nursing v. Merkley* (1997). A willful disregard for required reporting regulations resulted in denial of billing Medicare/Medicaid (CMS). This was a serious denial to the administrator of the long-term care facility's ability to be paid for services. Her appeal for judicial review resulted in confirmation of the board's finding that she willfully disregarded the state's mandatory reporting of an accident that results in patient harm (*Westin v. Shalala*, 1999). Disciplinary actions are also brought for lack of action when there is a duty to act. A nursing supervisor was disciplined for failing to prevent the witnessed abusive acts of a supervised employee. The board's discipline was on the supervisor's own act (or inactions) and not on the act of the supervised staff

(*Stephens v. Pennsylvania Board of Nursing*, 657 A. 2d 71 (Pa. 1995)).

■ INVESTIGATION AND DISCIPLINARY PROCESS

Anyone (patient, patient's family member, coworker, or employer) can file a complaint with the board of nursing. The board will notify the nurse in writing that a complaint has been filed and an investigation has been started, and the board may request a written response from the nurse. The response should be provided in an objective manner. Before submitting a response, the nurse should consult an attorney. Some nursing malpractice policies now cover attorney fees in disciplinary matters.

A schematic outlining the investigation and disciplinary process is provided in **Figure 3-2**.

■ ADMINISTRATIVE DUE PROCESS

The nurse has a constitutional right called "due process" during the administrative process. Due process ensures that nurses receive a hearing where they have the right to be heard and defend any charges brought against them before the board can terminate a "liberty" (e.g., the practice of nursing). Administrative due process guarantees nurses certain rights through the process (see **Figure 3-3**).

In certain situations, however, the board has the right to summarily revoke or suspend a nurse's license when the nurse presents an immediate danger to public safety. The practice of nursing, while a property interest under the Constitution, is a privilege granted by the state licensing board upon completion of criteria by the nurse. As such, this privilege can be limited by the board's duty to public safety.

■ CIVIL ACTIONS

Civil actions deal with disputes between individuals. Civil law is designed to monetarily compensate individuals for harm caused to them. Nurses can become involved in civil actions, such as malpractice actions, personal injury lawsuits, and workers' compensation. Nurses also can become involved as a witness in a patient's personal injury case against another person. Workers' compensation laws prevent employees from suing their employers for injuries received on the job. The cost of the injury and lost wages due to the injury must be settled through the workers' compensation benefits plan the employer provides for the employees.

Malpractice is the negligent conduct of a professional. It is defined by: (1) duty—established by a professional relationship;

If the board imposes a punishment, it can take one or more of the following disciplinary actions:

- Revocation of the nurse's license
- Suspension of the nurse's license
- Letter of reprimand (published in the board's reports; it means that action has been taken against the nurse's license)
- Letter of admonishment (in the nurse's file but isn't made public)
- Probation (fulfilling certain requirements to continue practice)
- Imposition of a fine

Figure 3-2   Board actions.

1. Right to due process
   a. Right to be informed of allegations
   b. Right to be heard (present your facts)
   c. Right to fundamental fairness in the process
2. Right to remain silent (speak to an attorney before speaking to investigator)
3. Anything you say will be used by the board to support the allegations against you
4. Right to retain an attorney (at your own expense)
5. Right to have your attorney present at all steps of the process including initial investigation through posthearing interviews

Figure 3-3   Rights of administrative due process.

(2) breach of duty—an act or omission in violation of the nursing standard of care; (3) a physical injury; and (4) causation—the nurse's breach of duty caused the plaintiff's injury. All four of these elements must be present and proven for the plaintiff to prevail. Even in the face of negligent acts by the nurse, the plaintiff must prove that the nurse's act caused the injuries.

In *Charash v. Johnson* (2000), a Kentucky appeals court found that the hospital was short staffed, but the plaintiff's estate failed to prove that it was related to the plaintiff's death. Likewise, a nurse who attempted four times to start an IV, contrary to hospital policy to make only two attempts, was not liable for the patient's nerve damage because the plaintiff was unable to prove the causal connection (*Coleman v. East Jefferson General Hospital*, 742 So.2d 1045).

Most plaintiffs (the person who initiates the lawsuit) will hire a lawyer to pursue a malpractice claim. To establish the claim, pertinent medical records and opinions of expert witnesses (nurses with experience in the same field of nursing who will testify as to the standard of care) will be obtained to support the allegations of malpractice. The parties then exchange information (discovery phase) about the plaintiff's claims of negligence and damages (injury and any costs incurred due to the injury) and the defendant's defense to such claims. Discovery is done through interrogatories, requests for production and depositions. An interrogatory is a document filed with the court in which one party asks questions of the other (see **Figure 3-4**). A request for production is a request in which one party asks the other to produce documents for the requesting party, such as medical records, operating room logs, or even specimen logs. The requesting party can use these documents to learn more facts about the case or identify potential witnesses to the event being litigated. The defendant nurse may also be required to give deposition testimony. A deposition is a legal proceeding where questions are asked and answered under oath and recorded by a stenographer.

When the discovery phase is complete, the case will either settle or proceed to trial. Any money paid to the plaintiff may come from the nurse's malpractice insurance policy or from the nurse if the judgment amount exceeds the policy amount, the nurse is uninsured, or the malpractice carrier has

Interrogatories that may be asked in a typical nursing malpractice case:

- The nurse's credentials, license education, and employment history
- Policies and procedures related to the incident
- Journal articles on the subject of the case
- Transcription requests for illegible entries or names of providers in the medical record
- Names of all employees or the patient's family or visitors who may have witnessed the incident
- Defenses to liability the defendant plans to bring
- Names of expert witnesses the defendant will use
- Make a request for admission, usually around undisputed facts such as confirmation of employment at time of the event, shift worked, title

Figure 3-4   Typical interrogatory questions.

denied coverage. Malpractice coverage is denied when the nurse acted outside the scope of employment.

▪ REFERENCES

Charash v. Johnson, Ky. App. LEXIS, 42 (Ky. App. April 21, 2000).

Coleman v. East Jefferson General Hospital, 742 So.2d 1045 (La. App. 1999).

Nevada State Board of Nursing v. Merkley, 940 P.2d 144 (Nev. 1997).

Stephens v. Pennsylvania Board of Nursing, 657 A. 2d 71 (Pa. 1995).

Westin v. Shalala, 845 F.Supp. 1446 D. (Kan. 1999).

Chapter 4

Standards of Care

Katherine Dempski

A Definitions

Standard of care: degree of care, skill, and judgment practiced by a reasonable nurse; may be established by expert testimony

National standard: under same or similar circumstances	vs	Locality rule: in the same or similar area
Standards: authoritative statements that evaluate the quality of practice	vs	Guidelines: outline for professional conduct (usually based on scientific evidence or expert opinion)
Procedure: step-by-step guide on implementing a policy	vs	Policy: plan for meeting agency goals
Ordinary negligence: act or failure to act that is below standard of care	vs	Gross negligence: negligent act that is a reckless disregard for human life
Nursing negligence: unreasonable nursing care or conduct for the circumstances	vs	Nursing competency: level of care required for a nurse to avoid disciplinary action

B Sources for the standard of care

1. Professional organizations (e.g., ANA, American Association of Critical Nurses)
2. Nursing literature (e.g., journals, periodicals)
3. Agency policy, procedure, and bylaws (must be updated to reflect changes in standards)
4. Federal administration codes (e.g., nurse-patient ratios for federally funded institutions)
5. Joint Commission on Accreditation of Hospital manual
6. Court decisions (sets precedents for future cases)
7. Experts and expert testimony (e.g., published authors, nursing professors)
8. State statutes and administrative regulations (e.g., Nurse Practice Act)
9. PDR or medication packet inserts in an adverse drug event or wrong drug event
10. Medical equipment cases vendor recommendations for use and maintenance, or national organizations that make recommendations on safe use of medical devices

In most states, the professional standard of care is defined by statute or case law. When they breach the standard of care, nurses can be liable for nursing negligence in a civil court. They also can face the restriction or revocation of their nursing license in an administrative proceeding by the licensing board. Having a definition of the standard of care gives a clearer view of when nursing negligence has occurred and allows the injured party to be compensated for the harm done. It also allows the nurse to avoid a nursing malpractice claim when a bad result occurs despite due care by the nurse.

■ NATIONAL STANDARD OF CARE VERSUS THE LOCALITY RULE

The national standard of care (see **Figure 4-1A**) is the degree of care, skill, and judgment exercised by a reasonable nurse under the same or similar circumstances. A nurse has the duty to practice nursing using the standard of care. This does not require the nurse to render optimal care or even possess extraordinary skill. Likewise, the rule that a nurse must exercise best nursing judgment does not necessarily hold the nurse liable for an error in nursing judgment. However, the nurse's error in judgment must not be below the standard of care. Good nursing care does not guarantee the patient a good result.

The *locality rule* holds that a nurse must practice with the degree of skill and care possessed by other nurses in the same or similar area (locality). How a nurse in a rural emergency department performs will be compared to nurses in other rural areas. The locality rule is followed in a minority of states.

The *national standard of care* holds a nurse in a rural community hospital to the same standard of care as a nurse in a metropolitan medical center given the similarity of the situation. The national standard takes into consideration that the emergency department at a metropolitan medical center has more resources and technology than a rural emergency department. The majority of states follow the national standard.

The national standard (or locality rule in a minority of states) is used in a malpractice civil action, whereas a nursing board disciplinary action looks for a nurse's level of competency. State regulations define the level of competency required of a nurse. Falling below the level of competency can result in a disciplinary action by a state board even when no harm was done to a patient.

■ HOW THE STANDARD OF CARE IS APPLIED

A nurse is liable for nursing malpractice when the nursing standard of care is not followed. As the definition implies, the standard for nursing conduct varies in each situation. For example, an emergency department nurse draws blood from a 45-year-old woman. The nurse does not put the side rails up on the stretcher. As the nurse walks away to send the blood to the lab, the woman faints and falls from the stretcher. The patient sues the nurse. Both parties to the suit admit expert testimony and the emergency department's policy and procedure manual. The emergency room department manual states that side rails must be used for all children, elderly, and confused or unconscious patients. Expert testimony confirms that side rails are often necessary for children and the elderly because patients in these age groups fall from stretchers more frequently and are injured severely even from minor falls. The jury may determine that the nurse did not violate the standard of care in that situation because the nurse had no indication that the patient was at risk for falling.

If the same facts are presented but the patient is an 80-year-old, the situation changes. Now the nurse does have some indication that the patient is at risk for falling, and the standard of care changes for that situation. Most likely the nurse will be found to have breached the standard of care required for this situation.

The standard of care is not a cookbook of step-by-step ways to conduct oneself professionally in any given situation. It requires the nurse to be aware of any harm that may befall the patient and to take reasonable steps to prevent that harm. The standard of care comes from many sources (see Figure 4-1B). The nurse is accountable to know the standard as developed through these multiple authoritative sources.

Failure to meet standards can be grounds for licensure discipline actions. The method a nurse used in holding NICU infants (under the arms and dangling or by the back of the neck) caused her license to be revoked. The standards used by the board were established by the standards of the professional organization and certification standards for that specialty (*Mississippi Board of Nursing v. Hanson*, 1997).

■ NURSE PRACTICE ACT

Each state has a nurse practice act (NPA) that defines the practice of nursing and determines whether nurses stay within their scope of practice. The scope of practice varies in each state. An agency's policies and procedures must not expand the scope of nursing practice. **Figure 4-2** shows how to determine when an act falls within the scope of practice.

■ STANDARDS OF CARE IN SPECIALTIES

Specialists are held to the standard of other similarly situated specialists. The conduct of a nursing specialist, such as a pediatric nurse practitioner, will be compared to that of other similarly situated pediatric nurse practitioners. When specialists have the responsibility of the same procedure, some states allow each specialty to be an expert on the standard of care for that procedure. For example, in a malpractice action against a pediatric nurse practitioner, a nurse midwife may explain to the jury the standard of care in neonatal resuscitation because both may perform that procedure under their state's NPA.

■ MAJORITY VERSUS MINORITY VIEWS

There is a generally recognized course of treatment for each diagnosis within each specialty. The phrases "schools of thought," "best medical judgment," and "respectable minority"

Determination activity falls within scope of nursing practice; nursing activity should meet all criteria:

1. Is the activity consistent with nursing practice act scope of practice as well as rules and regulations?
2. Are there board guidelines regarding this activity? (Look to FAQ page on state board Web site.)
3. Are there standards of nursing practice from professional organizations, nursing literature, or nursing research?
4. Do your colleagues and peers accept this activity as a nursing activity?
5. Do you have the required knowledge and have you demonstrated competencies in this activity?
6. Is this a valid order in accordance with institutional policies, protocols, and procedures?
7. Are you prepared to assume accountability for this activity?

Figure 4-2   Determining scope of practice.

Source: New Jersey State Board of Nursing. (2005). *Seven step decision making model: Algorithm for determining scope of nursing practice.* Retrieved September 11, 2008, from http://www.newjersey.gov/lps/ca/nursing/seven.htm

recognize that within each specialty there are alternative treatments for each diagnosis that are professionally acceptable to meet the standard of care.

■ EXPERT WITNESSES

Nursing malpractice is a professional negligence suit that requires an expert opinion as to the standards of care within the nursing profession and how it was breached. Therefore, expert nursing testimony in case law establishes the standard of care in that set of circumstances. The issue of physicians acting as experts on nursing standards was addressed by the Illinois Supreme Court. The court ruled that only a nurse is qualified to establish the standards for the nursing profession (*Sullivan v. Edward Hosp.*, 2004).

■ ACCREDITATION STANDARDS

Accrediting bodies, such as The Joint Commission, have set standards for practice in accredited institutions. Effective communication among the healthcare team and with patients is just one example of a standard set by The Joint Commission. The need for all patients to participate in their own healthcare decisions requires effective communication, including providing information that is appropriate to the patient's age, understanding, and language. Therefore, elements of performance (standards) include a needs assessment that addresses learning abilities and cultural beliefs. As with most requirements in accreditation, self-evaluation must be performed by collecting data on the patient's perception of care (patient satisfaction surveys) to address the patient's healthcare education needs. Initial orientation and ongoing staff training in communication and cultural diversity must be in place for compliance.

■ REFERENCES

Mississippi Board of Nursing v. Hanson, 703 So.2d 239 (Miss. 1997).

Sullivan v. Edward Hosp., 806 N.E.2d 645 (Ill. 2004).

Chapter 5

Defenses to Negligence or Malpractice

Susan J. Westrick

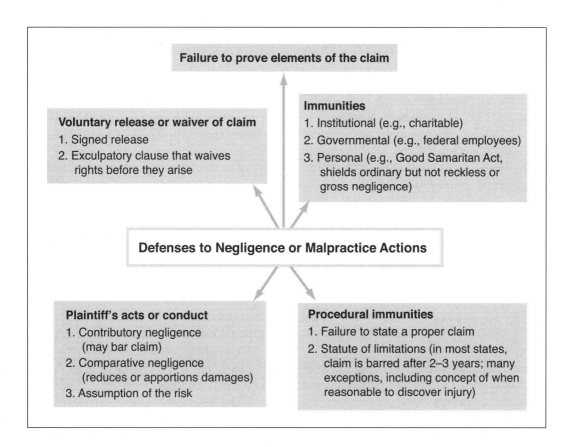

After a lawsuit is filed against a nurse, various defenses (see **Figure 5-1**) can be raised. These defenses may absolve the defendant completely or may limit the plaintiff's (or patient's) claim. They are based on various statutes or common-law doctrines, and more than one can be raised against a claim.

■ FAILURE TO PROVE ELEMENTS OF CLAIM

In negligence or malpractice actions, four elements must be proved for a successful claim: (1) a duty to the plaintiff, (2) a breach of the

duty or failure to act reasonably, (3) damage or resultant injury to the plaintiff because of this breach of duty, and (4) proximate (or legal) causation between the breach of duty and the resultant injury. Failure to prove even one of these elements will cause the plaintiff's claim to fail and thus would be a valid defense.

■ VOLUNTARY RELEASE OR WAIVER OF CLAIM

In the process of settling a claim, a patient may sign a release absolving the defendant of

19

all future claims or limiting claims based on the incident in question. Another means of voluntarily relinquishing rights is for a patient to have signed an exculpatory agreement or clause, serving as a release to future claims before they arise. The court may overrule these agreements if it feels that patients have been coerced or misinformed about their rights.

■ IMMUNITIES

An immunity from suit will act as a shield in case of a lawsuit. Examples of these are statutes or common-law doctrines that may apply to governmental or charitable-organization employees. However, many of these doctrines, especially charitable immunity, have been eroded over the years to allow legitimate claims to go forward. Most healthcare institutions are in reality profit-making organizations, even if part of their mission is charitable.

An example of federal immunity is the Federal Tort Claims Act (FTCA). Under this act the exclusive remedy for patients' claims while under the care of employees in governmental institutions is against the government and not the employees themselves. The government is substituted for the defendant, and individual employees, including nurses, are protected. There are some exceptions to this rule. Also limited under the act is the right of active military service personnel to bring claims against the government. The rationale for this is that these service personnel receive free medical care and disability pensions and that this is their exclusive remedy. However, civilian recipients of military medical care may sue the federal government, and military personnel may sue civilian medical caregivers.

Each state has its own statute called the Good Samaritan Act or Law, which provides for some form of personal immunity for acts or omission of medical care rendered by a volunteer who in good faith provides emergency medical assistance. Each state further defines

what constitutes an "emergency," but it usually involves potential loss of life or limb so pressing that action must be taken. These acts encourage citizens and healthcare practitioners to assist in emergencies without fear of civil or criminal liability for their actions if a mistake is made. However, it is important to recognize that most often one is protected from ordinary negligence only and not from gross negligence or reckless behavior. Nurses who render assistance are expected to follow accepted standards of nursing as guidelines. This doctrine applies when there is no nurse–patient relationship that would imply a duty of care under the circumstances (e.g., when a nurse is rendering care as a volunteer).

The court addressed the issue of negligence as applied to volunteer activities in the case of *Boccasile v. Cajun Music Limited* (1997). A physician and nurse Champoux were volunteering in a first-aid station at a festival attended by over 1000 people. An attendee began to have symptoms related to a food allergy. The doctor left the station to attend to him and eventually administered an EpiPen of epinephrine. The patient, Mr. Boccasile, continued to have symptoms, required CPR at the scene, and died the next day after transport to the hospital. In a wrongful death action, the decedent's widow claimed gross negligence on the part of both the physician and nurse Champoux. The Supreme Court of Rhode Island affirmed the lower court's grant of summary judgment for the defendants and against the plaintiff. The physician and nurse Champoux contended they were protected as volunteers under the state's Good Samaritan Act. The act protects from liability any care given voluntarily and gratuitously unless it is gross, willful, or wanton negligence. The plaintiff did not produce any credible evidence to support what the standard of care should have been in this situation, nor any evidence that the defendants' conduct failed to meet that standard, and thus the grant of summary judgment was upheld. Even though the plaintiff did not win this case, it underscores the importance of who may be liable for volunteer activities and whether a caregiver's individual liability insurance policy will cover volunteer acts. Many individual liability policies for nurses do cover any negligence or malpractice claim related to volunteer service, while employer policies typically do not.

In almost all states there is no duty to render emergency assistance to strangers, but it could be argued that health professionals have an ethical duty to do so. In Vermont, in an exception to this rule, persons are required to provide reasonable emergency assistance as long as it poses no danger to themselves.

■ PLAINTIFF'S NEGLIGENCE OR CONDUCT

Contributory Negligence

Another valid defense that can bar or limit the patient's claim of negligence against a nurse is the plaintiff's conduct, which can be viewed by the court as contributory negligence and in some jurisdictions is a complete bar to recovery of damages. The idea behind this is that the patient contributed to his or her own injury by not acting as a reasonably prudent person would in the circumstances and thus should not profit. Examples include patients not following instructions, not following warnings about side effects from medications, providing false information that led to improper treatment, and failure to return for appointments for follow up. Nurses must carefully document patients' failure to follow instructions or to keep appointments.

Comparative Negligence

Some jurisdictions have not held to the strict standards of contributory negligence but have adopted a more flexible approach that incorporates comparative negligence. Using this doctrine the court would apportion the per-centage of the injury from the plaintiff's own negligence to reduce any damage award. This puts responsibility on both persons to act reasonably under the circumstances. In some jurisdictions this rule is modified so that when the patient's negligence exceeds that of the defendant, the defendant's recovery of damages is barred altogether.

Assumption of the Risk

This defense incorporates the idea that the patient voluntarily assumes the risk of treatment and therefore has no claim against any resultant outcome that he or she specifically agreed to. It is conceptually similar to the informed-consent doctrine. It should be pointed out that the patient never assumes the risk of negligent treatment by a health professional, so in this situation, the defense may be of limited use if actual negligence can be shown.

■ PROCEDURAL DEFENSES

Failure to State a Proper Claim

Failure to state a claim upon which relief can be granted may incorporate various flaws in the plaintiff's action (e.g., failure to show that a nurse–patient relationship existed or the claim does not allege or prove negligence but rather some other type of claim against the nurse).

Statute of Limitations

Most states have enacted statutes of limitations that limit the time in which a plaintiff may file an action for negligence or malpractice. Many of these are limited to a 2- or 3-year period. The actual time it takes for the case to come to trial may be several years, but the claim must be filed within the statutory period.

Various exceptions to the statute of limitations have evolved and vary from state to state. A generally accepted one is that the time limit may be extended to when the patient would reasonably have known of the injury (e.g., a patient had radiation treatment that caused fertility problems 10 years later). Nurses need to be aware of this when considering malpractice insurance needs because claims may arise many years later.

Some states have a statute of repose, which sets absolute time limits for claims to be made. These cover the "should have known" concept and may apply to cases involving diagnoses of cancer.

Another way of working around the statute of limitations is for the patient to claim the action as ordinary negligence, rather than malpractice, because the time limit may be longer. Also, the claim may be asserted as a contract claim that may not be affected by the statute.

■ REFERENCE

Boccasile v. Cajun Music Limited, 694 A. 2d 686 (1997).

Chapter 6

Prevention of Malpractice

Katherine Dempski

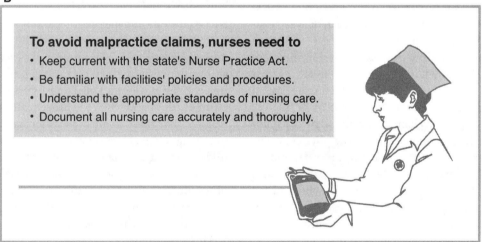

A

Common Areas of Nursing Malpractice
- **Inadequate assessment of the patient** — failure to monitor and assess a change in a patient's condition and report the change to the patient's physician
- **Medication errors** — transcription errors, administration errors
- **Inadequate training for assignment** — accepting and performing an assignment that the nurse is not competent to perform and failing to recognize own limitations
- **Patient falls** — leaving patient "at risk for falls" unattended
- **Faulty equipment**
- **Inadequate communication** — failing to notify the physician of changes in patient's condition, failing to adequately document in the patient's medical record, failing to advise nursing supervisor of situations where patient injury may occur, such as inadequate physician response
- **Failure to follow proper policy and procedure**

B

To avoid malpractice claims, nurses need to
- Keep current with the state's Nurse Practice Act.
- Be familiar with facilities' policies and procedures.
- Understand the appropriate standards of nursing care.
- Document all nursing care accurately and thoroughly.

A nurse is negligent when the nursing care fails to meet the appropriate standard of care. Nurses named as defendants in a malpractice claim face potential financial loss and adverse psychological effect. Nurses should be aware of situations that are potential liability prob-

lems (see **Figure 6-1A**) and take steps to avoid them (see Figure 6-1B).

■ PHYSICIAN'S ORDERS

When orders are illegible, unclear, incomplete, against agency policy, may cause harm to the patient, or are beyond the nurse's training, the nurse must discuss the orders with the physician. Illegible, unclear, and incomplete orders should be clarified, and no assumptions should ever be made. Nurses have a duty to clarify medication orders and not to administer medications that may harm the patient whether by interaction with other medications or by incorrect dose. When questioning a medication order, nurses should use the many resources available such as the pharmacist, a reliable drug reference, supervisors, physicians, and if necessary, a physician's supervisor or colleague.

Following a physician's order to discharge a patient did not shield a nurse from partial liability of the patient's death. A patient who complained of severe abdominal pain was diagnosed as having a urinary tract infection, and a discharge order was given by the physician without a physical examination. The nurse was concerned about the discharge order enough to consult with the nursing supervisor but took no further action. A few hours after discharge, the patient was readmitted with ruptured appendicitis, developed adult respiratory distress syndrome, and eventually expired. In the subsequent suit against the physician and hospital, the nurse testified that she was concerned over the order but was following the chain of command by discharging the patient by order of the physician. The court stated the nurse had an independent duty to use her professional judgment and not follow an order she knew or should have known was not within the standard of care and could foreseeably be harmful to the patient (*NKC Hospitals, Inc. v. Anthony*, 1993).

Nurses have a duty to be the patient's advocate and to know self-limitations. When questioning or not following a physician's orders, the nurse should discuss the concerns with the physician and the nursing supervisor. Following the agency's chain of command policy is necessary in this difficult situation. A collaborative team effort will offer the best reso-

lution to legal and ethical concerns. A nurse's duty to question a physician's orders extends to when the order "obviously" will result in harm to the patient and not when there is a reasonable difference in medical opinion (*Daniels v. Durham County Hosp. Corp.*, 2005). The Daniels' brought a claim against the physician and nurses on several legal theories following the death of their newborn post–mid-forceps delivery. The appellate court upheld the lower court finding that the nurses were not negligent in questioning the physician's order for mid-forceps delivery because it was not obvious negligence to disobey. Nurses are not qualified to resolve medical disputes regarding medical diagnosis and treatment. They should collaborate with the healthcare providers in determining appropriate care but may not prescribe medical treatment or make a medical diagnosis. To do so would be to step outside the scope of nursing practice as defined in most states.

■ INDEPENDENT DUTY

Nurses have an independent legal duty to the patient to make an accurate and thorough nursing assessment. The nurse must exercise this independent duty to investigate and inspect the patient's status and go up the chain of command when the nurse reasonably believes that the patient may suffer harm by following orders. Nurses have been held liable under this independent duty when they knew (or should have known) that the physician's order did not match up with the assessment and patient complaints and the patient suffered harm from the nurse's inaction.

This independent duty was recognized by the court to include the nurse's duty to recognize and intervene to protect the patient from discharging in an unsafe and dangerous condition in *Poluski v. Richardson Transportation* (1994). An independent transport service was used by an acute care facility to transfer a patient to a rehabilitation center. The transport employee negligently placed the patient in a wheelchair without the proper leg support for a surgically repaired leg. The acute care facility staff supplied the transport employee with a sheet to rig a support for the leg. The nursing staff, including the supervising nurse, all waved good-bye to the patient, never stopping the transporter or questioning the inappropriate leg support. The patient sued the transport company when her leg was irreparably damaged, and the transport company named the acute care nurses as codefendants. The nurses' defense was that the patient was "discharged" and no longer under their duty of care. The court found the nurses shared liability for failing to stop the negligent form of transport as an "independent duty" separate from a physician, which includes the duty to protect patients from foreseen harm. The nurses had the skill and knowledge to protect the patient and failed to act (intervene) on an improper discharge method on hospital premises.

■ DELEGATION OF TASKS

Delegation is the transfer of responsibility for performing an activity while retaining accountability. Nurses delegate tasks to unlicensed assistive personnel (UAP) daily and should be familiar with the UAP's training and competency level. Delegating a task outside the UAP's level of competency or improper delegation increases the risk of professional liability. An *improper delegation* is the delegation of a licensed activity as defined in the state's NPA. To prevent liability in this area, the nurse should be aware of the NPA's and the ANA's position statements on delegating tasks to UAP. (See Chapter 10, Delegation to Unlicensed Assistive Personnel.)

■ MEDICATION AND TRANSCRIPTION ERRORS

Administering medication incorrectly is one of the most common areas of nursing negligence. This includes giving an incorrect dose, using the incorrect route, and improperly administering an injection. Improper placement of a decimal point can turn a dose into 10 times the ordered amount, and the nurse can be held liable for the error when the drug is administered.

Most transcription errors occur due to assumptions made by nurses when they are unable to read illegible handwriting. Frequent errors occur when transferring the order to the medication administration records. Most institutions have computerized methods that remove this step from the process, thereby decreasing some human error. When nonprofessionals transcribe orders, legal liability remains with the nurse.

■ PROFESSIONAL RESPONSIBILITY AND LIMITATIONS

Nursing negligence occurs frequently when a nurse takes on an unfamiliar nursing procedure or assignment. The standard of care does not change for an inexperienced nurse. Professionalism requires knowing one's limitations and taking steps to avoid patient harm. The nurse should follow agency policy for going up the chain of command for assignment change or utilize available resources, such as experienced nurses or supervisors, for guidance with unfamiliar procedures. When a nursing error is made, it is the professional responsibility of the nurse to use skill and expertise to intervene and minimize the harm done to the patient.

When a nurse agrees to an employed position that requires a license or degree of skill less than the nurse is licensed for (a registered nurse employed as a licensed practical nurse or a nurse practitioner employed as a registered nurse), the nurse will still be required to hold the skill and knowledge of the advanced license and may be held legally liable to the higher standard (despite the job description) should there be patient harm.

State nursing board Web sites are excellent references, and most offer FAQ pages regarding licensing concerns and acts which fall within or out of the scope of practice.

■ COMMUNICATION WITH PATIENTS

Many negligence cases against healthcare providers have some element of poor communication between the provider and the patient. Patients who feel that the healthcare providers were attentive, caring, concerned, and truthful are highly unlikely to visit a malpractice attorney's office claiming injury due to negligence.

■ PROPER USE OF EQUIPMENT

The standard of care requires nurses to identify areas of risk of injury to their patients and take steps to avoid the harm. This includes the proper use of medical equipment including restraints (see **Figure 6-2**). Manufacturers' instructions must be followed, and when malfunctioning equipment is identified, the appropriate authority should be notified to have it removed for maintenance. Nurses have been found liable for failing to correctly use medical devices. For example, in *Estate of Chin v. St. Barnabas Medical Center* (1999), two inexperienced nurses sought the assistance of a third nurse to hook up nitrogen and fluid irrigation tubes of a hysteroscopy. In *Steinkamp v. Caremark* (1999), a nurse negligently pulled back a needle, shearing off the catheter tip, despite the manufacturer's warning.

■ PERFORMING NURSING PROCEDURES

Nurses have a duty to perform nursing procedures correctly. Surgeons were once considered to be responsible for all negligent acts that occur during surgery (known as "captain of the ship" policy). Surgical nurses now have their own liability for incorrect sponge and needle counts. Nurses who are independent contractors to an agency also carry their own liability. Accordingly, agencies are not held responsible under the corporate liability theory for the contracting nurse's negligence.

■ DIFFICULT PATIENTS

Difficult patients who are more likely to sue are typically uncooperative, immature, dependent, and hostile to the medical staff. Unfortunately, it is this difficult personality that makes most healthcare providers turn away, act aloof, or react in a hostile manner. Providing nursing care to this type of patient is unnerving. However, to avoid potential harm

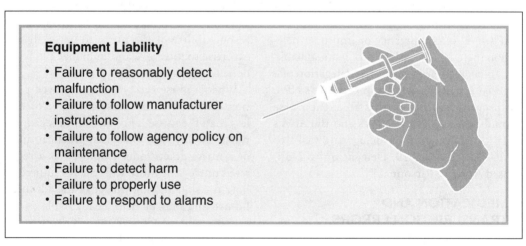

Equipment Liability

- Failure to reasonably detect malfunction
- Failure to follow manufacturer instructions
- Failure to follow agency policy on maintenance
- Failure to detect harm
- Failure to properly use
- Failure to respond to alarms

Figure 6-2   Equipment liability.

(and a malpractice suit), it is in everyone's best interest to continually provide the standard of care despite personality conflicts.

This may require the nurse to assist the patient in identifying the source of the mistrustful and hostile feelings toward the healthcare staff. Providing consistent, polite, and attentive patient care and explaining all nursing procedures may help diffuse the hostility. The nurse is not expected to accept insults and should set limits on inappropriate patient behavior. A multidisciplinary team approach is recommended. Most institutions now have behavioral management teams to be proactive.

Documentation is a key factor in diffusing potential liability claims. Document the patient's concerns and complaints and how those concerns are being addressed, without labeling the patient or complaining about the patient's behavior. The documentation should reflect the nurse's role as patient advocate and that policies and procedures are being followed. An incident report or other internal review document is the proper vehicle for documenting staff safety concerns or inappropriate behavior.

■ RISK MANAGEMENT

Risk management departments are responsible for improving quality of medical care by identifying potential risks and injuries to patients, staff, and visitors. Risk management teams consist of members from various departments and are coordinated through a trained risk management expert. Risk management teams collect information on and evaluate patient complaints, poor medical outcomes, and safety hazards. Data is collected from patient complaint forms, incident reports, utilization review reports, and other internal reporting systems. Risk management teams may also offer staff safety education to improve medical care and are a valuable resource on medical–legal issues.

■ CONTINUING EDUCATION

Continuing education to update assessment skills is the most valued tool a nurse has in preventing nursing negligence. Maintaining appropriate credentialing and reading professional journals keeps nurses informed about standard of care updates. Agency policies and procedures must be updated to reflect the current standard of care. Nurses who are members of the policy and procedure committee or a professional journal club take an active stand in updating their skills and preventing nursing malpractice.

■ REFERENCES
Daniels v. Durham County Hosp. Corp., 171 N.C. App. 535 (2005).

Estate of Chin v. St. Barnabas Medical Center, 734 A.2d 778 (NJ 1999).

NKC Hospitals, Inc. v. Anthony, 849 S.W.2d 564 (Ky. Ct. App. 1993).

Poluski v. Richardson Transportation, 877 S.W.2d 709 (Mo. Ct. App. 1994).

Steinkamp v. Caremark, 3 S.W.3d 191 (Tex. Ct. 1999).

Chapter 7

Nurses as Witnesses

Susan J. Westrick

Testimony Guidelines for Nurse Witnesses

1. Don't guess.
2. If you don't know the answer, say so.
3. If you don't remember, say so.
4. Be sure you understand the question.
5. Ask for clarification of the question as necessary.
6. Take your time; think before you answer.

PLUS

Fact Witnesses	Expert Witnesses	Witness to Documents
7. Prepare nursing notes in a timely manner. 8. Don't sign another nurse's notes. 9. Testify only to firsthand knowledge.	7. Review records before agreeing to be an expert witness. 8. Be certain the case is in your area of expertise. 9. Be thorough.	7. Assess capacity of the patient. 8. Don't sign if you believe the patient does not understand. 9. Check with your employer first.

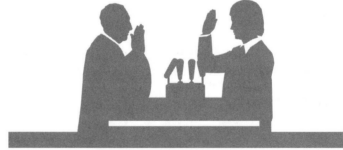

■ FACT WITNESSES

The nurse's role as a fact witness is to testify, in verbal or written form, about facts he or she has personally observed. A fact may be an action performed, an event, or an occurrence and can include the patient's condition, actions of others, the patient's environment, nursing practices, or documentation practices. The nurse may be a witness for either the plaintiff (the party bringing the lawsuit) or the defendant (the party being sued). In most instances, the testimony will be rendered at a deposition or at trial. A deposition is a question-and-answer session wherein one party to a lawsuit acquires information known only to the other party. Questions are first asked by the attorney for the party attempting to gather information. The witness answers the questions after taking an oath to tell the truth. When the attorney who asked the questions is finished, the other attorney may ask questions that relate to the questions and answers already addressed. Then the first attorney may ask additional questions, and so on.

A court reporter is present and creates a stenographic record of all of the spoken words. Occasionally the deposition is videotaped.

The process of rendering testimony as a fact witness at trial is similar to that of a deposition. It will take place in a courtroom or hearing room before a judicial authority, usually a judge but possibly a magistrate or hearing officer. It may also take place in front of a jury. **Figure 7-1** illustrates various types of witnesses and testimony guidelines for nurses.

■ EXPERT WITNESSES

An expert witness is one who has superior knowledge of a subject by virtue of education and experience. A nurse, through nursing education and specialized experience in nursing, is well qualified to serve as an expert witness at a deposition or trial. However, the focus of the testimony is not on the nurse's direct observations but on nursing care issues. The nurse may be called as an expert to opine as to the care that is the subject of the lawsuit or to testify to a standard of care.

Hence, qualifications and credentials will be at issue prior to the court's recognizing the nurse as an expert witness. The attorneys who represent all parties may agree or "stipulate" to the nurse's qualifications. If they do not so stipulate, the attorney who wishes to present

the nurse as an expert witness will have to prove to the court that the nurse is qualified. The attorney may do so through submission to the court of the nurse's résumé or curriculum vitae or other such written material.

The nurse will have the opportunity to review the medical records prior to participation as an expert witness. When reviewing them, the nurse should keep in mind his or her role in the case (e.g., as an expert for the plaintiff or for the defendant or as being impartial). If the nurse is an expert witness for either party, questions directly relating to the specific case will be asked. It is expected that the opposing party will offer expert testimony that differs from the nurse's opinion. Therefore, the nurse must be familiar with the specific records relative to the case and be prepared to substantiate any opinions.

If the nurse is testifying as to a standard of care, general questions will be asked about any area of expertise (e.g., critical care, home care, obstetrics). When this expertise is established, hypothetical questions will likely be asked. A hypothetical question is one that describes the issues similar to the case without identification of any specific person. The questioner will then inquire as to whether the care described in the hypothetical question deviated from the standard of care. The nurse will opine as to whether or not there was a deviation from the standard of care and must be able to substantiate any opinion in reliance on education and specialized experience.

It is imperative that the nurse be aware of any conflicts of interest that may arise out of serving as an expert witness. A conflict of interest is a situation in which there is a clash between professional, financial, or ethical interests of the witness. Such conflicts of interest will have a negative impact on the nurse's credibility because they create, at best, the appearance of a bias, if not an actual bias. As soon as a potential conflict of interest becomes apparent to the nurse, it should be brought to the attention of the party that has retained the nurse's services.

■ QUALIFICATION AS AN EXPERT WITNESS

Recently, courts have addressed the question of whether a physician can testify as to the standard of care for nursing actions. In *Sullivan v. Edward Hospital* (2004) the Supreme Court of Illinois held that a physician, board certified in internal medicine, is not qualified to testify as an expert witness on the applicable standard of care for nurses regarding preventing patient falls. The plaintiff's physician expert witness stated that he had observed many nurses practicing over the years and thus was familiar with these standards of care. This was not persuasive to the court because an expert witness must be familiar with the specialized knowledge and skill as previously noted. The court noted that nursing has evolved over the years as a profession with a specialized body of knowledge, code of ethics, standards, and professional regulation. The American Association of Nurse Attorneys (TAANA) submitted an amicus brief (or friend of the court) that assisted the court in articulating its position. Portions of the TAANA position paper on "Expert Testimony in Nursing Malpractice Actions" and the amicus brief were cited within the court's opinion.

■ TESTIMONY IN CRIMINAL CASES

Nurses may sometimes be called to testify in a criminal proceeding. The nurse may give testimony in cases involving child, adult, or sexual abuse, and if qualified, the nurse could be an expert witness in these situations. Nurses in the emergency room may hear patients' statements regarding who is at fault for their injuries, and these statements may be admissible in court if the patient is later unable to provide the testimony. This is in spite of the fact that this second-hand testimony would normally be excluded as hearsay. There are exceptions to the hearsay rule. In *State v. McHoney*

(2001) the nurse had the patient nod to indicate the initials of the person who was responsible for her grave injuries. The patient died shortly thereafter. The nurse testified at the trial as to the patient's actions during her care, and this was admitted under an exception to the hearsay rule. Other times, the nurse's documentation of the patient's statement could be admitted as evidence. As with other testimony and documentation, all statements should be factual and recorded or presented in the patient's own words when possible.

■ WITNESS TO DOCUMENTS

Because of the nurse's proximity to patients, he or she may be asked to serve as a witness to legal documents. Some examples include, but are not limited to, a last will and testament, deed, living will, power of attorney, or appointment of healthcare agent. Although patients or family members may request the nurse to sign these documents as a witness, it is best not to do so because it may create ethical conflicts later.

The legal requirements for the execution (signing) of legal documents vary from state to state. Nonetheless, a nurse who is a witness to the execution attests to the capacity and adult age of the person signing, that the person is acting voluntarily, authenticity of the signature, and that he or she saw the other witness sign the document. The nurse could be called to testify at a later hearing if problems occur regarding circumstances of the signing.

The patient's capacity to sign a legal document refers to the ability to understand the nature and effect of the act. Determining the patient's capacity to sign a legal document does not involve extensive expert evaluation but rather observation and assessment. To assist the witnesses, the attorney who conducts the execution will ask the patient a series of questions about the document and the patient's understanding, agreement, and willingness to sign it. The patient should be able to name the document and state that he or she read it and agrees with the contents. If the patient's condition prevents him or her from reading or speaking, the attorney may ask a series of yes or no questions, and the patient may respond through body language. Common sense prevails in accordance with the patient's condition.

The nurse's familiarity with the patient affords the nurse a unique role as a witness to the execution of legal documents. If the nurse knows that confusion or medications may affect the patient's capacity, he or she must inform the attorney before the document is signed. If the nurse is not satisfied that the patient understands and agrees with the document, the nurse should not sign as a witness.

Nurses should check with their employers prior to serving as a witness to legal docu-ments. Some employers have policies regard-ing this issue, and the nurse should comply with any such policy. The policy may require that employees not sign legal documents as a witness to avoid any ethical conflicts.

■ REFERENCES

State v. McHoney (2001), S.E.2d, S.C. 2001, WL 283241.

Sullivan v. Edward Hospital (2004), 806 N.E.2d 645 (Ill. 2004).

The American Association of Nurse Attorneys. (2004). TAANA position paper on expert testi-mony in nursing malpractice actions. *Journal of Nursing Law, 9*(4), 18–25.

Wright, L. D. (2003). Physician expert testimony on the standard of care for placement of an intra-venous line. *Journal of Nursing Law, 9*(3), 43–44.

Chapter 8

Professional Liability Insurance

Susan J. Westrick

A Checklist/Features

- Ask to see your employer's policy.
- Examine your own policy.
- Determine policy coverage and limits.
- Check provisions related to settlement, exclusions, indemnification, and limitations of coverage.
- Determine type of policy (claims made or occurrence).
- Keep coverage in effect after you leave job if covered by a claims made policy, or obtain a tail policy.
- Note rights and obligations of insured and insurer.
- Notify insurer of name or address changes, any change in job status or responsibilities, or any potential claims against you.

Claims Made Policy	vs	**Occurrence Policy**
Must be in effect when the claim is made.		Effective if the policy was in effect at time the incident occurred (applies to previous incidents even if claim is made years later).

B Individual Coverage   vs   Employer Coverage

- Usually covers volunteer work as RN.	- Covers actions only if within the scope of employment.
- Covers state board action against your license.	- May not cover intentional torts.
- Covers representation by your own attorney.	- Represented by employer's insurance company or hospital attorney.
- Consider if in high-risk areas of practice.	- May not cover for claim filed after your employment is terminated.
- May be required as a condition of employment.	- Policy limits may not be high enough to cover all claims.

Nurses are at risk for liability if a malpractice claim against them is successful. One way to shift the risk of this liability is to buy professional malpractice insurance so that the insurer pays the claim. Malpractice attorneys increasingly name individual practitioners in lawsuits as well as the agencies for which they work. Professional liability insurance protects nurses against covered claims in the course of their professional duties. This includes claims arising from real or alleged incidents including negligence or malpractice. The cost of legal defense and settlement costs in addition to the limits of liability of the policy are covered. Many employers tell their employees they are covered for such claims by the employer's insurance. This may be true under most circumstances, but there are risks and disadvantages involved in relying solely on the policy of the employer. Increasingly, institutions are self-insured, and nurses need to find out the implications of this for their individual malpractice coverage. Self-insurance does not shift the risk of loss to a third-party insurance company, but rather the risk is retained within the organization, usually by trust funds set aside for this purpose. Nurses are accountable to know the terms, conditions, and exclusions of their own or the employer's policy (see **Figure 8-1A**).

■ TYPES OF POLICIES

The insurance agreement sets out the terms of the policy and specifies the rights and responsibilities of the nurse (or agency) as the insured and the insurance company as the insurer. The agreement is a contract governed by contract law and by many special regulations determined by state and federal laws. Two basic types of policies are available:

1. Claims made: The policy must be in effect when the claim is made. If a claim is made years later and the policy is no longer in effect, the policy will not cover the claim. A tail policy may be purchased to cover a gap in coverage when one changes jobs or retires.
2. Occurrence: As long as the policy was in effect when the incident occurred, even if the claim is made years later, the policy will still cover the claim. This preferred type of coverage is broader but is usually more expensive.

■ POLICY PROVISIONS AND COVERAGE

Each policy should be examined individually to determine its features. Every policy will state the limits of coverage (e.g., $1 million coverage per incident or $3 million coverage maximum per year). Excess judgments are any amount of damages that are above the policy limits. These become the responsibility of the nurse and are payable from personal assets. This can include the claimant's right to future wages.

Limitations and exclusions should be noted carefully. Professional liability insurance policies do not cover criminal acts, acts that are outside the scope of practice, or acts in settings other than those stated in the policy. Agency policies will not likely cover the nurse's conduct if it rises to the level of creating an extreme risk for the patient, such as an extreme overdose, because this is considered to be reckless behavior. Volunteer activities not associated with employment would not be covered unless specifically mentioned in the contract. Likewise, a nurse's actions outside the scope of the state NPA would not be covered.

Because employer policies are usually limited to malpractice claims or professional negligence, acts of ordinary negligence or actions by a state board of nursing against a nurse's license are not typically covered. Nurses' individual malpractice policies increasingly cover some of these areas not covered by employer policies, especially state board actions, and this is one advantage of having an individual policy (see Figure 8-1B). A nurse's individual policy most likely would cover attorney's fees even if the nurse is wrongly accused of misconduct by the state board. Punitive damage awards are usually excluded from coverage because the purpose of these damages is to punish the wrongdoer. Also, damage awards can exceed employer policy limits, leaving the nurse's personal assets at risk if there is no individual liability insurance in place.

Most insurance policies give the insurer the right to settlement of a claim or lawsuit without the consent of the insured. In some cases if the insurer refuses a reasonable settlement offer, it may later be liable for any judgment and award of damages, even if the amount of damages is above the policy limits. Sometimes nurses do not want to settle a claim because they will not be allowed to present their side of the alleged negligent incident. However, the cost of litigation is very high, and it is often in the best interest of all parties to settle the claim or lawsuit.

■ RESPONSIBILITIES OF THE INSURED

As described in the following list, the insured agrees to cooperate with the insurer in processing all claims.

1. The insurer must receive timely notice of any claim against the nurse. In fact, it is best to notify the insurer of any potential claim or untoward incident so that if an investigation is required it can be done in a timely manner.
2. The nurse must provide the insurer any change of address, name, or work status.
3. The insured must pay the premiums when due to ensure continuance of the policy.
4. The nurse must cooperate with the insurer in handling the claim and must be truthful in all dealings.

■ RIGHTS OF THE INSURED

The insured has the right to have claims processed in a timely and competent manner. The insurer has the duty to defend the claim and provide an attorney who works for or on behalf of the insurance company. The insurance company also pays court costs, settlements, and damage awards for liability up to the limits of the policy.

■ REASONS FOR INDIVIDUAL PROFESSIONAL LIABILITY INSURANCE

Many nursing organizations recommend that nurses carry individual professional liability policies to ensure protection of the public, who have the right to recover damages when claims are valid. Nurses are increasingly named in lawsuits as plaintiffs' attorneys seek damages from all who are involved. The doctrine of respondeat superior, which makes the institution responsible for the acts of employees, will not automatically relieve named defendants (nurses) when liability is found. In addition, although it is not often used, the employer can exercise the right to indemnification against the nurse, especially if the employer's interest is adverse to the nurse's. Indemnification means that the employer can try to recover the damages it was responsible for on behalf of the employee. This right of indemnification usually involves the healthcare agency that seeks reimbursement from the nurse's individual policy.

Nurses with individual policies will be provided an attorney who will represent their interests, not the employer's, and their defense costs will be covered. Other benefits typically include payment of lost wages and other reasonable reimbursable expenses that are not usually part of employer malpractice policies. Other issues to consider are that the employer's policy limits may not be high enough to protect a nurse and all of his or her coworkers, and the policy may not cover a nurse if a suit is filed after he or she leaves the place of employment.

■ EFFECT OF AN INDIVIDUAL LIABILITY POLICY

Many insurance policies are written with provisions to designate the policy as either "primary" or "secondary." Secondary policies are used as payment after any primary insurance coverage. Issues related to which policy should cover, and to what limits, is a frequent cause of litigation between the parties when there is not agreement as to payment for an award of damages. Although it is sometimes the nurse's individual professional liability policy that is at issue, the nurse is not directly involved in the lawsuit because it is typically between the insurance companies.

For example, in *Travelers Indemnity Company v. American Casualty Company of Reading, PA* (2003) an underlying malpractice action by a patient resulted in a $4.5 million dollar settlement against doctors, nurses, and a hospital. The hospital's insurer (Travelers) carried both a primary and an "excess" policy. Travelers paid first as a primary policy but then brought a lawsuit to have the nurses' individual malpractice insurance (American Casualty) pay to their limits before the "excess" policy of Travelers had to pay toward the large settlement. The patient had sued two physicians and 10 nurses who were employed at the hospital and alleged that the prenatal and postnatal treatment of his wife and son, born in 1985, was negligent. Three of the nurses had individual professional liability insurance policies with American Casualty; two policies had a $500,000 limit and one policy had a $1 million limit per incident. Travelers contended that these individual policies should pay as "other insurance" before the excess liability policy covered by Travelers paid on behalf of the hospital. The Illinois appeals court agreed with Travelers and ruled that the nurses' individual policies were also "primary" policies, within the meaning of the insurance contracts, and that the Travelers excess policy (covering the hospital and its employees) should only be required to pay after the limits of the American Casualty policies were exhausted.

Another case that illustrates the complexities of coverage of individual liability policies is *St. John's Regional Health Center v. American Casualty Company of Reading, PA* (1992). In this case American Casualty, as the nurse's insurance company, appealed a summary judgment holding them liable for indemnification of St. John's Regional Health Center (St. John's) for a $375,000 settlement paid on behalf of nurse Lierz. Nurse Lierz was required to purchase an individual policy in the amount of $500,000 per incident as a condition of her employment. This was also required for employees as a precondition of the hospital joining the pooled liability fund. The payment for the settlement came from funds pooled by several hospitals that were operated by the Sisters of Mercy Health System. At the time of the lawsuit, nurse Lierz asked both St. John's and American Casualty to defend her. American Casualty refused, and St. John's settled the suit. St. John's then sought reimbursement from American Casualty as the nurse's individual policy insurer. Nurse Lierz's individual policy had a clause stating that it covered only after any "other insurance," and her insurer wanted the pooled funds, a form of "self-insurance," to cover the claim as the "other insurance." The appeals court agreed with St. John's that the pooled liability funds would not be "other insurance" and that the intent of having the nurse buy her own individual liability policy was to have that policy cover first. Therefore, the nurse's insurer was responsible for indemnifying the hospital for payment of the settlement on behalf of nurse Lierz.

An Ohio court refused to allow a nurse's professional liability insurance policy to cover a claim for personal injury after the nurse was killed in a motorcycle accident. The executor of her estate sought a declaratory judgment to allow the policy to cover for uninsured/underinsured motorist (UM/UIM) benefits because there was a policy provision that covered personal injury. However, the court found that the policy provided coverage for personal liability and personal injury under certain circumstances that did not include liability arising out of use of a motor vehicle. Although the policy did not have an exclusion for claims arising out of automobile accidents, it did not cover liability arising out of the use of a motor vehicle. The court of appeals upheld the summary judgment in favor of the insurer and declined to transform the professional nurses' liability policy into a motor vehicle liability policy. (*Debbie Hiller, Executor of the Estate of Nora Price, Deceased, et al. v. OHIC Insurance Company, et al., American Casualty of Reading, PA,* 2006)

Whether or not to have an individual professional liability policy or rely on an employer's policy is an individual decision. The nurse must be sure to check employment policies about whether it is required to carry an individual malpractice policy as part of the employment agreement. Nurses need to consider their employment or work status, potential risk of lawsuits, personal financial situation, and professional ethical concerns.

Professional liability insurance policies are offered by insurance companies that are affiliated with professional organizations, such as the ANA, or are advertised in major nursing publications. As illustrated in the foregoing cases, when there is overlap in coverage with institutional and individual policies, the insurance companies determine which policy, or whether both policies, will cover. Because individual policies are available at reasonable rates and there are many advantages to having individual coverage, it is prudent to follow this course of action.

■ REFERENCES

Debbie Hiller, Executor of the Estate of Nora Price, Deceased, et al. v. OHIC Insurance Company, et al., American Casualty of Reading, PA, 2006 Ohio 4536; 2006 Ohio App. LEXIS 4490 (2006).

St. John's Regional Health Center v. American Casualty Company of Reading, PA, 980 F.2d 1222; 1992 U.S. App. LEXIS 31584 (1992).

Travelers Indemnity Company v. American Casualty Company of Reading, PA, 337 Ill. App. 3d 435; N.E.2d 582; 2003 Ill. App. LEXIS 274; 272 Ill. Dec. 43 (2003).

Chapter 9

Refusing an Assignment/ Patient Abandonment

Susan J. Westrick

Conditions to Allow Refusal of an Assignment

1. Nurse lacks the knowledge or skill to give competent care.
2. Nursing actions outside the scope of the NPA are expected.
3. Health of the nurse (or her fetus) is directly threatened by the nature of the assignment.
4. Nurse has not been oriented properly to the unit and safety is jeopardized.
5. Conscientious objection on clearly stated and documented moral, ethical, or religious grounds.
6. Nurse is fatigued to the extent that it could interfere with nursing judgment and create a safety risk for patients.

Steps to Follow When Refusing an Assignment

1. Express specific reasons for refusal to a supervisor.
2. Explore alternatives such as reassignment, buddy system, or sharing tasks with another staff member.
3. Document specifics of the incident in personal notes, including who was notified.
4. Be willing to adhere to properly implemented floating or crosstraining policies.
5. Make sure that other staff are available to care for patient to avoid charge of patient abandonment.

Acceptance of Assignment with Reservation or under Protest

1. Fill out any forms for this purpose.
2. Clearly document the facts of the incident on agency records and personal notes.

Refusing a patient assignment presents a dilemma for the nurse. Many nurses do not want to disrupt patient care or the work environment, but in some instances they have an ethical and legal duty to refuse an assignment. Abandonment occurs when the nurse refuses to care for the patient and no one else is available to do so; it involves negligence. Avoiding charges of patient abandonment is a prime consideration, and the nurse needs to be on solid ground when circumstances warrant such refusal (see **Figure 9-1**).

■ LEGAL AND ETHICAL FRAMEWORK

Negligence Law

Negligence theory provides guidance in terms of professional responsibilities to patients. Nurses have a duty to provide reasonably prudent care to patients in the same or similar circumstances. If a nurse refuses a patient assignment and a later charge of negligence or professional malpractice is brought, the impact of the refusal will be considered. If harm to the patient results, a charge of negligent abandonment may be sustained. Conversely, if a nurse accepts an assignment for which he or she is unprepared and harm results, the same outcome of negligence may be found.

Nurse Practice Acts/State Boards of Nursing

The nurse must also be aware of the scope of practice as defined in the state's NPA when deciding whether to accept or refuse an assignment. If the assignment includes undertaking tasks that are outside its scope, then there is a legal duty to refuse the assignment. Nurses can be subject to disciplinary procedures by the state board of nursing for any violations of the act. Many state boards have also provided guidance to nurses either through regulations, guidelines, or position statements relating to patient abandonment, refusing assignments, or other staffing issues.

Code of Ethics

Another important frame of reference is the ANA (American Nurses Association, 2001) Code of Ethics for Nurses, which requires nurses to use informed judgment when deciding to accept a patient assignment or when making assignments to others. Nurses are expected to use individual competence and qualifications in seeking consultation from qualified nurses or for accepting responsibilities. The code specifies that nurses are responsible for nursing judgment and action and that

they are accountable for their decisions related to patient care assignments. Assignments are to be accepted or rejected based on education, knowledge, competence, and level of experience. Nurses must also provide care to patients regardless of their social or economic status or their health problems. Professional codes of ethics may be used in malpractice cases to help establish the standard of care that should have been followed in a particular situation.

Position Statements and Research

The ANA has issued a position statement titled "The Right to Accept or Reject an Assignment" (1995). This publication outlines duties and responsibilities for nurses that are grounded in both the ANA Code of Ethics and state nurse practice acts. Overall this document articulates the ANA's belief that nurses should reject any assignment that puts patients or themselves in serious, immediate jeopardy, even when there is not specific legal protection for rejecting the assignment. The duty to safeguard clients is the basis for the nurse not to provide care for which he or she is unqualified. Another document that influences acceptance of patient assignments is the ANA position statement on "Assuring Patient Safety: Registered Nurses' Responsibility in All Roles and Settings to Guard Against Working While Fatigued" (2006). This statement cautions nurses to consider level of fatigue when accepting assignments, especially when the assignment involves working extra hours beyond regularly scheduled shifts or as a result of mandatory overtime. Underscoring this position statement is the Institute of Medicine's (IOM) 2004 report, which found that when nurses work excessive hours, especially in excess of 12 hours in direct patient care, there is an increase in patient care errors. In another study, it was found that the likelihood of making an error was three times higher when nurses worked shifts lasting 12.5 hours or longer (Rogers et al., 2004). Another ANA position statement on "Opposition to Mandatory Overtime" (2001) recommends against use of this strategy to solve staffing problems and cautions that it should only be used in emergency situations and not as a staffing pattern.

These position statements and research studies reflect some of the staffing issues that have arisen due to the nursing shortage and other factors that have led to understaffing. While institutions are required to have adequate numbers of competent staff to ensure patient safety, nurses are often put in a position of facing a dilemma when asked to care for patients under less than ideal situations.

Legislation and Regulation

As an attempt to help solve some of these staffing problems, many states have statutes that limit mandatory overtime. California has established nurse-patient ratios for certain healthcare settings in an effort to assure adequate numbers of staff members. Some nurse practice acts have passed regulations and guidelines to further assist nurses and clarify issues related to staffing. On the national level, the Patient Safety Act of 2005 addresses safe levels of staffing.

Also, there are federal and state "conscientious objection" statutes that allow nurses to refuse to care for patients based on moral, ethical, or religious objections. These "conscience clauses" were originally passed to protect against religious objections but now have been extended to grant healthcare providers the right to refuse for many other moral or ethical reasons. There are restrictions and conditions under which these refusals can be made, and alternative care must always be provided for the patient.

In an Illinois case, a nurse tried to use the Illinois Conscience Act to assert that she was wrongfully terminated (*Free v. Holy Cross Hospital*, 1987). Nurse Free had refused to evict a bedridden patient from defendant hospital on ethical grounds. The court held that the statute did not protect her because her concerns were ethical but not "sincerely held moral conviction…arising from what are traditionally characterized as religious beliefs."

Another strategy to minimize staffing dilemmas is to negotiate for specific nurse–patient ratios in collective bargaining agreements (CBA) and to limit mandatory overtime. Nurses are encouraged to support legislative and other solutions to ensure safe care of patients, and they must be thoroughly familiar with standards set by state and professional organizations.

■ FACTORS TO CONSIDER IN ACCEPTING OR REFUSING AN ASSIGNMENT

The following areas should be considered when deciding to accept or refuse a patient assignment:

1. Knowledge and skill: Nurses who are unfamiliar with a particular patient's nursing care needs have an ethical duty not to care for that patient. This is based on concerns for patient safety and the need for all patients to receive competent care. An inexperienced nurse who is caring for a complex client can jeopardize the patient, and consideration should be made to change the assignment or provide support by a more experienced nurse. Any care that involves tasks outside the scope of the NPA should be considered a valid basis for refusal.

2. Health and fatigue level of the nurse: According to standards set by the ANA, a nurse is expected to provide care to any patient who needs care when doing so presents no more than a minimal risk to the nurse. For example, a nurse who is pregnant can refuse to care for a patient if doing so poses a direct threat to the fetus. However, when there is no direct threat and the healthcare worker can be protected through standard precautions, refusal to care for patients (e.g., patients

with AIDS) has not been upheld by the courts. In individual cases it could be established that a particular patient is uncooperative and therefore does pose a direct threat to the nurse's safety. Nurses are cautioned not to work while fatigued or ill because this puts patients at risk.

3. Orientation to unit: Lack of orientation to a unit can present issues of patient safety. For example, not knowing where emergency equipment is kept can be hazardous, and not being familiar with routines of the unit can impact on quality of care and safety.

4. Availability of other staff: If another staff member is available to provide care, this may be the best solution. However, if the unit is understaffed, the only alternative may be for the nurse to provide the care to the patient. If problems occur later, the court will likely view the situation in the context of what was reasonable under the circumstances.

5. Modification of assignment: It may be possible to share the patient with another nurse or to provide only the part of the care that the nurse is competent to provide. For example, a nurse who is floated to a coronary care unit from a general unit may only be able to handle some nursing interventions but not the specialized intervention related to assessing cardiac monitors. Because many errors that occur with nurses who are floated to unfamiliar practice settings are related to medication administration, the nurse should not be asked to administer unit-specific medications. A buddy system may be another way to share an assignment.

6. Conscientious objection: Nurses should always seek positions where they know they will not frequently be assigned to care for patients who would have procedures they would object to, such as in abortion clinics. The nurse is cautioned that alternative care must always be available for the patient, otherwise a charge of

patient abandonment could be sustained. Advance notice of any objections should be given whenever possible so that the nurse manager can find alternative staff.

■ ACCEPTANCE OF ASSIGNMENT WITH RESERVATION OR DESPITE OBJECTION

A nurse may need to accept an assignment even though there are valid reasons for not doing so. The nurse may risk being fired or subjected to other action by the employer. An important step in this situation is for the nurse to specifically state to the supervisor why the assignment should not be accepted. A statement such as "I have never worked with patients receiving chemotherapy" provides clear information about the basis for refusal. The nurse should document the incident in his or her personal notes, including facts about the conditions of accepting the assignment with reservation, who was notified, and any alternative solutions the nurse offered, such as trading assignments with another staff member.

The nurse needs to put the organization on clear notice of the situation (e.g., understaffing) to most likely shift the liability to the corporation (corporate liability) in case a negligence action is brought later. It is the responsibility of nursing management and the agency or corporation to ensure that adequate numbers of qualified staff members are available to care for patients.

Some state nurses' organizations provide a form that can be filled out and filed with the supervisor. The form usually has check-off boxes to indicate the specific basis for refusing the assignment or accepting the assignment despite reservations, such as not being oriented or having too high a nurse–patient ratio. The nurse should keep copies of all written memos or forms that are submitted to supervisors. An example is a form titled "Acceptance of Assignment Despite Objection." State nursing organizations or collective bargaining agents typically collect these forms to establish trends related to staffing.

■ AVOIDING CHARGES OF PATIENT ABANDONMENT

By accepting an unreasonable assignment, the nurse risks responsibility for any negative consequences. Whether this is fair or not is an unsettled question, and the nurse must decide what to do while weighing the risks and benefits.

In all cases the nurse needs to consider patient abandonment. It is proper to refuse patient assignments for valid reasons, but the nurse must be sure the patient is not abandoned. The nurse cannot refuse an assignment for moral or religious reasons if there is no one else to care for the patient. Doing so is considered to be patient abandonment and would constitute negligence on the part of the nurse. To prevent potential problems, a nurse should not work in areas where conflicts between personal beliefs and patient care frequently occur.

A disciplinary action by the regulatory board for nurses was upheld by the court in the case of *Husher v. Commissioner of Education of the State of New York* (1992). Nurse Husher was found guilty of unprofessional conduct in abandoning her professional employment. These charges stemmed from her walking off her assigned nursing unit after her 7:00 a.m. to 3:00 p.m. shift without informing the remaining staff on the unit. She had earlier been informed by the supervisor that she would need to stay beyond her shift until properly relieved because she had the least seniority. This procedure was in keeping with a valid overtime policy that she was aware of. Nurse Husher informed the staff she was going to the nursing supervisor's office and that she would be available for emergencies. Instead, she left the hospital, leaving 29 patients unattended by an RN, three of whom were intubated and on respirators in the care of nurse's aides, orderlies, and a respiratory therapist. The hearing panel of the regulatory agency found her guilty of professional misconduct and suspended her license for 1 year. The court upheld the determination of the hearing panel and found that her actions constituted gross misconduct.

While many state boards have now clarified what constitutes patient abandonment as compared to employment abandonment, the Husher case is an example of both. The regulatory board may not necessarily discipline a nurse's license under their definition of patient or employment abandonment, but the employer is free to make an adverse employment decision, including termination, even if there is no state board action. A situation involving patient abandonment places the nurse at risk for both.

In *Eyoma v. Falco et al.* (1991), the issue of patient abandonment could have been raised in finding nurse Falco 100% liable for the patient's injuries in a wrongful death lawsuit brought by his estate. The patient, Mr. Coker, was in the postanesthesia recovery (PAR) room under the care of nurse Falco after having routine gallbladder removal surgery. According to the doctor, he had asked nurse Falco to "watch his respirations" because he had received narcotics. The nurse claimed that she was asked to watch the patient's breathing but not that he had received narcotics. After the doctor left the recovery room, she asked another nurse to watch the patient. She then left the recovery room to care for another patient. Falco admitted that she never got a verbal response from the other nurse, and when she returned, no one was near the patient. When the doctor later returned to the PAR to check on the patient, nurse Falco said he was "fine." However, the doctor then realized that the patient was not breathing. Coker had suffered a respiratory and then cardiac arrest resulting in brain damage. Mr. Coker later died at a nursing home. The jury, having been instructed to find either or both the doctor or nurse liable, found nurse Falco 100% liable, which was upheld by the appeals court. They found that she breached the standard of care in not properly monitoring the patient in the PAR, leaving the patient without verifying that he would be monitored (improper delegation), and failing to recognize that the patient had stopped breathing. It could also be viewed that because of the improper delegation to the other nurse that nurse Falco abandoned her duties to the patient by leaving him in a dangerous situation without proper care.

■ CROSS TRAINING AND FLOATING

Employers generally have the right to expect nurses to "float" to similar types of units as long as they have proper training and support. The recent trend, and The Joint Commission (JCAHO) requirement, is to cross train employees for other jobs to reduce the need to refuse assignments due to lack of training or skill. A nurse may risk being fired for unreasonably refusing to float to other units or for severely criticizing an employer's policies for cross training. In an era of nursing shortages in many areas of practice, nurses will face issues of refusing or accepting patient assignments on a more frequent basis.

In *Waters v. Churchill* (1994) a public employee nurse complained about cross training and other staffing policies and was fired for disruptive speech and activity in the workplace after an investigation by the employer. There was evidence that Churchill dissuaded another employee from transferring to her department by making negative statements about policies, her supervisor, and conditions in general. Some of these conversations took place during a dinner break and were overheard by other employees. These employees eventually reported the overheard statements to defendant Waters, who was nurse Churchill's immediate supervisor. After she was fired, Churchill sued her employer and supervisor claiming her termination violated her right of free speech based on the first amendment to the US Constitution. On appeal to the US Supreme Court, the judgment of the Court of Appeals for the Seventh District in Churchill's favor was reversed. The case was remanded to determine if the employer's firing of Churchill for disruptive speech was a pretext for firing her for other reasons. The court did determine that the government as employer (and not as sovereign) has a right to restrict

speech in the workplace, as in this case, after a reasonable investigation. The employee's speech is not protected if it is determined that it is disruptive, even if part of the speech could be viewed as protected.

This case reminds nurses that appropriate forums should be used to express workplace concerns about policies and staffing and that it may not matter if these statements are made on one's own time, such as during a dinner break. In this case the statements were overheard by other employees and still could be considered disruptive. These kinds of statements, depending on their content and context, will not automatically be protected as exercising one's right to free speech.

■ UNDERSTAFFING AND PATIENT SAFETY

Nurses have sometimes refused to care for patients because of concerns about high nurse–patient ratios or being asked to care for patients outside their area of expertise. Generally, these objections are not upheld when challenged, and nurses are usually advised to provide care but to follow guidelines established for acceptance of assignment despite objection or with reservation.

In *James Johnson v. St. Clare's Hospital & Health Center* (1997), nurse Johnson was discharged after he refused to accept assignments to a floor he considered to have too high a nurse–patient ratio. His reason for this refusal was that he asserted that he needed to avoid stress and high nurse–patient ratios because of medical conditions, including being a recovering alcoholic and suffering from autoimmune hepatitis. He made claims for wrongful discharge as based on discrimination under the Americans with Disabilities Act (ADA) and the Rehabilitation Act. According to the employer, when he was hired nurse Johnson was told he may be required to "float," that is, to work on other units when necessary. Johnson offered no medical evidence to support his stress allegations. He did follow up one of these refusals to float with a memo stating that, "When I realized that my assignment on 4 mc was more than I could safely handle I notified my supervisor and did not accept the assignment." This written statement made no mention of any disability or illness. It was also noted that Johnson did not file a "Notice of Unsafe Staffing" form, the established procedure for addressing inadequate staffing, because this would have required him to work the shift and "grieve" to the union about staffing levels afterward.

Nurse Johnson was suspended for this incident and for refusing another assignment under similar circumstances where he again thought the staffing was inadequate. He was discharged for these actions, and he then submitted a letter requesting accommodations for his disability due to being asked to "... perform duties beyond my abilities and beyond contracted nurse/patient ratios...that not only endangers my health but the health of patients." The hospital appropriately responded to his letter but refused to reinstate him. The letter stated that he was terminated from his position for "... gross misconduct which included insubordination and abandonment of your duties." The court upheld the hospital's discharge, finding no case of ADA discrimination, partially due to the plaintiff having no medical evidence that he is "handicapped." His "say-so" that his status as a recovering alcoholic requires him to avoid work stress caused by too high a nurse–patient ratio was not enough to overcome the employer's right to fire him.

This case points out the need to voice concerns in writing about accommodations needed in the workplace before being confronted with situations that would require the accommodation. Most importantly, the employer does not merely take the employee's word that an accommodation is needed and what that may be; medical evidence is required. Also, the employee must follow established workplace procedures to deal with understaffing situations, especially when governed by a union contract that specifies what the procedures are.

In another case, a nurse refused an assignment because it would require her to work in an area "not within her area of expertise" (*Janet Whittier v. Kaiser Foundation Hospitals*, 2007). Plaintiff nurse Whittier claimed she refused this assignment pursuant to her rights under a collective bargaining agreement (CBA) and that the "float policy" based on the basis of seniority created patient care problems. She was disciplined for this refusal and for poor documentation of pain management of a patient. Whittier did not file a grievance regarding this action but instead sought a transfer to another part of the hospital. A later incident involved her leaving her work station to escort a patient to an appointment, after which she was placed on administrative leave and later terminated. Nurse Whittier filed a lawsuit asserting a violation of public policy. The US District Court of California found that her public policy claim failed because she did not identify any express statutes or public policy that would fall within the Labor Management Relations Act (LMRA) as based on asserting rights under the CBA. Furthermore, the court found her claim under the LMRA to be time barred by the 6 month statute of limitations in which to file a claim.

Inadequate staffing was an issue in the case of *Pamela Robbins v. Provena Hospitals, Inc.* (2003). Nurse Robbins was the cochair and later chair of the Illinois Nurses Association (INA), the exclusive bargaining agent for registered nurses at the medical center owned by the defendants. Part of Robbins's lawsuit alleging retaliatory discharge was based on a public policy exception for "duty to report," which included complaints about the adequacy of staffing. When she met with officials from the Illinois Department of Public Health (IDPH), they inquired as to whether the staffing concerns resulted in delays in patient treatment. If this were true, the medical center's right to participate in and receive reimbursement for Medicare or Medicaid related services would be jeopardized. After this, Robbins and other nurses changed the "assignment despite objection" (ADO) forms to expressly notify the medical center about delays in patient treatment as a result of inadequate staffing. These forms were also submitted to supervisors to comply with an Illinois law that requires nurses to "report unsafe, unethical, or illegal care practice or conditions to the appropriate authorities." The nurses subsequently filed hundreds of ADOs for the following year alleging delays in patient treatment and unsafe staffing levels. In addition, Robbins organized public legislative hearings on the Patient Safety Act, proposing penalties for facilities that refused to give nurses a role in determining staffing levels. Nurse Robbins also circulated a petition addressed to the IDPH (signed by over 160 nurses) demanding an investigation into staffing, which was confiscated by the employer. She was later terminated for these and other activities that the defendant medical center alleged violated an agreement prohibiting nurses from engaging in strikes and work stoppages. Part of nurse Robbins's claim was also based on the False Claims Act (FCA) that prohibits defrauding of the federal government. Because she did not give her employer specific notice of allegations of false claims under this act, her lawsuit was dismissed. She could not show a retaliatory claim under the FCA.

This case underscores the need to not only gather information of the specific nature to validate claims against an employer but also the need to strictly comply with any requirements under a statute. The use of ADO forms can be an effective strategy to collect information for state nurses associations, state regulatory agencies, and to inform the public. However, this may not be enough to overcome the right of employers to make employment decisions on valid grounds, and nurses who actively pursue these claims run the risk of adverse employment decisions.

■ REFERENCES

Agency for Healthcare Research and Quality. (2006). *The patient safety and quality improvement act of 2005*. Overview, June 2006. Retrieved October 26, 2008, from http://www.ahrq.gov/qual/psoact.htm

American Nurses Association. (1995, July 2). *ANA position statement: The right to accept or reject an assignment*. Washington, DC: Author.

American Nurses Association. (2001). *Code of ethics for nurses with interpretive statements*. Washington, DC: Author.

American Nurses Association. (2001, October 17). *ANA position statement: Opposition to mandatory overtime*. Washington, DC: Author.

American Nurses Association. (2006, December 8). *ANA position statement: Assuring patient safety; registered nurses' responsibility in all roles and settings to guard against working while fatigued*. Washington, DC: Author.

Blyth, D. (2007). Do you know what constitutes patient abandonment? *Nursing Management*, *38*(8), 8–10.

Brous, E. (2002). How to handle that staffing predicament. *RN*, *65*(5), 67–70.

Eyoma v. Falco et al., 247 N.J. Super. 435; 589 A.2d 653; 1991 N.J. Super. LEXIS 130 (1991).

Free v. Holy Cross Hospital, 505 N.E.2d 1188 (1987).

Higginbotham, E. (2002). When your beliefs run counter to care. *RN*, *65*(11), 69–72.

Husher v. Commissioner of Education of the State of New York, 591 N.Y.S.2d 99 (A.D. 3 Dept. 1992).

Institute of Medicine (IOM). (2004). *To err is human: Building a safer health care system*. Washington, DC: The National Academy of Medicine.

James Johnson v. St. Clare's Hospital & Health Center, 1997 U.S. Dist. LEXIS 22492 (1997).

Janet Whittier v. Kaiser Foundation Hospitals, 2007 U.S. Dist. LEXIS 17129 (2007).

Pamela Robbins v. Provena Hospitals, Inc., 2003 U.S. Dist. LEXIS 10692 (2003).

Rogers, A., et al. (2004). The working hours of hospital staff nurses and patient safety. *Health Affairs*, *23*(4), 2002–2012.

Waters v. Churchill, 511 U.S. 661; 114 S.Ct. 1878; 128 L.Ed.2d 686; 1994 U.S. LEXIS 4104; 62 U.S. L. W. 4379 9 I.E.R. Cas. (BNA) 801 (1994).

Chapter 10

Delegation to Unlicensed Assistive Personnel

Susan J. Westrick

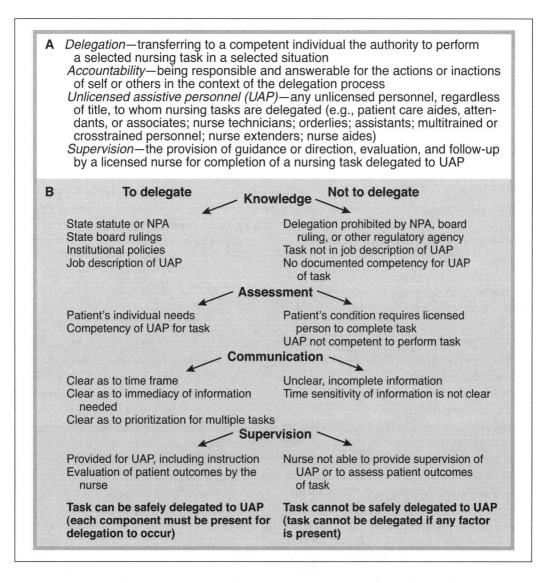

A *Delegation*—transferring to a competent individual the authority to perform a selected nursing task in a selected situation

Accountability—being responsible and answerable for the actions or inactions of self or others in the context of the delegation process

Unlicensed assistive personnel (UAP)—any unlicensed personnel, regardless of title, to whom nursing tasks are delegated (e.g., patient care aides, attendants, or associates; nurse technicians; orderlies; assistants; multitrained or crosstrained personnel; nurse extenders; nurse aides)

Supervision—the provision of guidance or direction, evaluation, and follow-up by a licensed nurse for completion of a nursing task delegated to UAP

B

To delegate	Not to delegate
Knowledge	
State statute or NPA	Delegation prohibited by NPA, board ruling, or other regulatory agency
State board rulings	Task not in job description of UAP
Institutional policies	No documented competency for UAP of task
Job description of UAP	
Assessment	
Patient's individual needs	Patient's condition requires licensed person to complete task
Competency of UAP for task	UAP not competent to perform task
Communication	
Clear as to time frame	Unclear, incomplete information
Clear as to immediacy of information needed	Time sensitivity of information is not clear
Clear as to prioritization for multiple tasks	
Supervision	
Provided for UAP, including instruction	Nurse not able to provide supervision of UAP or to assess patient outcomes of task
Evaluation of patient outcomes by the nurse	
Task can be safely delegated to UAP (each component must be present for delegation to occur)	**Task cannot be safely delegated to UAP (task cannot be delegated if any factor is present)**

In an era of professional nurse shortages in all settings, effectively working with assistive personnel to implement the nursing process is a necessary and continuing part of nursing practice. Optimum use of all levels of personnel is a reality to meet financial and other constraints in healthcare settings. As the licensed caregiver, the nurse is responsible and accountable for the quality of care that patients receive. The nurse may delegate or assign tasks to an unlicensed caregiver, but accountability in terms of outcomes for the patient is retained by the nurse. Unlicensed assistive personnel (UAP) act for the nurse in implementing selected patient care activities but do not act in place of the nurse. The critical thinking, professional judgment, and decision making by the nurse can never be delegated. See the definitions in **Figure 10-1A**.

■ LEGAL FRAMEWORK FOR DELEGATION

The first frame of reference to ensure proper delegation (see Figure 10-1B) is the statute or nurse practice act (NPA) that defines the scope of practice for nurses in a particular state. These statutes generally follow the model set forth by the American Nurses Association (ANA), which defines the practice of nursing by a professional nurse as the process of diagnosing human responses to actual or potential health problems, including supportive and restorative care, health counseling and teaching, case finding and referral, and collaborating in the implementation of the total healthcare regimen. The definition set forth in the statute limits what the nurse can delegate by defining what nursing practice itself is.

Other authoritative references include any state board rulings on the use of UAP and position papers from the National Council of State Boards of Nursing (NCSBN) or the ANA. The NCSBN and ANA have issued a Joint Statement on Delegation (2006) that reviews terminology, policy considerations, principles, and resources for delegation. The core philosophy of this document is that delegation is an essential skill for nurses and that patient safety is the paramount consideration. Some specialty nursing organizations, such as the Emergency Nurses Association (ENA), have also issued position statements. The ENA position statement on the "Role of Delegation by the Emergency Nurse in Clinical Practice Settings" (1998) suggests activities that should and should not be delegated. Although these position papers are not legal

references, they are viewed as authoritative sources for determining standards within the profession. These standards related to delegation would be reviewed if a case of malpractice or licensure discipline against a nurse involved a question of improper delegation.

Similarly, the ANA Code of Ethics for Nurses provides guidance for nurses when delegating tasks to other healthcare workers. Central to the code is the idea that the nurse retains accountability for the delegated task. Also specified is that nurses who are in management and administrative roles are responsible to maintain an environment that supports proper delegation, including policies, job descriptions, and competency validation for UAPs and helping nurses develop skills related to delegation.

■ GUIDELINES/SITUATIONS FOR DELEGATION

The following factors should be considered by the nurse in any decision to delegate:

- Delegable task: The nurse first should determine if the task is properly delegable. For example, giving medications or interpreting clinical data cannot be delegated because these are licensed functions. However, it is generally agreed that routine tasks (e.g., taking vital signs) or personal care activities (e.g., bathing) for stable patients with predictable outcomes can be assigned to UAP.
- Patients' needs: The nurse is responsible for individual patient assessment and determination of nursing care needs. Therefore, even though an intervention, such as giving a bath, may be routine, the nurse may need to complete this task for certain patients if further assessment or health teaching is needed. The nurse should not to delegate any task that would jeopardize patient safety.
- Competency of UAP: Job descriptions for UAP should clearly specify their responsibilities. UAP should have a record of documented competencies to

perform tasks and should have participated in a formalized educational program that provided instruction. However, it is the duty of the nurse to ensure that UAP are competent in particular situations (e.g., they may not be able to measure blood pressure properly even though there is documentation that they can). It is the nurse's responsibility to determine ability and provide proper instruction for UAP or complete the task himself or herself. The nurse must provide supervision for UAP and serve as a resource. The sole criterion for determining who should complete a task in a particular situation is patient safety, as determined by the nurse.

- Communication: Clear directions must be given to UAP so that the task can be completed properly. For example, the nurse should not say, "I need a finger stick done on Mr. Jones." A better instruction would indicate the immediate need for a blood glucose measurement and the need to report the value to the nurse immediately, who will determine if insulin is needed. It is suggested that the nurse obtain "minireports" throughout the shift to clarify data obtained and to provide any supervision necessary for UAP. Communication is an ongoing process and involves the opportunity for the UAP to ask questions and express any concerns about performing the delegated task.

- Supervision/Evaluation: As part of the nurse's duty to supervise UAP, the nurse is responsible for evaluating their performance. This is an opportunity to provide positive and constructive negative feedback as well as supervised practice of a skill if needed. The ability to set priorities for completion of tasks is an essential skill needed by UAP and often requires guidance by the nurse. This duty also involves surveillance and monitoring of the UAP activities to ensure positive and expected patient outcomes.

■ THE PROCESS OF EFFECTIVE DELEGATION

The nurse uses critical thinking and professional judgment in deciding when delegation is appropriate. Delegation occurs on a case-by-case basis with the nurse assessing the individual patient's needs and circumstances. It is not a to-do list for certain job classifications and is a process that needs ongoing assessment and evaluation of factors, such as complexity of the task, stability of the patient's condition, predictability of outcomes from the intervention, and the abilities of the staff to whom the task will be delegated. There are many positive benefits of delegation, including opportunities for leadership, instruction, team building, and mentoring staff members. In addition, the nurse is given time to perform more skilled nursing functions consistent with role expectations. The NCSBN also considers that the organization must provide the environment and support for nurses for effective delegation in terms of sufficient resources, policy development, competency validation of UAP, and skill mix of staff members. Proper and effective delegation involves: (1) the right task, (2) the right circumstances, (3) the right person, (4) the right direction/communication, and (5) the right supervision. In all situations, the nurse's professional judgment and critical thinking determine what can be delegated safely to UAP or others.

■ LIABILITY ISSUES IN DELEGATION

Improper Delegation and Nurse Liability

The nurse can be liable for improper delegation in several circumstances. One example is when a task that should not be delegated (e.g., medication administration) is assigned to UAP. Another example is when the nurse delegates a task to UAP who are not competent to perform the task. While nurses can generally rely on documented competencies of UAP, there may be information that the nurse knows or should have known to indicate UAP are not competent in a particular situation. Another example of improper delegation occurs when the nurse does not provide the required supervision for UAP. The nurse should always be available for questions or further instruction. Delegation can also occur laterally to another caregiver, as in the Eyoma case where the nurse improperly delegated the care of a patient in the postanesthesia recovery room to another nurse (*Eyoma v. Falco*, 1991). Nurse Falco asked another nurse to watch her patient while she left the room but did not get a response from the other nurse. Thus, the other nurse did not acknowledge the delegation, and nurse Falco was found liable for the patient injury resulting from improper delegation and patient abandonment.

Proper Delegation without Nurse Liability

If the nurse has delegated properly, UAP can be individually liable for their actions. One example is when UAP do not inform the nurse of an inability to perform a task or when UAP perform a task incorrectly, even after instruction and supervision. UAP who perform tasks that are beyond those delegated or are outside their competencies are liable for their own actions and for mistakes or adverse patient outcomes as a result of their actions. The liability of UAP is generally shifted to the institution as the employer.

Staffing Issues

Inadequate staffing is not a rationale for delegating tasks. In such an instance, the nurse needs to document his or her refusal to delegate a task as based on concern for patient safety and its effect on patient care. This should be forwarded to a supervisor who has the power to correct the staffing. By taking these steps, the nurse is shifting the liability to the institution for any untoward outcomes resulting from the situation.

■ CASE LAW RELATED TO DELEGATION AND WORKING WITH UNLICENSED STAFF

Many cases related to malpractice involve issues of nurses working with unlicensed personnel and whether the nurse provided proper instruction or supervision in the patient care situation. The cases do not often use the term "delegation" when referring to nurses working with UAP, but this is involved with most of the cases where the actions of both the nurse and the UAP are questioned. Cases are reported more frequently in nursing homes, long term care, and home care settings and often involve nurses' aides or home healthcare aides. The reality of utilizing increased numbers of UAP in the workplace in all settings is a trend that will likely continue.

Failure to Communicate and Report

In the case of *Milazzo v. Olsten Home Health Care, Inc. and Kathleen Broussard, RN* (1998), the plaintiff Milazzo suffered permanent injuries as a result of delay in treatment. Milazzo was a second day postop patient in the hospital recovering from placement of a shunt to relieve pressure in the ventricles surrounding her brain. Her family hired Buchanan as a "sitter" from the defendant agency to be with Milazzo over the night shift. Buchanan was also a certified nurses' aide and personal care attendant. Part of Buchanan's duties were to assist the patient Milazzo and report any significant changes in her condition. Nurse Broussard performed a neurological assessment at the beginning of the shift, according to the standard of care, and visited the patient, who was sleeping, about every 2 hours thereafter. At each of the patient visits, the nurse asked the sitter how the patient was doing, and the sitter always said "fine." Nurse Broussard told Buchanan to let her know if anything was wrong. However, at one point during the night, the sitter had called for the assistance of two unit nursing assistants to help her take the patient to the bathroom and then put her back to bed. At that time, Milazzo was unable to stand and was "leaning to the left" and required this extra assistance. Earlier, Milazzo had ambulated with just Buchanan's help and walked to the bathroom. Buchanan claimed she thought the nursing assistants would tell the nurse about Milazzo's change in condition, but no one reported this to nurse Broussard or to the patient's family. The sitter did write the change on the form at the end of her overnight shift and informed the patient's daughter, who had come to stay with her during the day. When examined by the physician that morning, Milazzo was unable to move her left side and was conversing inappropriately. Tests determined irreversible neurological damage and Milazzo required further cranial surgery. At trial it was determined that nurse Broussard had followed the standard of care but that the sitter Buchanan had been negligent in not reporting significant changes in the patient's condition. Earlier intervention would have resulted in a greater chance of recovery.

Even though the nurse was found not to be at fault for the patient's injuries, this case points to the need to clearly communicate with sitters and nursing assistants and to clarify reporting procedures.

Similarly, in *Molden v. Mississippi* (1998), two nurse's aides appealed the decision of the trial court in affirming the state department of health's finding of negligence and revocation of their nurse aide certifications. This decision was upheld by the Supreme Court of Mississippi. The court found that nurse aides Molden and Avery were negligent when a nursing home resident suffered second-degree burns after a whirlpool bath. Molden tested the water with her double gloved hand, gave the bath, and was assisted by Avery. After the patient's bath, Avery stated she told Molden to report to the treatment nurse that the patient's skin was peeling and that her toe was bleeding. Neither Avery nor Molden reported the patient's symptoms, but Molden told nurse Harrison that the patient was ready for the dressings for her decubitus ulcer. Nurse Harrison, an LPN, discovered that the patient's legs were very red and had blisters on them, which she reported to the charge nurse. The patient was taken to a hospital and treated for second-degree burns. Thereafter,

both Avery and Molden were reported to the health department who, after a hearing, revoked their certifications and placed them permanently on the Nurse Aide Abuse Roster.

Again, although nurses were not found at fault in this case, and the conduct of the nurse aides cannot be excused, it may be that policies related to checking bath water temperature should be clarified and reviewed with the staff. Unlicensed staff members can greatly benefit from periodic review and education regarding tasks that are routinely delegated to them.

Failure to Supervise/Check Assignment of Unlicensed Staff

In *Williams v. West Virginia Board of Examiners* (2004), nurse Williams appealed a decision of the nursing board to suspend her license for 1 year. Williams was employed as a nurse manager who supervised homemaker-health workers. As part of her duties, she was required to make periodic visits to the home when home health aides were present, review patient records, and update documentation of patients' problems and progress that was recorded in patient in-home files. A state health department inspector found deficiencies in several of these areas. On one occasion there were progress notes documented for the nurse manager's patient visit when home health aides were present at the patient's home at the same time, but the home health aides denied that nurse Williams had visited. Nurse Williams could not produce handwritten notes for the required paperwork to document other scheduled visits. Several clients also denied that visits from the nurse occurred as she had reported. The nursing board found that Williams was guilty of violating standards of the profession when she falsely documented visits. They placed her on probation and suspended her license for a year, which was upheld on appeal. Part of the defense for her actions was that she had an overly large caseload, but the health inspector found the nurse–patient ratio to be consistent with standards.

In another case of supervising unlicensed health assistants, nurse Hicks, a licensed practical nurse (LPN), was disciplined for patient neglect when a resident was found tipped over in his wheelchair and had not been returned to bed by nursing home assistants (*Hicks v. New York State Department of Health*, 1991). Part of nurse Hicks's duties were to ensure that nursing home residents were placed in bed and received appropriate care during her evening shift. Security personnel found the patient in the dark, half in his bed and half still restrained in his overturned wheelchair. There was evidence of urine and hardened feces dried on his skin when he was found, and this was documented in the nurse's record. The court upheld the health department's finding of patient neglect against nurse Hicks. The case was grounded on her failure to properly supervise the nursing assistants and ensure that their duties had been completed. Although the court did not use the term "delegated," the principle is the same where accountability remains with the licensed professional who assigns and supervises tasks to UAP.

Improper Delegation of Tasks

In *Singleton v. AAA Home Health* (2000), the physician orders specified that "skilled nurses" should pack the patient's four decubitus ulcers and change the dressing. The defendant home healthcare agency (AAA) provided caregivers. Nurses had performed the wound packing and dressing changes for over a year, but the wound worsened and the patient needed additional surgery 2 years later to assist in wound healing. At that time it was discovered that there was an old gauze in the wound that had not been removed. The wound continued to fail to heal, and a lawsuit commenced alleging that the failure to remove the old gauze caused delay in wound healing and further damage. At issue in the case was whether unlicensed "sitters" performed "wound care" and whether they were taught the packing procedure. There was documentation by the supervising nurse that she had instructed the sitters on how to pack the

wound, but the sitters denied this, stating that they only changed the outer layer of the dressings. None of AAA's nurses had observed sitters perform this wound care procedure. The plaintiff's expert witness testified that the standard of care required documentation of the number of gauzes used to pack in the wound and the number removed from the wound for each dressing change. In finding that the defendant breached its duty to the plaintiff, the court granted the plaintiff's motion for a judgment notwithstanding the verdict (JNOV) in favor of the plaintiff. Part of the finding for liability was based on the duty of skilled nurses who worked for the agency to properly implement the physician's orders for skilled nurses to pack the wound.

This case presents many issues related to the inadequate wound care that the patient received, including that it was not a delegable task (ordered to be performed by skilled nurses), whether the procedure was taught properly, and whether the task (even if properly delegated) was properly supervised. Based on facts presented in the Singleton case, it appears that none of these conditions or steps for safe and effective delegation took place.

In *Fairfax Nursing Home v. Department of Health and Human Services* (2002), a nursing home received substantial fines by the US Department of Health and Human Services (DHHS) for placing ventilator-assisted patients at great risk of harm. Inspectors found many violations of documentation, follow up, and inadequate care of these patients, several of which resulted in patient deaths. The nursing home was found to have lacked substantial compliance with regulations required for proper care of ventilator-assisted patients and lacked policies and procedures to protect them. Many patients were found to have ventilator-associated pneumonia that was inadequately diagnosed and treated. This presented a "risk of immediate jeopardy" that justified the severe fines and requirements to comply with standards. Among the cited deficiencies was a state surveyor's observation of a Fairfax employee's failure to use sterile technique while performing tracheostomy care and neglect in hyperoxygenating the patient before and after suctioning the tracheostomy. In some instances the suctioning procedure was performed by nurse's aides as unlicensed personnel. The overwhelming systemic nature of the problems in care of patients resulted in fines of over $3000 per day for 105 days by an administrative law judge, which was upheld on appeal.

Proper Delegation, Protocols, and Supervision

In *Hunter v. Bossier Medical Center* (1998), a hospital successfully defended a patient's medical malpractice action by presenting evidence that nurse aides and the registered nurse followed proper procedures and protocols. The patient Hunter was ambulated by two nurse's aides and then was standing near the wall in his room while his bed was being made by one of the aides. Hunter became lightheaded and was "eased to the floor" by the other nurse's aide. When nurse Montano entered the room and checked the patient, she found Hunter leaning up against the nurse's aide's legs, which was consistent with a patient who had been slid to the floor. Hunter was found to not have immediate injuries from the incident. After discharge, he later had some pain and other problems that he attributed to his "fall" in the hospital. Hunter claimed that he had lost consciousness and woke up with his leg bent under him. However, the medical review panel (MRP) found the testimony of the nurse's aides (who had 20 years of experience between them) and nurse Montano to be persuasive and placed importance on nurse Montano's medical chart notation that documented the events at the time. The nurse's aides also referred to a training manual and identified the page for the procedure they learned for "easing" a patient who is falling to the ground. Thus, the appeals court affirmed the jury's finding in favor of the defendant hospital.

This case underscores the importance of proper procedures, documented training, and supervision of nurse's aides. Along with the factual and objective documentation of the nurse that supported the finding that the standard of care was met in this case, the Hunter case illustrates that with these protections, safe and effective care for patients can occur when unlicensed personnel are utilized. Doing so will often determine whether the institution can successfully defend itself against malpractice claims.

■ REFERENCES

American Nurses Association. (2001). *Code of ethics for nurses with interpretive statements.* Washington, DC: Author.

American Nurses Association. (2008). *Guide to the code of ethics for nurses—interpretation and application.* Silver Springs, MD: Author.

American Nurses Association (ANA) and National Council of State Boards of Nursing (NCSBN). (2006). *Joint statement on delegation.* Retrieved October 26, 2008, from http://www.nursingworld.org/MainMenuCategories/ThePracticeofProfessionalNursing/InfoforNurses/ANANCSBNStatementonDelegationpdf.aspx

Emergency Nurses Association Position Statement. (1998). *Role of delegation by the emergency nurse in clinical practice settings.* Author.

Eyoma v. Falco, 247 N.J. Super. 435; 589 A.2d 653; 1991 N.J. Super. LEXIS 130 (1991).

Fairfax Nursing Home v. Department of Health and Human Services, 300 F.3d 835; 2002 U.S. App. LEXIS 16505 (2002).

Hicks v. New York State Department of Health, 173 A.D.2d 1057; 570 N.Y.S.2d 395; 1991 N.Y. App. Div. LEXIS 7225 (1991).

Hunter v. Bossier Medical Center, (1998) 31,026 (La. App. 2 Cir. 09/25/98); 718 So.2d 636; 1998 La. App. LEXIS 2626.

Milazzo v. Olsten Home Health Care, Inc. and Kathleen Broussard, RN, 97-30 (La. App. 5 Cir. 01/28/98); 708 So.2d 1108; 1998 La. App. LEXIS 193 (1998).

Molden v. Mississippi, 730 So.2d 29; 1998 Miss. LEXIS 443 (1998).

Singleton v. AAA Home Health, 00-00670 (La. App. 3 Cir. 11/02/00); 772 So.2d 346; 2000 La. App. LEXIS 2705 (2000).

Williams v. West Virginia Board of Examiners, 215 W.Va. 237; 599 S.E.2d 660; 2004 W.Va. LEXIS 67 (2004).

Part I Review Questions

1. A healthcare institution markets itself as a comprehensive care center able to coordinate and meet the community's healthcare needs. A patient goes to the emergency department where the nurses are employees but the physicians are independent contractors. The patient exhibits signs of an impending cerebral vascular accident (CVA; slurred speech, drooping facial expression, and one-sided weakness) with a congested cough and wheezing. He is discharged with the diagnosis of pneumonia. Which of the following may he bring a civil action against?

    (A) The nurses individually for failing to recognize and communicate the symptoms to the physician
    (B) The physicians, as independent contractors, for failure to diagnose and treat the CVA
    (C) The hospital under corporate liability for the action of the nurses as employees and the physicians as independent contractors
    (D) All of the above

2. When incorporating concepts of law and ethics in practice, the nurse must consider that:

    (A) Ethical codes do not have the force of law and will not be looked at by courts for guidance
    (B) Legal duties are often minimal, and ethical codes may require conduct beyond legal accountability

    (C) Fulfilling legal duties will prevent any ethical conflicts
    (D) Patients' wishes will always supersede ethical or legal codes

3. Which of the following would typically *not* be included in a state's Nurse Practice Act (NPA)?

    (A) Scope of practice guidelines
    (B) Definition of what constitutes practice outside the scope of nursing (e.g., the practice of medicine)
    (C) Definitions of what constitutes unprofessional conduct
    (D) Requirements for maintaining licensure

4. Mandatory licensure for RNs means that:

    (A) Anyone who works as a nurse for compensation must be registered with the state as an RN
    (B) Anyone can work as a nurse for compensation but cannot use the title RN unless registered with the state as an RN
    (C) Not only are nurses required to be registered but also they must be certified
    (D) A nursing license from a neighboring state would be recognized as valid in the state in which the nurse is practicing

5. A nurse administers potassium chloride to a patient by intravenous (IV) push, although the physician's order states it is

to be given by IV piggyback. The patient's cardiac monitor immediately shows a flatline and the patient dies. What type of actions might the nurse become involved in as a result of this error?

(A) Criminal action
(B) Civil malpractice action
(C) Administrative law action (disciplinary action)
(D) All of the above

6. The state board of nursing *cannot* take which of the following actions against a nurse?

(A) Suspension of the nurse's license for a period of time
(B) Censure of a nurse
(C) Placing a nurse on probation
(D) Imprisonment

7. The nurse administers pentobarbital to a patient when phenobarbital was ordered. There was no injury to the patient; however, the nursing supervisor reported the incident to the state board of nursing. The nurse is notified of the charges brought against her, and a disciplinary hearing is held. What is the role of the state board of nursing?

(A) To protect the public
(B) To uphold standards of nursing practice
(C) To investigate all complaints to determine if disciplinary action is appropriate
(D) All of the above

8. Standards of care are:

(A) The optimal degree of professional skill
(B) Used to show gross negligence and incompetence
(C) Used to determine what is negligent performance
(D) None of the above

9. Professional negligence occurs when a nurse:

(A) Provides nursing care that results in an adverse outcome
(B) Fails to provide the optimal level of nursing care
(C) Fails to respond as a reasonable prudent nurse
(D) Exercises an error in judgment

10. A home care nurse working for a proprietary agency instructed a patient to change his dressing every day and to observe the wound for signs of infection. When the nurse returned 2 weeks later, the original dressing was still in place. The wound showed signs of infection, and the patient required antibiotic therapy. The wound became worse and resulted in tissue damage. In a malpractice action against the nurse 1 year later, the patient claimed negligent supervision of the wound. A defense that would *most likely* be available for the defendant nurse to raise would be:

(A) Assumption of the risk
(B) Comparative or contributory negligence
(C) Charitable immunity
(D) Statute of limitations

11. A home care nurse visits a patient who had surgery 3 weeks ago. As part of the patient's care plan, he was instructed to perform range of motion exercises. However, he has not done so, and it is now 3 weeks later when the nurse visits. The patient is complaining that he is having difficulty walking and continues to have problems with his recovery for several months. If a lawsuit is later filed claiming malpractice against the nurse and physician:

(A) The patient is entitled to a recovery because his informed consent amounted to a contract for services that was not successfully fulfilled

(B) A defense that could be raised is contributory negligence

(C) The patient will not recover since he assumed the risks of failure when he signed the surgical consent form

(D) The nurse cannot be sued because she works for an agency

12. In most states, the Good Samaritan Act provides immunity from civil liability to:

(A) Volunteers providing emergency medical care when there is no legal duty to assist

(B) Professionals providing emergency medical care in emergency department or acute care settings

(C) Nonmedical volunteers for ordinary negligence and professional medical volunteers for gross (extraordinary) negligence

(D) None of the above

13. When providing care to patients, the nurse *increases* the risk of liability when:

(A) Refusing to implement an incomplete physician's order

(B) Administering predrawn and labeled injections prepared by another nurse

(C) Notifying a physician's supervisor when an order may be harmful to a patient

(D) Doing none of the above

14. A nurse is making rounds on the surgical floor when Ms. Clark, who just had a hysterectomy, says to him, "You people are wretched humans, you get pleasure out of using me as a pincushion." The nurse should:

(A) Identify her as a difficult patient and resolve to only enter her room when a nursing procedure needs to be done

(B) Defend himself by explaining the necessity of needle sticks for lab procedures and pain medications

(C) Offer her special attention, offer to work with her for a solution, and visit her when no nursing procedure needs to be done

(D) Ask another nurse to switch assignments because he has a personality conflict with the patient and does not want to antagonize her further

15. A nurse is a fact witness in a personal injury lawsuit. The attorney representing the plaintiff asks the nurse a question at a deposition about the plaintiff's injuries, but the nurse isn't sure if the attorney is asking about the state of the plaintiff's injuries on admission or on discharge to her nursing unit. The nurse should:

(A) Give as much information as possible to cover both possibilities

(B) Decide to answer about the state of the injuries upon admission

(C) Ask the attorney to be more specific

(D) Decide to answer about the state of the injuries upon discharge

16. A nurse is taking care of a patient who is "pleasantly demented." The patient is always smiling and agreeable to all suggestions but doesn't understand events as they happen. The patient's family arrives to visit with an attorney and requests that the nurse witness the patient's signing of a deed to her home so that the daughter will own the property for estate planning purposes. The nurse should:

(A) Check with her employer to determine if there is a policy about nurses witnessing documents

(B) Inform the attorney that the patient, although smiling and agreeable, doesn't understand things as they happen

(C) Refuse to witness the document

(D) Prepare written documentation of the events in the chart as soon as possible

(E) All of the above

17. A malpractice claim is brought against a nurse in the year 2000. The case involves an incident that occurred at a previous job in 1996. The nurse will be covered for this incident:

    (A) Only if the nurse is still working for the previous employer (employer's policy will cover)
    (B) If he or she was covered by an individual or employer occurrence policy at the time of the incident
    (C) If he or she was covered by a claims made policy in 1996
    (D) By her new employer's policy as long as it is an occurrence policy

18. The employer's malpractice insurance will generally cover the nurse's actions if the negligent act is:

    (A) Of an extremely reckless nature, such as to endanger a patient through outrageous conduct
    (B) Outside the scope of the NPA
    (C) Within the employee's job description
    (D) One that occurred when the nurse was off duty but constituted performing volunteer nursing duties

19. A nurse is asked to work a double shift on a unit he is unfamiliar with. The nurse should do all of the following *except:*

    (A) Determine whether he can safely provide care for the population of patients
    (B) Ask to be oriented to the unit
    (C) Request that a nurse who is familiar with the unit work with him
    (D) Refuse the patient assignment and file a complaint with the union

20. A nurse caring for several patients becomes ill while on duty and decides she cannot continue to work that day. To avoid a later claim against her for patient abandonment, she should:

    (A) Tell her supervisor that she is leaving
    (B) Inform both her coworkers and the supervisor that she needs to leave the work area due to illness
    (C) Go to a physician to get a note to validate her illness
    (D) Not worry about letting anyone know because her shift will be over in an hour anyhow

21. The nurse is assigned to a group of patients on the evening shift. A UAP is working with the nurse. Which of the following interventions can be assigned to the UAP?

    (A) Administer an antibiotic cream to a patient's arm after the UAP gives the patient a bath
    (B) Complete a health history and admission assessment on a patient because the patient is not in acute distress
    (C) Take vital signs on a patient who has had surgery 4 hours earlier
    (D) Monitor and adjust the patient's IV line after the nurse instructs the UAP how to perform this task properly

22. A patient assigned to a nurse fell while in the bathroom. The nurse had instructed the UAP to assist the patient with walking on an as-needed basis. Assuming that the patient should have been assisted and was not, who is legally liable for the patient's fall?

    (A) The nurse because he or she is in charge of the UAP
    (B) The UAP because direction was given by the nurse
    (C) Neither the nurse nor the UAP because each acted properly
    (D) Both the nurse and the UAP could be liable because each had an independent duty to the patient

Part I Answers

1. *The answer is D.*

   The nurses and physicians are liable for their part of the malpractice. The hospital is liable under corporate liability for the negligent acts of its employees (vicarious liability) and for the negligent hiring and retention of the negligent independent contractors (the physicians). The hospital will be held liable for any negligent emergency department policy and procedures that were followed in the treatment of this patient if those policies caused the patient's injury.

2. *The answer is B.*

   Ethical codes often go beyond legal requirements, which may only require a minimal standard of conduct. Answer A is incorrect because ethical codes are sometimes viewed by courts as evidence of the standard of care required in certain cases. Answer C is incorrect because ethical conflicts can still exist even if legal duties are implemented. For example, the nurse legally may be required to protect confidential information provided by a patient but know that revealing it to another person may protect him or her. Answer D is incorrect because the law supersedes patients' wishes, and ethical codes may do so in some cases (i.e., suicide).

3. *The answer is B.*

   The state statute or NPA does not define what is outside the scope of practice for nursing. Anything not defined in the statute as nursing is considered to be outside the scope of practice for nurses. Other practice statutes, such as for physicians, would need to be consulted for specifics as to what constitutes practice as a physician.

4. *The answer is A.*

   Mandatory licensure means that both the title and the functions of the nurse are protected in these states. All states have this type of licensure. Answer B defines a situation of permissive licensure. Answer C speaks to certification, which is a voluntary credential or in some cases may be required for advanced practice. Answer D refers to the idea behind multistate licensure, which has not yet been accepted by all states.

5. *The answer is D.*

   The state might bring negligent homicide charges against the nurse, subjecting the nurse to a criminal proceeding. The patient's family may bring a malpractice claim against the nurse, and the state board may bring disciplinary charges against the nurse.

6. *The answer is D.*

   The state board of nursing does not have the power to imprison a nurse. That can only occur when criminal charges are successful against a nurse, and this would not be handled by the state board but would be adjudicated by a criminal court.

7. *The answer is D.*

   The state board of nursing is empowered by the NPA to administer, establish, and enforce standards of nursing practice.

8. *The answer is C.*

   Standards of care are used as evidence of negligent professional performance. They are not the optimal level of performance nor do they define gross (or reckless) or even incompetent conduct.

9. *The answer is C.*

   Negligence is the failure to meet the definition of the standard of care. An error in nursing judgment or not providing extraordinary care does not necessarily violate the standard of care. Providing the reasonable degree of nursing care does not guarantee that a patient will not experience what is statistically an adverse result.

10. *The answer is B.*

    The defense of either contributory or comparative negligence would most likely be available to the nurse because the patient did not follow the instructions and thus did not act reasonably under the circumstances. He contributed to his own injury, which in some states would bar recovery of damages or in others would limit recovery of damages, assuming there was any negligence found against the nurse. Answer A is incorrect because the patient does not assume the risk of negligent treatment. Answer C is not correct because the agency is not a charitable entity, and this exception has been eliminated in most jurisdictions. Answer D is incorrect because the statute of limitation usually is 2–3 years.

11. *The answer is B.*

    The patient did not perform the exercises that were recommended and thus contributed to his own problems. This contributory negligence can be raised as a defense to any claim of negligence or malpractice. In some states this could be called comparative negligence. Answer A is incorrect because informed consent does not waive a valid claim for negligence and does not become a contract. Answer C is not correct because the patient does not assume the risk of negligence or malpractice. Answer D is incorrect because the nurse can be sued individually, although the agency as the employer would likely be sued as well.

12. *The answer is A.*

    The act applies to all volunteers (medical or nonmedical) to encourage assistance in emergencies when there is no legal duty to assist. B is incorrect because this does not apply to medical personnel when there is a healthcare provider–patient relationship. When a person comes into the emergency department, there is a patient relationship. C is incorrect because the act provides immunity for ordinary and gross negligence for nonmedical volunteers. Medical volunteers enjoy immunity for ordinary negligence but are held to a higher standard than nonmedical volunteers and are expected to perform without gross negligence under the circumstances. For example, nonmedical volunteers may not be expected to maintain an airway in an unconscious accident victim but medical volunteers would.

13. *The answer is B.*

    Administering any medication drawn up by someone other than the nurse who is administering the medication carries an increased risk of liability. The nurse who gives the medication is the last line of defense to prevent negligence when a dose is incorrect. Medications should be drawn up by the nurse who is giving the medication so that there is less chance for error or miscommunication. A and C are appropriate actions.

14. *The answer is C.*

    This nurse needs to build a trusting nurse–patient relationship. Offering the patient attentiveness and visits without making her feel like a "pincushion" may foster the nurse–patient relationship. The nurse should utilize supervisors and more experienced nurses if necessary and make it a team effort. Patients who have a satisfactory relationship with their nurse are less likely to sue should they be injured. A, B, and D will foster a distrustful relationship with the patient.

15. *The answer is C.*

    The nurse should not answer a question that he or she doesn't fully understand or one that is unclear. To do so presents inaccurate information. If she is asked the same or similar question at the trial but gives a different answer because she was confused at the deposition, her credibility will be diminished. It will appear as though she's changing her answers and is an unreliable witness. A, B, and D are incorrect for the same reasons.

16. *The answer is E.*

    A, B, C, and D are all appropriate actions for the nurse to take. The nurse should check with his or her employer to see if the nurse will violate policy if he or she agrees to witness signing of the document. Because the nurse knows the patient and her condition, the nurse should tell the attorney that although the patient appears to agree and understand, her condition makes that very unlikely.

Because the nurse cannot in good faith believe the patient has the capacity to understand the nature and effect of signing the deed, the nurse should not bear witness to the signing. Written documentation should be completed as close to the time of the events as possible to accurately record them.

17. *The answer is B.*

    The nurse will be covered for this incident if there is current coverage by his or her own occurrence policy. This type of policy covers back to when the incident occurred. Answer C is incorrect because the claim must be made when the claims made insurance policy is in effect. Answer A is incorrect because the nurse does not have to be presently working for the employer for the insurance to cover. Answer D is incorrect because a new employer's policy will not cover incidents from a previous job.

18. *The answer is C.*

    The nurse's actions generally are covered if they fall within the nurse's job description and scope of duties. Answer A is incorrect because these actions are so extreme that the policy does not cover them. When acting in such an extremely dangerous manner, the employee is deemed to be acting on his or her own behalf and not that of the employer. Answer B is incorrect because acts covered for malpractice must be within the scope of the NPA because the contract is covering for nursing actions. Answer D is incorrect because volunteer acts are not covered by the employer unless specifically stated.

19. *The answer is D.*

    The nurse would risk being fired for insubordination for refusing the assignment and filing a complaint without more of a basis to do so. A nurse who refuses an assignment needs to be on solid ground for doing so. Along with being familiar with the terms of employment on this issue, the nurse needs to have a reasonable basis for refusal. Answers A, B, and C list valid assessments and steps to take before deciding whether to accept the assignment. If these are not in place, the nurse could refuse the assignment. In no case should the nurse accept the assignment if the criterion in A is not met (i.e., nurse must be able to safely care for the patients).

20. *The answer is B.*

The nurse needs to inform both the supervisor and her coworkers of the situation so that adequate coverage for her patients will be provided. Answer A is not adequate because unless coworkers know of the situation, patients can be placed at risk. There was an action against a nurse by a state board of nursing for patient abandonment based on these facts. The nurse stated that she felt "so horrible" that she left without informing her coworkers, but she had informed her supervisor. This was not enough to avoid the charge of patient abandonment because she did not ensure coverage of her patients by coworkers. Answer C is not correct because validating the illness is not the issue. Answer D is not correct

because she is placing patients at risk even though it may be only a short time until the next shift.

21. *The answer is C.*

A UAP generally can be assigned routine tasks on a stable patient. The answer does not indicate that the patient has any special needs requiring nursing intervention. Answer A is incorrect because the UAP cannot administer medications. Answers B and D include actions that require nursing judgment and decision making, so they cannot be delegated to the UAP.

22. *The answer is D.*

Both the nurse and the UAP have independent duties to the patient to carry out care interventions. The nurse does remain accountable for the outcome of the intervention (i.e., the patient's fall), but the UAP could also be liable for not following proper instructions. If the UAP was trained to assist such patients and did not carry out the proper intervention, then the UAP would also be liable. It is also possible that the nurse's directions may not have been clear to the UAP, and the nurse could be liable for the improper delegation. The nurse is not automatically liable for all the UAP's actions. The particular facts and circumstances of the fall and the delegation to the UAP would need to be considered.

Liability in Patient Care

Chapter 11

Patients' Rights and Responsibilities

Katherine Dempski

Federal Regulation—CMS Patients' Rights

- The right to information: Patients have the right to receive accurate, easily understood information to assist them in making informed decisions about their health plans, facilities, and professionals.
- The right to choose: Patients have the right to a choice of healthcare providers that is sufficient to assure access to appropriate high-quality health care, including giving women access to qualified specialists such as obstetrician-gynecologists and giving patients with serious medical conditions and chronic illnesses access to specialists.
- Access to emergency services: Patients have the right to access emergency health services when and where the need arises. Health plans should provide payment when a patient presents himself/herself to any emergency department with acute symptoms of sufficient severity, including severe pain, that a prudent lay person could reasonably expect the absence of medical attention to result in placing that person's health in serious jeopardy, serious impairment to bodily functions, or serious dysfunction of any bodily organ or part.
- Being a full partner in healthcare decisions: Patients have the right to fully participate in all decisions related to their health care. Consumers who are unable to fully participate in treatment decisions have the right to be represented by parents, guardians, family members, or other conservators. Additionally, provider contracts should not contain any so-called "gag clauses" that restrict health professionals' ability to discuss and advise patients on medically necessary treatment options.
- Care without discrimination: Patients have the right to considerate, respectful care from all members of the healthcare industry at all times and under all circumstances. Patients must not be discriminated against in the marketing or enrollment or in the provision of healthcare services, consistent with the benefits covered in their policy and/or as required by law, based on race, ethnicity, national origin, religion, sex, age, current or anticipated mental or physical disability, sexual orientation, genetic information, or source of payment.
- The right to privacy: Patients have the right to communicate with healthcare providers in confidence and to have the confidentiality of their individually-identifiable healthcare information protected. Patients also have the right to review and copy their own medical records and request amendments to their records.
- The right to speedy complaint resolution: Patients have the right to a fair and efficient process for resolving differences with their health plans, healthcare providers, and the institutions that serve them, including a rigorous system of internal review and an independent system of external review.
- Taking on new responsibilities: In a healthcare system that affords patients rights and protections, patients must also take greater responsibility for maintaining good health.

Source: US Department of Health and Human Services. (1999) *The patient's bill of rights in Medicare and Medicaid.* (1999, April 12). Retrieved September 11, 2008, from http://www.hhs.gov/news/press/1999pres/990412.html

Over the years, several organizations have enumerated various patients' rights, the most prominent of which have come from the ANA, American Hospital Association (AHA), and the American Medical Association. These patients' bills of rights had no legal mandate for participation. Thereafter, CMS established patients' rights, which mandate that hospitals establish a process to promptly resolve a patient's grievance and establish procedures for confidentiality, privacy, safety, and the right to participate in one's own healthcare treatment plan (CMS Conditions of Participation: Patients' Rights, 2006). Without knowledge of these regulatory rights or rights established by state statutes, nurses cannot successfully protect and support those rights under regulatory mandates or prevent professional liability for patient harm when rights are deprived.

■ SOURCES OF PATIENTS' RIGHTS

Since the 1970s, society and the legal system have worked to provide the basis for what we now know as patients' rights. Beginning with the right to informed consent, other important issues evolved; the right to privacy (*Roe v. Wade*) and the right to refuse medical treatment (*In Re Karen Quinlan*) are two of the more renowned and established rights.

The Patient Self-Determination Act (PSDA) of 1990 also provided the legal means by which patients could, by law, obtain more control over their health care, treatment, and decisions pertaining to both. The act requires all providers who receive Medicaid funds to provide individuals with written information regarding their rights to make decisions about their medical care. Medical providers are also required to inform patients about their rights to establish advance directives at the time of admission.

In addition, the Advisory Commission on Consumer Protection and Quality in Health Care Industry issued a proposal for a national bill of patients' rights (Interim Report Nov.

1997; Final Report Mar. 1998). It was the responsibility of the commission to promote and assure healthcare quality and to protect consumers and workers in the healthcare system. The commission enumerated seven patients' rights and one responsibility. These rights are listed in **Figure 11-1**.

The Center for Medicare and Medicaid has the strongest patients' rights protections. CMS has the enforcement tools of suspending payments for participating institutions and civil monetary penalties. To receive payments under Medicare and Medicaid, the hospital must protect and promote patients' rights under the following standards:

1. Notice of rights
2. Exercise of rights
3. Privacy and safety
4. Confidentiality of medical records
5. Restraint or seclusion (including staff training requirements and death notification requirements)

These conditions of participation are summarized in **Figure 11-2**.

Accreditation by The Joint Commission also includes establishing procedures that ensure patients' rights. The right to be included in planning and treatment, informed consent (including before any pictures or filming for purposes other than diagnosis, identification, and treatment), information on providers who are responsible for care and treatment, and the right to refuse care. Respect for end of life decisions includes assistance with advance directives, documentation on executing a signed directive, and procedures for honoring organ donation wishes. Unexpected outcomes must be disclosed. Patients have the right to effective communication in a manner they understand, including interpretative services and access to advocacy programs. Confidentiality and privacy will be protected, and proper pain management procedures will be in place.

Certain elements for performance under patients' rights must be measured for success

1. Notice of rights: Inform patients or representative of patients' rights; establish process for prompt resolution of grievance including contact information. The process must have a time frame for response, and the resolution must be in writing with a contact name and steps taken to resolve the grievance and results of the grievance. Complaints regarding quality care must be referred to the quality control or improvement organization.
2. Exercise of rights: Patients have the right to participate in their own plan or care, make informed decisions, be involved in their own treatment, and be able to request or refuse treatment (not to be construed as a mechanism to demand medically unnecessary treatment). Patients have the right to formulate advanced directives and have the staff comply with those directives. Patients have the right to have a representative of his or her choice. Patients have the right to have a physician of his or her choice notified of hospital admissions.
3. Privacy and Safety: Patients have the right to confidentiality of medical records and the right to access information in their medical records in a reasonable time frame.
4. Restraints or seclusion: Patients have the right to be free of restraints or seclusion for coercion, discipline, convenience, or retaliation. Restraints and seclusion can only be used for immediate physical safety of the patient, staff, or others, and they must be discontinued at the earliest possible time.

Figure 11-2   Summary of CMS conditions of participation: patients' rights.

by the accredited institution. Success is determined by a quantifiable measure, like an audit of charts for pain management assessment, intervention, and reassessment or the signature of an interpreter on an informed consent form for a hearing impaired patient.

■ MENTAL HEALTH SERVICES

Recipients of mental health services have specific state statutory patient right protections: right to informed consent, access to medical records, confidentiality of medical treatment, privacy, and to be free of abuse or coercion. In addition, patients have the right to be free of being observed through one-way glass (or video- and audiotaping) without consent, and any threats made to a healthcare provider may require notification to the police and the person who is threatened. Notification of formal voluntary and involuntary admissions must be given.

■ ANA CODE FOR PROTECTING PATIENTS' RIGHTS

The ANA's "Code for Nurses with Interpretative Statements" sets forth the nurse's moral and professional obligation to patients based on a value belief system. The nurse needs to take into account the inherent rights of patients. The nurse has a responsibility to protect the patient's ability to manage his or her own health care and treatment. This philosophy of self-determination fosters and supports the patient's need for autonomy to the greatest extent possible. The ANA code for nurses requires that nurses treat and provide services to their patients with respect for the human dignity and uniqueness of each person by recognizing each patient's rights.

In conjunction with the mandate to protect and facilitate the delivery of medical care based on these rights, the nurse also has an obligation to the health profession to see that the patient is not acting in a manner that would thwart treatment or exacerbate a medical condition.

■ STATUTORY LAW

While patients' rights have far-reaching incentives for compliance in institutions that participate in Medicare/Medicaid payments or those accredited by The Joint Commission, state statutes that enumerate certain patients' rights may give a private right of action for liability when those rights are negligently deprived and patient injury occurs. Each state that codified patients' rights did so in a similar fashion as CMS and accreditation bodies. Some states' patients' rights laws are specific to certain organizations, such as long-term care or managed care organizations.

An administrator of her sister's estate brought several claims against the nursing home after she died of a salmonella outbreak, including negligence, civil conspiracy, and violation of the state patients' bill of rights. The violation of the bill of rights stemmed from failure to inform the decedent of her medical condition, failure to afford the decedent an opportunity to participate in her care, failure to inform her of her rights and assistance in exercising her patient rights, and failure to treat her with respect and consideration. The applicable statute states that any facility that negligently deprives a patient of a

right established in the statute is liable for injuries suffered as a result of the negligent deprivation. In this case, however, liability on this issue was never determined because the count alleged under the bill was brought past the statute of limitations. This case demonstrates that states do allow a private cause of action for violation of enumerated patient's rights (*Durkin v. First Healthcare Corporation et al.*, 1990).

■ REFERENCES

Advisory Commission on Consumer Protection and Quality in Health Care Industry. Interim Report Nov. 1997; Final Report Mar. 1998.

American Hospital Association. (1972). *A patient's bill of rights*. Chicago, IL: Author.

American Medical Association. (1998–1999). *Code of medical ethics*. Author.

American Nurses Association. (1976, revised 2001). *Code for nurses with interpretative statements*. Washington, DC: Author.

American Nurses Association. (1991). *Position statement—Nursing and the patient self-determination act*. Washington, DC: Author.

Annas, G. J. (1998). A national bill of patient's rights. *New England Journal of Medicine, 338*, 695–699.

CMS Conditions of Participation: Patients' Rights, 42 U.S.C. 1302 and 1395hh; 42 C.F.R. § 482.13 (Final Rule December 2006).

Durkin v. First Healthcare Corporation, et al., 1990 Conn. Super LEXIS 1445 (Oct 1990).

Chapter 12

Confidential Communication

Susan J. Westrick

A Disclosure Permitted

- With consent by patient, may be a signed waiver

- When information is necessary for other caregivers to care for patient

- If statutes require disclosure, e.g., child abuse reporting law

- If common law right exists to protect the public interest, e.g., safety of blood supply

- If duty to warn an identifiable victim in great danger warrants disclosure

- If court proceedings require disclosure

B Disclosure Not Permitted

- When nurse–patient communication is protected by a privileged communication statute or common law

- To relatives, spouse, or friends unless consent given by patient

- When information is requested by unidentified caller

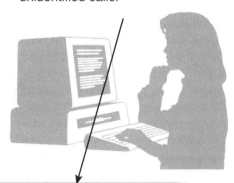

C Consequences of Disclosure without Permission

- Exposure to civil suits for breach of confidentiality or invasion of privacy
- Disciplinary action by state board of nursing
- Job loss since employer would have cause for discharge
- Fines for violations of HIPAA, or other penalties stated in privacy laws or legislation

Confidential communication involves any information a nurse obtains about a patient in the context of the nurse–patient relationship. When patients seek health care, they have a legitimate expectation that information about them will be kept confidential. By ensuring confidentiality, healthcare providers promote a desirable policy of full disclosure of information by patients. This full disclosure is necessary to treat patients adequately. Maintaining confidentiality of information also protects healthcare providers from legal and ethical challenges to unauthorized release of information.

■ LEGAL AND ETHICAL FRAMEWORK

Professional codes of ethics for nurses serve as the ethical basis to keep patient confidences. Explicit language in the ANA *Code of Ethics for Nurses* (2001) prohibits such disclosure. The American Nurses Association (ANA) has a position statement on privacy and confidentiality that is available on their Web site. Privacy rights are grounded in the US Constitution and have been made explicit in many federal and state statutes. For example, the federal Privacy Act of 1974 protects the confidentiality of patient records of those treated in federal governmental agencies or hospitals such as veteran's hospitals.

Various patients' bills of rights speak to the issue of confidentiality of patient information. Standards set by The Joint Commission and agency policies and standards all contain expectations of maintaining patient privacy. In addition, patients are protected from breach of confidentiality and assurance to the right of privacy under tort or negligence law.

■ HEALTH INSURANCE PORTABILITY AND ACCOUNTABILITY ACT (HIPAA)

The federal Health Insurance Portability and Accountability Act of 1996 (HIPAA) has expanded patients' rights to confidentiality concerning protected health information (PHI) held by any healthcare organization or covered entity, including physician offices, pharmacies, insurance companies, and any business associates of these entities. The privacy rules and regulations of HIPAA, as enacted by the Department of Health and Human Services, became effective in April 2003. The HIPAA legislation contains provisions to ensure that PHI is not released to any third party without the patient's permission (with certain narrow exceptions). Persons using the covered entity also have a right to know how their PHI is being used by the healthcare organization and who has access to it. Information can only be shared with those who have a "need to know" in the healthcare arena. This federal privacy rule preempts all state laws governing the treatment of PHI unless those laws are more stringent in safeguarding one's privacy rights.

Other key provisions require organizations to have special protections and safeguards for information stored by computers or electronically transmitted such as by fax machines. The act also contains significant fines and criminal charges in some instances for those who violate the privacy provisions of HIPAA.

Increasingly, covered entities are employing compliance officers to ensure that they are following HIPAA privacy rules. These individuals, who are sometimes nurses, are responsible to implement policies and procedures that are in line with the requirements of the act. An example of a policy to comply with HIPAA is having nurses use two identifiers to verify who is calling about patient information, such as asking callers for the patient's mother's maiden name and the last four digits of a patient's Social Security number. Complaints about privacy and confidentiality issues are generally directed to the hospital's risk management department.

In *Keshecki v. St. Vincent's Medical Center et al.* (2004), the plaintiff-patient filed a medical malpractice suit against defendant healthcare providers. Defense counsel discussed the patient's medical condition with her treating physicians. These physicians had been subpoenaed by the defense attorneys, but the plaintiff's attorney objected to these conversations on the basis of the patient's right to privacy. The Supreme Court of New York ruled that HIPAA and its regulations have changed the rules regarding ex parte (nonparty to the litigation) communications with a plaintiff's treating physician and that there should have been an authorization from the patient to allow this. Therefore, the court granted the motion for a protective order prohibiting the defense from using the plaintiff's treating physician as an expert witness or from using any of the improperly obtained information, namely that which was obtained without a proper authorization signed by the patient.

In another case involving ex parte communication, the US District Court ruled that defendants could conduct an interview with a nurse practitioner about the relevant events in the litigation and the plaintiff's medical condition (*Martin Bayne v. Shawanda M. Provost, Stephen Meehan et al.*, 2005). Plaintiff Martin Bayne, who has Parkinson's disease, sued the defendants based on a violation of his civil rights under 42 U.S.C. § 1983 and false imprisonment. One of his home care nurses, Linda Cardamone, a nurse practitioner and nonparty to the action, had visited Mr. Bayne earlier in the day in question and later spoke to him on the phone. Based on that conversation, nurse Cardamone made another phone call seeking assistance for the patient on the grounds that he had threatened to commit suicide. Defendants Provost and Meehan, New York state troopers, responded and took Mr. Bayne from his home. According to the plaintiff, they did so without conducting an investigation or mental health determination and took him to the hospital in an ambulance. The next day Mr. Bayne was released from the hospital with no finding of suicidal ideation.

As part of discovery in preparation for the trial, the defendants submitted to the plaintiff a HIPAA waiver so that they could have access to all of his medical records, but the plaintiff amended this to allow only written records but no authorization to discuss matters related to his medical condition. In finding for the defendants, the court stated that federal rules apply to the case, and the plaintiff had placed his medical condition at issue by bringing the lawsuit. Therefore, the defendants were entitled to a qualified protective

order and authorization to interview nurse Cardamone regarding the plaintiff's medical condition. The court also placed restriction on the use of the protected health information (PHI) only for the litigation and issued an order to return or destroy it at the end of the litigation. It was also noted that nurse Cardamone was not compelled to participate in an interview with defendants against her wishes nor to occur outside the presence of her attorney if she wished to have one present.

In *Giangiulio v. Ingalls Memorial Hospital* (2006), the defendant brought an appeal of a court order granting the plaintiff's motion to compel discovery of a nonparty's (NP) medical information. The Illinois Appeals court upheld the motion only as to information that did not involve the NP's identity as a recipient of mental health treatment but not to disclosure of other information. The complaint alleged that Giangiulio was a victim of a criminal assault by another patient during her stay at the hospital, and the alleged attacker was not named as a defendant in the lawsuit. The court found that HIPAA did not act as a bar to disclosure of some of the information in the interrogatories (written questions requesting information in the pretrial discovery process) or to the production of the requested knife.

■ PRIVACY AND CONFIDENTIALITY IN SITUATIONS INVOLVING SENSITIVE PATIENT INFORMATION

Healthcare organizations must be certain to have policies and procedures in place to ensure confidentiality and privacy of patient information, especially highly sensitive data, such as HIV status or reproductive information. These policies must be clearly understood by the staff and strictly followed to avoid even unintended mistakes in this area. Of particular concern is heightening staff awareness that confidential medical information cannot be released to anyone, including family members, without the patient's explicit permission. The case of *Randi A.J. (Anonymous) v. Long Island Surgi-Center* (2007) illustrates these concepts. The 20-year-old plaintiff–patient had undergone an abortion at defendant surgi-center (Center) and had specifically instructed the staff that any messages should be left on her cell phone, not her home telephone, so that her parents (who strongly opposed this procedure) would not know. On the preoperative history and patient questionnaire, the listed home phone number was crossed out, and her cell phone and work numbers were provided. However, administrative personnel at the Center used her insurance information to generate preprinted labels that were prominently affixed to nearly every page of her medical record with contact information listed as the patient's home telephone number.

· Part of the patient's blood tests were still pending after the procedure, and it was not known whether she would require an injection of RhoGAM for blood Rh incompatibility within 72 hours. The next day after the procedure, the blood test results were not on her chart, although they had been received in the office. A nurse at the Center used the contact information on the preprinted label on the corner of the Center's follow-up form to make a call to the patient's house. Her mother answered and the nurse later testified that she was aware she was not speaking to the patient but to her mother. Even so, the nurse asked her mother if her daughter had any vaginal bleeding and that she needed to know her blood type and Rh type. The nurse did not explicitly mention that the patient had an abortion, but from this information her mother concluded that her daughter had an abortion.

The appeals court upheld damages for past and future emotional distress awarded to the plaintiff–patient. This was based on liability for a breach of patient confidentiality in violation of a New York statute protecting confi-

dential medical information. However, a new trial was held on the issue of the $300,000 punitive damages award against the Center because the court ruled that evidence of no prior breaches of this type by the Center should have been presented to the jury as relevant to the case. Punitive damages are generally awarded as a deterrent to prevent particularly egregious conduct in the future or for reckless disregard for another's rights. Part of the evidence supporting the award of the punitive damages related to the fact that the Center did not have a clear policy to protect patients with sensitive confidential information and that there was confusion among nurses and other staff members about how such a situation should be handled when a patient requests that calls only be made to a certain phone number. Of particular concern to the court was the fact that the Center nurse knowingly had a conversation with someone other than the patient about highly sensitive, confidential information. Additionally, the Center had a policy that employees could be terminated for such conduct, but the nurse had not been disciplined.

This case illustrates the need to have all procedures conform to confidentiality standards and to coordinate all steps in the recordkeeping and documentation process. Office procedures should be periodically reviewed and staff informed of the need to strictly follow protocols.

■ DISCLOSURE PERMITTED

There are several exceptions to the general rule of nondisclosure of confidential information (see **Figure 12-1A**):

- *Patient permission to release information:* The patient may give verbal or written permission to release information. The written waiver states that the patient waives the right to keep the information confidential but should be specific as to what specific information can be released and to whom. Agencies usually have printed forms to be used, and a copy should always be placed in the patient's healthcare record.

- *Other healthcare workers or agencies:* Relevant information can be shared with other caregivers or agencies that have a legitimate right to know the information. Caution should be exercised in disclosing only the information necessary for care.

- *Statutory or other legal duty to report:* Some types of information are required to be reported to public health agencies or other authoritative bodies (e.g., a statutory duty to report gunshot wounds or suspected child or elder abuse and mandatory reporting of some communicable diseases). Information can be released to insurers or other agencies, such as workers' compensation boards, after claims are filed. If there is any question as to disclosure, the nurse should check agency policies or with a supervisor before any information is released.

- *Common law or public interest:* There have been extreme situations where the court has supported release of confidential patient information when it is in the public interest or is required for the safety of other patients (e.g., disclosing names of blood donors when the safety of the blood supply has been endangered). In other cases, regulations or laws permit disclosure of contagious diseases when a contact person's health is in danger. Nurses need to exercise caution in using this exception and be aware of specific exceptions permitted for the patient's situation; for example, one cannot assume that a spouse has an automatic right to know information about his or her spouse. Even though patients should be encouraged to reveal information that puts others at risk, they may have a right to withhold sensitive information (e.g., about sexually transmitted diseases). This situation presents an ethical dilemma for the nurse, and the physician, supervisor, or risk manager may need to be consulted. The common law has protected at-risk individuals when their direct safety is threatened.

- *Duty to warn:* In some very narrow circumstances, nurses may have a professional duty to disclose confidential information to protect an identifiable victim. Nurses should document repeated serious threats against another, but their duty could extend beyond documentation. They may have a legal and ethical duty either to report this to appropriate authorities or in some exceptional cases to warn the intended victim.

■ DISCLOSURE NOT PERMITTED

In some situations, confidential information should not be disclosed (see Figure 12-1B):

- *Privileged communication:* Some jurisdictions have statutes that provide patients the right of privileged communication with certain healthcare providers, which sometimes includes nurses. Confidential information learned in the context of the nurse–patient relationship may be protected against disclosure in legal proceedings. This legal privilege belongs to the patient and usually is exercised if the patient has the expectation of privacy in the circumstances. Because not all jurisdictions include nurses in the group of confidential caregivers, one needs to follow specific state statutes where the nurse is practicing; an attorney will advise the nurse regarding this should the situation arise. The information does not necessarily refer to just medical information but could be anything revealed during care, even criminal activity or dishonesty.

- *Release to relatives or friends or in telephone conversations:* The nurse needs to follow the general rule of nondisclosure of confidential information in almost all situations. Only general information about the patient's condition can be provided. Information should not be released to relatives, spouses, visitors, or others without explicit permission from the patient. One should not inadvertently tell another patient in the room of another patient's diagnosis. As a general rule, no information should be revealed over the telephone because the nurse does not know to whom he or she is talking. The nurse should advise the caller to contact the patient's family directly.

■ CONSEQUENCES OF DISCLOSURE OF CONFIDENTIAL INFORMATION

The following are among the consequences that may occur if confidential information is disclosed (see Figure 12-1C):

- *Exposure to civil suits:* For unauthorized release of information, a nurse may be held liable to a patient in a tort action for breach of confidentiality. A *tort* is a civil wrong resulting from breach of a legal duty to another that may be intentional or negligent (nonintentional). The nurse's employer may also be held vicariously liable or liable under a theory of corporate liability.

  Another tort that can be the basis of liability is *invasion of privacy*. This tort protects persons from public disclosure of private facts and has been the basis for liability for release of medical information. Disclosure of an especially sensitive medical fact (e.g., a diagnosis of AIDS) could lead to an award of punitive damages against the defendant. This tort can include publication of photographs of the patient released without his or her permission.
- *Disciplinary action by the state board of nursing:* Violation of ethical codes or negligence in performing ordinary duties can be the basis of a disciplinary proceeding

against a nurse. It is well recognized that patient information should be kept confidential, and there is an expectation of privacy in nurse–patient interactions.
- *Job loss:* A nurse could be discharged from his or her job as a result of a proven breach of confidentiality related to the care of patients.
- *Fines based on violations of the HIPAA:* Anyone who releases confidential protected health information can be subject to substantial fines or possible criminal charges by the government.

■ CONFIDENTIALITY IN AN ERA OF INFORMATION TECHNOLOGY

Caregivers need to be especially vigilant to protect patients' privacy and confidentiality rights in an era of expanded information technology and electronic transmission of patient information. If it is necessary to send patient information by facsimile (fax) to another caregiver or agency, the cover sheet and each page should be stamped "Confidential." This shifts the burden to the receiver to maintain the fax communication as confidential. HIPAA legislation requires that safeguards be in place with any electronic transmission of information.

Many institutions have computers in the hallways for the convenience of the staff. The nurse needs to be careful that while documenting care, private patient data is not visible to passersby. Privacy computer screens can assist in this situation. Patient care lists on clipboards and notebooks should not be carelessly left in patient rooms or within view of others. Nurses need to be constantly watchful for unintended disclosure of private information in all areas of practice.

■ BEST PRACTICES TO COMPLY WITH HIPAA AND PRIVACY LAWS

- Use cover sheets on patient care documents and personal notes in the workplace.

- Destroy any working documents, personal notes, or patient care summaries with any patient identifiers and place them in designated collection bins before leaving the workplace.
- Do not display any patient information in plain view of visitors or other patients.
- Use caution and common sense in discussing any patient diagnostic or treatment information in a multibed room or when visitors are present. Remember that curtains are not walls.
- Do not disclose or discuss any protected health information where it could be overheard, even if names are not used (cafeteria, elevator).
- Verify callers before any patient information is given over the telephone. Use two identifiers, such as the last four digits of the patient's Social Security number and mother's maiden name.
- Do not disclose any confidential medical information to family members or others without the patient's permission.
- Use cover sheets and a confidentiality statement on any documents that are faxed.
- Implement strict privacy and access policies concerning computer use and electronic transmission of patient data.

- Educate staff regarding the use/misuse of any confidential patient information, and implement written policies that prohibit unauthorized use.
- Require employees to sign a confidentiality statement as a condition of employment.
- Periodically review policies and procedures to ensure compliance with privacy laws and HIPAA regulations.

■ REFERENCES

American Nurses Association. *Position statement on privacy and confidentiality.* Retrieved October 26, 2008, from http://www.nursingworld.org/Main MenuCategories/HealthcareandPolicyIssues/ ANAPositionStatements/EthicsandHuman Rights/PrivacyandConfidentiality.aspx

Giangiulio v. Ingalls Memorial Hospital, 365 Ill. App. 3d 823; 850 N.E.2d 249 Ill. App. LEXIS 313; 302 Ill Dec. 812 (2006).

Keshecki v. St. Vincent's Medical Center et al., 5 Misc.3d 539; 785 N.Y.S.2d 300; 2004 N.Y. Misc. LEXIS 1476 (2004).

Martin Bayne v. Shawanda M. Provost, Stephen Meehan et al., 359 F.2d 234; 2005 U.S. Dist. LEXIS 6935 (2005).

Randi A.J. (Anonymous) v. Long Island Surgi-Center, 2007 N.Y. Slip. Op. 6953; 46 A.D.3d 74; 842 N.Y.S.2d 558; 2007 N.Y. App. Div. LEXIS 9965 (2007).

Chapter 13

Competency and Guardianship

Susan J. Westrick

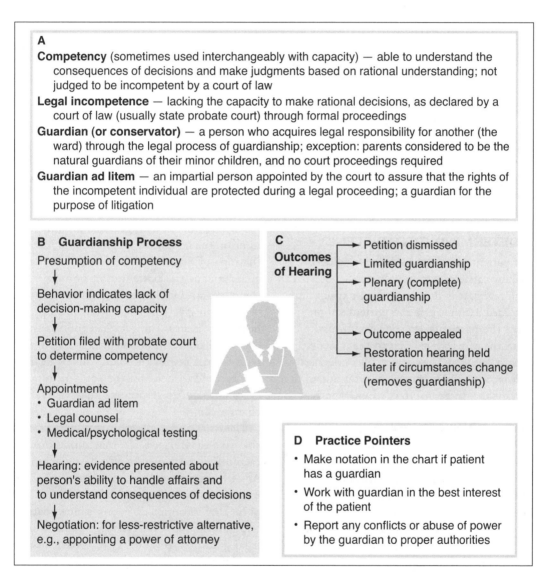

A

Competency (sometimes used interchangeably with capacity) — able to understand the consequences of decisions and make judgments based on rational understanding; not judged to be incompetent by a court of law

Legal incompetence — lacking the capacity to make rational decisions, as declared by a court of law (usually state probate court) through formal proceedings

Guardian (or conservator) — a person who acquires legal responsibility for another (the ward) through the legal process of guardianship; exception: parents considered to be the natural guardians of their minor children, and no court proceedings required

Guardian ad litem — an impartial person appointed by the court to assure that the rights of the incompetent individual are protected during a legal proceeding; a guardian for the purpose of litigation

B Guardianship Process

Presumption of competency
↓
Behavior indicates lack of decision-making capacity
↓
Petition filed with probate court to determine competency
↓
Appointments
• Guardian ad litem
• Legal counsel
• Medical/psychological testing
↓
Hearing: evidence presented about person's ability to handle affairs and to understand consequences of decisions
↓
Negotiation: for less-restrictive alternative, e.g., appointing a power of attorney

C
Outcomes of Hearing
→ Petition dismissed
→ Limited guardianship
→ Plenary (complete) guardianship
→ Outcome appealed
→ Restoration hearing held later if circumstances change (removes guardianship)

D Practice Pointers
• Make notation in the chart if patient has a guardian
• Work with guardian in the best interest of the patient
• Report any conflicts or abuse of power by the guardian to proper authorities

Any nursing care must be consented to, and to give the requisite consent, a person must be competent. Most patients give verbal or implied consent when the nurse implements typical and routine patient care activities. However, there are situations when the patient is temporarily incapacitated to give consent (e.g., an illness creating a loss of consciousness or dementia). In these situations consent is often presumed, unless there is evidence (e.g., an advance directive) that a patient would not want the type of care he or she is receiving. In other situations there is a legal determination that a person is incompetent, and a guardian is appointed to act for that individual. See the definitions in **Figure 13-1A**.

■ PRESUMPTION OF COMPETENCE

In all states, adults older than 18 years are presumed to be competent to make decisions about their medical care. This overriding presumption of competency serves to guide interactions with patients in healthcare settings but can be overcome by presenting proof to the court that the person lacks the capacity to make decisions. Those who question the competency of the individual have the burden to present clear and convincing proof that the person lacks this capacity. The court would then make the determination that the person is incompetent.

■ DETERMINING COMPETENCY

For patients who temporarily lack a decision-making capacity (e.g., heavily sedated or with a high fever), it is proper to render usual nursing care. However, if the patient might not want the particular care or the family questions the care that is given to the patient, it is best to document this objectively in the healthcare record and bring it to the attention of the physician. An example is when a patient is receiving chemotherapy, but the family does not agree that this is the best course of treatment. When a patient is temporarily or permanently incapacitated, the court may appoint a temporary guardian to help determine what is best for the patient. Nurses should use caution when there is a potential conflict between the family members' wishes and the patient's best interest. Nurses have a duty to act in the best interest of the patient and to fulfill their role as a patient advocate.

■ GUARDIANSHIP PROCESS/DETERMINATION OF COMPETENCY

The determination of a patient's competence centers on the person's decision-making capacity and not merely on his or her medical

diagnosis. Figure 13-1B outlines the guardianship process, and Figure 13-1C shows the possible outcomes of the hearing.

If incapacity is determined and the person is declared to be incompetent, a guardian is appointed by the court. The guardian is often a family member, but if none is available, the court may appoint a close friend or an impartial individual. The court determines the type of guardianship, plenary or limited. If plenary (or complete) guardianship is awarded, the guardian has control over all the individual's (now referred to as a *ward*) affairs. A limited guardianship is less restrictive and may be applied only to the individual's financial affairs or medical decisions. The court could also appoint a temporary guardian for a period of emergency, sudden, or prolonged illness.

For all patients with guardians, clear notations on the healthcare record should identify the type of guardianship, name of the legal guardian for the patient, and how to reach the guardian by phone or mail because this person can give consent for all medical and healthcare issues. The guardian continues the role until the ward is not incapacitated, perhaps for the rest of the ward's life. A hearing can be held to petition the court to remove the guardianship if circumstances warrant a change.

The issue of guardianship was addressed in the case of *Marjorie L. Tyler, Anna Rhine v. Huron Valley Sinai Hospital* (2006). Plaintiff Anna Rhine was an elderly woman who suffered from senile dementia and was incapable of making informed decisions. Rhine's daughter, plaintiff Marjorie Tyler, served as Rhine's legal guardian. In 2002 Tyler took Rhine to the defendant hospital's (Huron) emergency room because her mother was lethargic. Tyler expected that her mother would be examined, diagnosed, treated, and sent home. However, the examining physician recommended admission to the hospital due to dehydration, and could not determine anything in Rhine's medical history to account for this, so neglect was considered as part of the medical diagnosis. Another daughter of Rhine's also came to the ER, and both sisters wanted the patient to be discharged with an IV or allow her to stay in the ER. After the physician said that this was not feasible, the sisters caused a "ruckus," and allegedly there was yelling between Rhine's daughters and the nurses, and the sisters were abusive to their mother. After calling security and eventually the police, a nursing supervisor offered three options to Tyler and her sister: (1) admit Rhine to Huron, (2) show guardianship proof and take Rhine AMA (against medical advice) from Huron, or (3) arrange for the transfer of Rhine to Botsford Hospital (Tyler said she wanted her mother to be transferred there) or another facility. Tyler admitted she was informed of these options at least five times.

Tyler was aware that she needed guardianship papers to have legal authority to make decisions on her mother's behalf and that the defendants offered her and her sister the opportunity to remove their mother from Huron AMA upon presentation of proof of guardianship, but they rejected this offer. At one point Tyler said she was going to her car to get the papers, but instead she left the hospital. After this a deputy sheriff testified that the other sister, Wozny, became belligerent, refused to leave, and struck the officer, resulting in handcuffing and an arrest for trespassing and being a disorderly person. The appeals court affirmed the trial court in granting summary judgment for the defendant hospital Huron on the plaintiff's claims of false imprisonment and the intentional infliction of emotional distress. The court ruled they did not provide sufficient proof to support either claim and agreed with the trial court that the hospital was justified in insisting that Tyler produce guardianship papers, even though Rhine had been hospitalized at Huron before. The trial court had observed that guardianships can and do change over time. The plaintiff's claim for false imprisonment failed as well because the option of transfer AMA was offered upon valid proof

that Tyler had the authority to make this decision on behalf of her mother.

This case illustrates the need to follow strict protocols and procedures related to guardianship and the need for guardians to have current proof of their status. In all situations, nurses and caregivers must act in the best interest of the patient and as the patient's advocate, as they did in the Tyler case. Even so, caregivers may have to defend their actions when allegations of improper procedures are made in lawsuits and decisions are challenged by patients or family members.

In another lawsuit, the conservator for Mary Denittis was named as a defendant, along with the plaintiff Colman's employer, for claims of negligence and battery (*Corrine Colman v. Notre Dame Convalescent Home, Inc. and Gail Kemp, conservator of the person of Mary Denittis and Mary Denittis*, 1997). The plaintiff employee suffered injuries as a result of being struck by defendant Denittis, who suffers from senile dementia and was declared incompetent. Defendant Gail Kemp was appointed as her conservator. The court allowed the battery claim to go forward noting that liability for such acts may be consistent with common law principles that say liability should fall on the one who caused the act where one of two innocent parties must suffer loss from the act done. However, the court denied the plaintiff's claim for negligence, finding that there is no duty of care arising between an institutionalized patient and her paid caregiver. The court allowed summary judgment for the defendant on that claim.

■ SITUATIONS WHERE GUARDIANS MAY BE PRESENT

- Minors: Parents are the natural guardians of children less than 18 years old. If the parents are divorced, the custodial parent is the legal guardian unless the court determines otherwise. Some minors are considered to be emancipated if they are married or living apart from their parents and may be able to make their own decisions, including health care.

- Elders: Elder patients frequently have guardians. These elders may be in extended care facilities or in the home. Concerns about an elder's decision-making capacity should be brought to the attention of either family members or agency personnel, such as nurse managers or social workers. The nurse should document objectively on the patient's record the assessment data relevant to this concern and what referrals were made. If an abusive situation is involved, proper authorities, such as elder protection services, need to be notified.

- Psychiatric patients: Just because a patient has a psychiatric illness or is involuntarily committed to a psychiatric facility does not mean the person lacks decision-making capacity. These patients can still refuse treatment and make their own decisions unless certain circumstances arise. The question for the court becomes one of whether the person is capable of understanding refusal or consent to a procedure and the consequences of that decision.

- End-of-life decisions: Although the court may appoint a guardian for a person who is unable to make end-of-life decisions, it is increasingly common for persons to execute written documents called advance directives that delegate to others this responsibility: a durable power of attorney, which delegates to a named person the authority to make certain decisions if the patient later becomes incompetent; a durable power of attorney for health care, which would apply only to healthcare decisions as determined by state statutes; and a living will, which allows the patient's wishes to be carried out, usually in situations of terminal illness or persistent vegetative state. Other times the court may direct a guardian to use substituted judgment in the best interest of the ward that is consistent with the ward's values and preferences.

■ IMPLEMENTING PROCEDURES RELATED TO COMPETENCY, CONSENT, AND GUARDIANSHIP

In all cases the nurse acts in the best interest of the patient and is aware of the duty to work with any guardian on the patient's behalf. If a healthcare provider encounters a patient who lacks decision-making capacity and there has been no legal determination of who will act on behalf of the patient, guidance should be sought through policies and procedures in the agency. If these are lacking, a nurse manager or administrator should be notified for direction. Most state statutes indicate who would give consent in these situations, and agency policies need to be consistent with them. The typical order of next of kin to consult for consent or end-of-life decisions is: (1) spouse, (2) adult children, (3) parents, (4) grandparents, (5) adult brothers and sisters, and (6) adult nieces and nephews. Healthcare practitioners must carefully follow any order and priority for consent because disagreements may arise, even among those in the same classification.

Guardianship proceedings are *not* initiated lightly, and one is not appointed unless a real need is determined by clear and convincing evidence; serious consequences result from a determination of incompetence. Guardianship intrudes on a person's autonomy and diminishes his or her privacy. However, the goal of guardianship is to protect the individual and to protect his or her assets. Even so, the guardian could potentially abuse the responsibility. If the nurse observes abuse of the situation, the nurse cannot ignore his or her role as a patient advocate (see Figure 13-1D).

■ REFERENCES

Corrine Colman v. Notre Dame Convalescent Home, Inc. and Gail Kemp, conservator of the person of Mary Denittis and Mary Denittis, 968 F. Supp. 809; 1997 U.S. Dist. LEXIS 9790 (1997).

Marjorie L. Tyler, Anna Rhine v. Huron Valley Sinai Hospital, 2006 Mich. App. LEXIX 869 (2006).

Chapter 14

Informed Consent

Katherine Dempski

Informed Consent

Information:	description of procedure risks and benefits of procedure reasonable alternatives and their risks and benefits
How much information:	material risks and benefits reasonable person would want to know before undergoing or refusing procedure (majority view) or material risks and benefits reasonable physician would consider (minority view)
Assessment of patient competence:	communicates understanding of procedures and information given

---

Historically, lack of consent to medical treatment entitled a patient to sue for battery. *Battery* is the unlawful or unauthorized touching of another. Informed consent is now recognized as a professional standard of conduct, and negligence for lack of informed consent is the basis for liability. Informed consent is a communication process between patient and provider and not a mere exercise in obtaining a patient signature on a form. **Figure 14-1** is a summary of the information necessary in the informed consent process. Accreditation standards, CMS requirements, and state laws specific to informed consent all govern this process, and institutions must put in place an informed consent policy that is practical for patients and practitioners and compliant with regulatory and legal standards.

■ ACCREDITATION AND REGULATORY STANDARDS

The Joint Commission accreditation standards on informed consent consist of three elements (Patient Rights, RI 2.40). First, hospital policies must outline procedures that require informed consent and the process used, such as a written consent form. The institution must go by applicable state requirements on certain procedures (such as blood product administration), but in general, invasive procedures and procedures requiring anesthesia need informed consent. The process must be obtained and documented in the record under the hospital policy to meet the second standard. The third element requires the informed consent to contain a discussion on proposed treatment, risks, benefits, likelihood that the intervention will achieve its goal, and alternatives, including risks.

All information in the medical record is protected health information under HIPAA and state confidentiality laws. An informed consent policy should address confidentiality and the need for providers to be aware of relevant information needed to safely treat the patient.

CMS "Patients' Rights" states that patients have the right to make informed decisions regarding their health care (42 C.F.R. 482.13(b)(2)). A properly executed informed consent must be in the medical record before surgical procedures (unless an emergency exists), and the medical staff must specify which procedures require specific informed consent and who may obtain the consent (42 C.F.R. 482.51 (b)(2)). A properly executed consent form contains the same elements as required by The Joint Commission with these additional elements:

- Description of proposed procedure and anesthesia to be used
- Probable consequences of refusing proposed and alternative treatments or procedures
- List of practitioners who will perform significant tasks other than the primary surgeon, including graft harvesting, dissecting, altering or removing tissue, and implanting devices

A patient gives informed consent when the following three elements are met:

1. Information: The patient should be informed of the risks and benefits associated with the treatment, the risks and benefits involved in refusing treatment (including that refusing a procedure does not mean that all other medical care will be withdrawn), the probability of a successful outcome, alternatives to the procedure, and the credentials of the person who will perform the procedure. It would be difficult to make the patient aware of every conceivable risk and benefit to a procedure or treatment. Therefore, the patient should be informed of all the material risks and benefits of the procedure a reasonable person would want to know when deciding to undergo or refuse the treatment or the most common risks, depending on the state statute.

2. Voluntary consent: For consent to be voluntary, the patient must not be under any influence or coercion. Nurses are often responsible for administering medications prior to procedures and should verify that informed consent was obtained before medicating because a sedated patient cannot give voluntary consent (and may lack the competence to do so).

   A patient's voluntary consent to treatment can be expressed either in writing (by a signature) or verbally (and documented by the person obtaining the consent). Voluntary consent also can be implied by a patient's actions, for example, when a person holds up an arm for a needle stick. On the other hand, silence by a person does not constitute consent to treatment in a situation where a reasonable person would speak up before receiving the treatment.

3. Competence: A patient must be competent to give informed consent to a procedure. Competent patients can communicate choices, understand relevant information concerning treatment, and appreciate the situation as it applies to them. The Joint Commission requires policies for obtaining informed consent from surrogate decision makers. All information given to the patient would be given to the surrogate (which may be determined by guardianship, advance directives, next of kin, or medical healthcare power of attorney).

■ OBTAINING CONSENT

The physician who performs the medical or surgical procedure is responsible for obtaining informed consent (see **Figure 14-2**). Advanced-practice nurses are responsible for obtaining informed consent prior to performing any risky or invasive procedure that falls within their scope of practice. The patient's consent is usually evidenced by the patient's signature on a consent form. Individual state statutes may require that consent be in writing. Institutional policies should reflect any specific state requirements, and anyone responsible for obtaining informed consent must be aware of these requirements.

Nurses at the bedside are responsible for explaining all nursing procedures to the patient. The patient's consent is implied when the procedure is explained and the patient allows the nurse to begin nursing care. Procedures that are not invasive or risky do not require informed consent. Of course, what is risky and invasive needs to be defined, and the nurse should be aware of the policy on informed consent.

A nurse should never be delegated the responsibility of obtaining informed consent for a medical or surgical procedure being performed by a physician. Even when the nurse is aware of the risks involved in a medical procedure, the nurse may not be aware of the risks specific to that patient or know the exact procedure the physician has planned. The nurse who obtains informed consent under these conditions runs the risk of misleading the patient and all the legal liability that follows.

When a procedure is performed at the hospital by the patient's private physician, the private physician, not the nurse, has the duty to obtain the consent unless the hospital imposed a duty upon itself to obtain the consent. This issue was before one court. The private physician performed a high forceps delivery, and the infant died a few days later from injuries sustained. The plaintiffs placed into evidence the patients' right to be fully informed and make decisions on medical care. The court held that the plaintiff-patient did not present evidence that the defendant hospital and nurses took on the duty to

---

1. Hospital policy must describe:
   • Procedures, treatments requiring consent, and emergency care exceptions to these procedures and treatments (such as loss of life or limb if treatment is delayed to obtain consent)
   • Process to obtain consent (written forms or documentation in progress note)
   • Documentation in medical record
   • Circumstances for surrogate decision maker
2. Informed consent must be obtained and documented according to policy.
3. Consent must contain the following:
   • Nature of proposed procedure, treatment, or intervention
   • Potential risks, benefits, and side effects, including problems related to recovery
   • Likelihood that the procedure will achieve goals
   • Alternatives to proposed procedure, treatment, and care, including the risks and benefits
4. When indicated, any limitation on confidentiality must be stated.

Figure 14-2   Informed consent accreditation elements.

obtain the consent (*Daniels v. Durham County Hosp. Corp.*, 2005).

■ WITNESSING CONSENT

The nurse's role in the informed-consent process usually involves witnessing the consent, that is, observing the patient consent to the procedure by signing the consent form. In some cases a court may ask the witnessing nurse to identify the signature or explain the circumstance under which the consent was obtained or ask the nurse if the consent was given voluntarily.

Witnessing consent at the bedside often means that the patient will ask the nurse some questions regarding the procedure or outcomes. The nurse should answer questions regarding the nursing care involved in the procedure. Questions regarding medical care should be referred to the physician. The nurse should document the patient's concerns and how they were addressed.

■ LACK OF CONSENT: THE NURSE'S RESPONSIBILITY

The nurse should always notify the physician prior to a procedure if a consent form is not in the medical record. The Joint Commission National Patient Safety Goals require surgical time-outs, which include verifying that the consent is in place and discussing the procedure to be performed with the whole surgical team and patient. The nurse would be expected to follow the institution's policy when consents are not in the medical record, including notifying the physician involved and the nurse's supervisor. The physician's supervisor may need to be notified as well.

The nurse's duty to report withdrawal of consent was the issue in *Isaac v. Jameson Memorial Hosp.* (2002). The patient verbally withdrew consent for sterilization to be performed, but the nurse did not notify the physician. The court held the hospital responsible under the theory of respondeat superior

and corporate negligence. The hospital was liable for negligence, not the physician who performed the procedure.

■ EMERGENCY EXCEPTION TO INFORMED CONSENT

Most state statutes on consent for medical treatment include an exception to informed consent in an emergency. Each will define an emergency, but in general, the requirements for this emergency exception to apply are:

1. The healthcare provider must reasonably believe that a delay in treatment because of waiting for the patient's consent would result in serious bodily injury or death.
2. The patient is unconscious or otherwise incapable of giving consent.
3. No one available has the legal authority to act as the patient's guardian, agent, or the next of kin.
4. A reasonable person would consent under the circumstances.
5. The healthcare provider has no reason to believe that this particular patient would refuse treatment. For example, the healthcare provider may have to reconsider a blood transfusion if it were known that the patient has certain religious beliefs against such treatment even in an emergency situation.

When an emergent cesarean section was performed under general anesthesia, and the neonatal team resuscitated the infant for over 24 minutes, leaving him with permanent disabilities, the parents sued for negligence and failure to obtain informed consent for the resuscitation. The father remained in the postcare birthing area and not in the surgical room. The neonatal team leader sent the nurse out to give the father updates but never spoke to him or informed him of the likelihood of the outcome. The parents testified that they would not have consented to the 24 minutes of resuscitation but would have requested it be discontinued after several minutes. The defendant hospital and providers claimed an emergent situation with no practical time to obtain consent from the father who was not "readily available" within the meaning of the state statute outlining exceptions for informed consent. The court held judgment in favor of the defendant physicians and hospital, recognizing that an emergency situation occurred, and that it was not practical to obtain consent. For the purpose of that state statute, "readily available" means more than physical proximity; there must be sufficient time and opportunity for discussion and deliberation (*Stewart-Graves et al. v. Vaughn et al.*, 2007).

■ INCOMPETENT PATIENTS

Incapacity to consent may come from a temporary condition, such as sedation or unconsciousness, or it can be more long term, such as a mental illness. A patient's incompetence to consent to a medical procedure must be determined by a physician according to the healthcare agency's bylaws and applicable state law. Consent to treat incompetent patients must come from someone with legal authority to do so. The patient may have designated a medical decision maker through an advance directive or healthcare power of attorney. In the absence of a predetermined decision maker, the state statutes will determine a surrogate for end-of-life decisions or the next of kin in an emergency. Each state designates the order of authority for the next of kin, such as parents may consent for an unmarried adult child, a spouse may consent for a spouse, or an adult child can consent for a parent.

■ LIMITATIONS TO INFORMED CONSENT

Informed consent is not unlimited, and healthcare providers can be liable for extending consent to further treatment not explained and consented to by the patient. During a surgical procedure, the surgeon would be expected to treat any emergency situation that arose unless the patient informs the surgeon otherwise. The best informed consent covers an emergency situation without being overly broad and thus not valid.

■ SPECIAL INFORMED CONSENT

Many states now have HIV statutes that require a healthcare provider to give specific information to the patient when obtaining informed consent, such as counseling and confidentiality. Specific documentation is required; therefore, healthcare providers must be aware of these state statutes.

Specific federal laws outline informed consent requirements in experimental treatments. It is a detailed consent form, and the patient must be allowed to withdraw from the experiment at any time.

■ RELIGION

Competent adults may refuse medical treatment (even life-saving treatment) for religious reasons without medical or legal interference. Courts may become involved (by appointing a temporary legal guardian for healthcare decisions) when a minor may suffer serious bodily harm or death. When time is critical, judges have been awakened during the night by hospital legal counsel and the patient's legal counsel to hear arguments on both sides to grant or deny medical treatment orders.

■ MINORS

In most states, 18 years is the age of majority. The general rule is that a parent or legal guardian must give consent for medical treatment of a minor. However, there are statutory exceptions to this. Many states allow minors to consent to medical testing and treatment of sexually transmitted diseases, human immunodeficiency virus (HIV) infection, mental health, substance abuse, and pregnancy.

Emancipated minors may also consent to their own medical treatment. The American Academy of Pediatricians recommends that competent children over age 13 years be part of the consent process.

One irony of consent laws is when a minor is the parent of a child who is in need of medical care, the minor may consent for the treatment of the child but not her own treatment, depending on state consent statutes. While some states recognize the minor parent as the one to give consent for the child, others require that the minor parent be emancipated by another fact, such as living independently or in military service. Absent a recognized statute authorizing the minor parent's consent, the adult parent or guardian of the minor parent may be the one to give consent for the minor's child, but in emergent situations where the adult is not readily available, the minor parent may give consent. Institutions should have consent policies defining each of these situations and follow the state's consent for minor statutes.

There is an emergency exception when the child requires immediate lifesaving care, or even when delay of treatment would cause pain and suffering, where a reasonable parent would consent to the procedure and treatment. Statutes are specific on defining emergencies and require due diligence in contacting the parent or guardian when possible and consulting a mature minor. (**Figure 14-3** lists specific scenarios for emergency exceptions in consent for minors.)

Sexual Assault

Several states have statutes that authorize providers to treat minors for sexual assault with a minor's consent to treatment and education on sexually transmitted diseases. Parental notification is required unless the parent is the suspected abuser. Absent a specific state statute to treat, the institution should have a guideline for treating minors in this situation under the mature minor exception or emergency exception.

Mature or Emancipated Minor

When parental involvement is excluded due to the relationship between the minor and parent, the provider may take into consideration factors the state statute has codified,

- A parent is not present or available by phone: Do not treat unless there is an emergency.
- A parent is not present or available by phone: If state child services has custody, obtain consent from child custody unless there is an emergency.
- A parent is not present or available by phone: If the patient is not in state custody and there is a question of child abuse, seek a medical treatment order or treat in an emergency.
- A parent is available but refuses treatment, and the refusal amounts to a question of abuse or neglect: Seek a medical treatment order.
- A parent is available but refuses treatment that puts the child at immediate risk of harm, and there is no suspicion of abuse or neglect: Seek a medical treatment order.

Figure 14-3   Treatment of minor patients.

such as emotional maturity of the minor and his or her ability to understand the risk of treatment. The minor may be emancipated by state law. Each state may define "emancipation," but in general, an emancipated minor lives separately from the parent with no financial support from the parent, is married, is in the military, has a child, or is emancipated by judicial proceedings. The court maintains the original documentation of the emancipation with the minor being issued copies for proof. Not every state includes each of these exceptions.

Confidentiality and Notification to Parents

Statutes may also permit disclosure to parents of mature or emancipated minors, such as when follow-up treatment is necessary or hospitalization is prolonged or complicated. Disclosure of testing for pregnancy and sexually transmitted diseases may not be allowed. Furthermore, the statute may require the minor's permission to disclose. Absent a permissive statute for disclosure, the provider should seek the minor's permission for parental disclosure.

Reproductive Exception

To encourage treatment without fear of parental punishment, some states have enacted statutes that permit providers to treat minors for STDs, educate minors about contraception, and dispense contraception to minors.

Drug and Alcohol

To encourage minors to seek treatment there are state statutes which allow minors to consent for treatment without parental consent.

Mental Health Exception

State statutes vary, but some states permit minors who are capable of participating in mental health treatment to consent to outpatient treatment. Minors of a certain age may consent to inpatient treatment. Statutes may specifically limit minor consent for certain medications and procedures.

■ REFERENCES

Abbott, K. M. (1996). Minors and consent to treatment: A policy proposal for the health care provider. *Journal of Nursing Law, 3*(2).

Calloway, S. D. (2006). Consideration of standards and guidance related to informed consent. *American Society of Healthcare Risk Management, 26*(3).

Daniels v. Durham County Hosp. Corp., 171 N.C. App. 535 (2005).

Isaac v. Jameson Memorial Hosp., 59 Pa. D. & C. 4th 375; 2002 Pa. Dist. & Cnty. Dec. LEXIS 112 (2002).

Stewart-Graves, et al. v. Vaughn, et al., 170 P.3d 1151; 162 Wn.2d 115 (Wash. 2007).

Roberson, A. (2007.) Adolescent informed consent: Ethics, law and theory to guide policy and nursing research. *Journal of Nursing Law, 11*(4), 191–196.

Chapter 15

Refusal of Treatment

Katherine Dempski

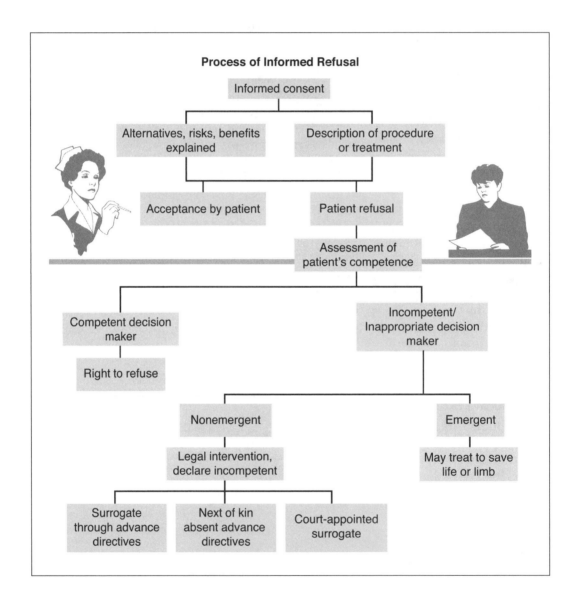

Process of Informed Refusal

Informed consent

Alternatives, risks, benefits explained

Description of procedure or treatment

Acceptance by patient

Patient refusal

Assessment of patient's competence

Competent decision maker

Incompetent/ Inappropriate decision maker

Right to refuse

Nonemergent

Emergent

Legal intervention, declare incompetent

May treat to save life or limb

Surrogate through advance directives

Next of kin absent advance directives

Court-appointed surrogate

Patients have control over what is done to their bodies and minds as long as they have not been determined to be incompetent. However, nurses must be aware that even though a patient has the right to refuse medical care, this refusal must be an "informed refusal." **Figure 15-1** demonstrates the process for informed refusal.

■ RIGHT TO REFUSE TREATMENT— GENERALLY

In 1990, the US Supreme Court, in the case of *Cruzan v. Director, Missouri Department of Health*, recognized that individuals have a constitutionally protected liberty interest in refusing unwanted medical treatment.

■ PATIENT SELF-DETERMINATION ACT

As a result of the Cruzan case, Congress passed the federal Patient Self-Determination Act (PSDA) of 1990. This law mandated that every hospital, nursing home, healthcare agency, and health maintenance organization (HMO) that receives Medicare and Medicaid funds must provide adult patients with a statement of rights under state statutory law to make health choices, including the right to refuse treatment and to execute an advance directive.

■ PATIENTS' BILL OF RIGHTS

Following the enactment of the PSDA, individual states (if they had not already done so) created or modified their own patients' bill of rights (Patients' Bill of Rights, 1999). Nurses should review the pertinent bill of rights available at the healthcare institution or by state law.

■ INFORMED CONSENT

Informed consent is the process by which a fully informed patient participates in choices about his or her health care. The essential parts of this decision-making process include discussions about: (1) the nature of the medical decision or procedure; (2) reasonable alternatives to the recommended intervention; (3) the relevant risks, benefits, and uncertainties related to each alternative; (4) assessment of patient understanding; and (5) the acceptance of the intervention by the patient.

For the consent (or refusal) to be valid, the patient must be competent to make the deci-

sion, and the consent (or refusal) must be voluntary. It is important that the patient understand the healthcare provider's reasoning process for the recommendation. The discussions should be carried out in lay terms.

■ ASSESSMENT OF PATIENT'S COMPETENCE

In most cases, it is clear whether a patient is able to comprehend the information and is therefore considered to be competent. However, in some situations, it is not so clear. Patients in a healthcare setting are often extremely anxious and fearful. This should not be confused with a person's ability to make reasonable decisions. There are a number of different legal standards in which a person's legal competence could be judged. However, generally an assessment should be made of the patient's ability to: (1) understand the situation (i.e., does the patient know where he or she is and why he or she is in the hospital); (2) understand the risks associated with the procedure; and (3) communicate a decision based on that understanding.

When a patient's competence is unclear, a psychiatric consultation may be helpful. Again, just because a patient refuses treatment does not in and of itself mean the patient is incompetent. Treatment refusal may be a sign that the healthcare provider should further pursue the patient's beliefs and understanding about the decision, as well as his or her own understanding.

If the patient is demonstrated to be incapacitated or incompetent to make healthcare decisions, a surrogate decision maker must speak for the patient. Specific procedures defined by each state's law must be followed to appoint a surrogate decision maker if the patient did not appoint one prior to becoming incompetent.

When a competent adult becomes incapacitated by accident or disease, chances are the person has left a living will or health care by proxy, which gives evidence as to the person's decision regarding medical care. However, when an adult never had the mental capacity to make medical decisions, the right to refuse medical treatment becomes complicated. Some states have case law on the doctrine of substituted judgment, which utilizes all the facts and circumstances to come to a decision on how the incompetent person would decide if he or she is competent.

A Massachusetts court settled the issue of a third party seeking to terminate life sustaining treatment in a fatal form of leukemia in a 67-year-old man, Mr. Saikewicz, who had the mental age of a toddler and would not understand the side effects of the treatment. He had lived in an institution his whole life, and his two remaining relatives refused to be involved. Noting that the rights of incompetent persons include the right to refuse potentially lifesaving treatment, the court relied on the doctrine of informed consent and the right to privacy and adopted the "substituted judgment" standard, which determines how the incompetent person would decide if he or she were competent. It requires utilizing guardian ad litem, healthcare providers, and ethicists. In this case the pain of the treatment, the low chance of remission, and Mr. Saikewicz's inability to cooperate should be taken into consideration as part of substituted judgment (*Superintendent of Belchertown State School v. Saikewicz*).

Ideally, the doctrine of substituted judgment uses the surrogate decision maker's knowledge of the patient's beliefs, ethics, and any decisions or conversations the patient may have had prior to the incompetence and then uses that to determine how the patient would have decided. This is more difficult to apply when the patient has never achieved a state of competency, as the preceding case demonstrates.

■ MINORS

With respect to minors, the decision maker is presumed to be the parent or guardian.

The exceptions to informed consent laws, allowing minors to consent to drug and alcohol treatment or mental health treatment without parental consent, do not extend to a right of the minor to refuse the same treatment that has been consented to by the parent. The courts would look to whether the minor was able to make an informed decision to refuse.

In *Department of Health and Rehabilitative Services v. Straight*, the Florida Appellate court affirmed the parental right to place a minor child in a drug treatment program without the minor's consent or judicial review. The applicable state statute provides for the parent to apply to the courts for involuntary placement but does not restrict the right of a parent to place a minor in treatment regardless of consent. The court cited the Supreme Court's decision that the due process clause did not require preconfinement hearings in all cases in which parents wished to hospitalize their children in treatment programs. The court held the parents' right to care, custody, and management of children gives the decision power to the parent, and when child does not agree, the power does not automatically transfer to the state (*Parnham v. J.R.*, 1979).

A parent's refusal of lifesaving treatment for their child may be overruled by a court order. The court will look to whether the parent is acting in the best interest of the child. A medical treatment order and temporary guardian may be put in place.

Institutional polices should include the involvement of the ethics committee and legal counsel to determine judicial review.

■ INFORMED REFUSAL

Although the patient has the right to refuse medical treatment, the nurse's duty to the patient does not end at documenting "patient refuses." The nurse has a legal duty to ensure that the patient's decision to refuse treatment is an informed one. Patient teaching on the risks of refusing treatment is an essential element to the patient's right to refuse. A nurse who documents in the medical record "patient refuses treatment" has not completed the duty owed to the patient. The documentation must reflect the teaching that was presented to the patient and that the patient refuses with an understanding of the risks.

In *Hackathorn v. Lester Cox Memorial Center,* a nurse was liable to a patient for the burns he received from a heating pad despite the nurse's attempts to assess his back. The patient was admitted for a herniated disk. The nurse documented that she asked the patient to "roll over" so she could assess his back for heating pad burns. He refused several times. When the pad was removed, he had several serious burns that required treatment, and it caused a delay in surgery for the herniated disk. The nurse claimed contributory negligence by the patient for his own injuries (based on his refusing the nursing assessment). The court found that the nurse did not complete her duty by informing the patient of the risk of heating pad burns and the need for periodic assessment. Furthermore, the nurse could not prove (through documentation) that the patient was even

capable of rolling over for a back assessment upon her request. Therefore, the patient's refusal was not "informed" and did not contribute to his own injuries. The nurse should have documented that the patient was educated on the benefits of complying and was physically capable of complying with the nurse's request, yet he refused with knowledge of the risks for burns.

■ REFERENCES

Abbott, K. M. (1996). Minors and consent to treatment: A policy proposal for the health care provider. *Journal of Nursing Law, 3*(2).

Cruzan v. Director, Missouri Department of Health, 497 U.S. 261 (1990).

Department of Health and Rehabilitative Services v. Straight, 497 So.2d 692 (Fla. Dist. Ct. App. 1986).

Department of Health and Rehabilitative Services v. Straight, 497 So.2d 692: (1986); 503 So. 326 (1987) (petition dismissed for Florida Supreme Court review).

Hackathorn v. Lester Cox Memorial Center, 824 S.W.2d 472 (Mo. 1992).

Parnham v. J.R., 442 U.S. 584 (1979).

Patients' Bill of Rights, 42 C.F.R. § 482.13 (1999).

Superintendent of Belchertown State School v. Saikewicz, 370 N.E.2d 417 (Mass. 1977).

Chapter 16

Pain Control

Katherine Dempski

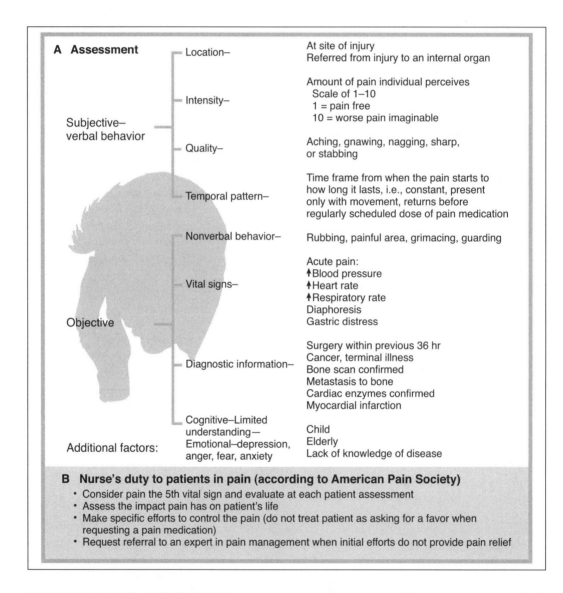

A Assessment

Subjective–verbal behavior

Location– At site of injury / Referred from injury to an internal organ

Intensity– Amount of pain individual perceives / Scale of 1–10 / 1 = pain free / 10 = worse pain imaginable

Quality– Aching, gnawing, nagging, sharp, or stabbing

Temporal pattern– Time frame from when the pain starts to how long it lasts, i.e., constant, present only with movement, returns before regularly scheduled dose of pain medication

Nonverbal behavior– Rubbing, painful area, grimacing, guarding

Objective

Vital signs– Acute pain: / ↑Blood pressure / ↑Heart rate / ↑Respiratory rate / Diaphoresis / Gastric distress

Diagnostic information– Surgery within previous 36 hr / Cancer, terminal illness / Bone scan confirmed / Metastasis to bone / Cardiac enzymes confirmed / Myocardial infarction

Additional factors: Cognitive–Limited understanding— / Emotional–depression, anger, fear, anxiety — Child / Elderly / Lack of knowledge of disease

B Nurse's duty to patients in pain (according to American Pain Society)
- Consider pain the 5th vital sign and evaluate at each patient assessment
- Assess the impact pain has on patient's life
- Make specific efforts to control the pain (do not treat patient as asking for a favor when requesting a pain medication)
- Request referral to an expert in pain management when initial efforts do not provide pain relief

■ SOURCES FOR STANDARDS

The nurse's duty to provide appropriate pain management for patients is derived from several sources. Professional standards include the ANA position statement on pain management as part of the nurse's role in end-of-life decisions to administer effective dose of medications that are prescribed for symptom control and to advocate for the patient when prescribed medications insufficiently manage pain. Titration for adequate control is ethically justified. In 1992 and 1994, the Agency for Health Care Policy and Research (AHCPR), now known as the Agency for Healthcare Research and Quality (AHRQ), released guidelines for both acute pain management and cancer pain management. The American Pain Society also has position statements on treatment at the end of life and pain assessment as a fifth vital s ign. These authoritative references would likely be cited by courts in establishing what would be the proper standard of care in these situations.

In 2001, The Joint Commission made a standard that every patient has the right to have their pain assessed and treated. Additionally, some states have passed legislation in the form of statutes called pain relief acts. These acts generally specify that neither disciplinary nor state criminal prosecution shall be brought against healthcare providers for the therapeutic treatment of intractable pain.

■ PAIN DEFINED

Pain is one of the most compelling reasons why people seek medical care. Pain is a protective mechanism that alerts the person to potentially harmful stimuli.

There are three types of pain. *Acute pain* occurs immediately after an injury and continues until the healing is completed. If acute pain is not managed effectively, it can progress to a chronic state. *Chronic pain* lasts for a prolonged period of time, usually for more than 6 months, and is often associated with depression. *Malignant pain* can be described as intractable and is often associated with cancer.

■ ASSESSMENT

A nurse is responsible for assessing subjective and objective data (see **Figure 16-1A**). A physical assessment, including a review of the patient's vital signs, is essential. The nurse

should also assess the emotional response to pain and the results of diagnostic tests that confirm painful events, such as a bone scan that confirms metastasis of cancer to the bone.

■ TREATMENT

The most common approach of pain management is the use of analgesic medication. The physician orders analgesics; however, the nurse is responsible for administering the drugs, evaluating their effectiveness, and notifying the physician if the relief of pain is inadequate. In a hospital setting, the nurse:

- Determines if and when an analgesic is given because most analgesics are ordered on an as-needed basis (prn)
- Selects the appropriate analgesic when more than one is prescribed
- Knows the drug's potency, absorption, and pharmacokinetics
- Evaluates the effectiveness of the medication
- Observes for side effects
- Reports to the physician when a change in medication is needed

In the nonhospital setting, the nurse is responsible for advising the patient about analgesic use.

The Acute Pain Management Guidelines (AHCPR, 1992) include a collaborative interdisciplinary team approach, individualized pain management plan with patient and family input, an ongoing assessment, use of medication and nonmedication treatments, and institutionalized policies on pain management.

■ POSTOPERATIVE PAIN

Postoperative pain is treated according to specific guidelines. Narcotics should be given around the clock immediately postop as determined by the interdisciplinary team, not prn. Analgesics should be given before or as soon as pain returns and before activity, such as ambulation or incentive spirometer use.

■ LIABILITY ISSUES

Some people believe that administering large doses of morphine constitutes assisted suicide or euthanasia. It is the position of the ANA that relieving pain, even if it hastens death in a terminally ill person, is the ethical and moral obligation of the professional nurse; it is not euthanasia or assisted suicide. This position must be consistent with the patient's wishes.

Nurses need to continually update and implement current standards of care. Agency policies need to be consistent with these so that the nurse's legal duty to provide pain relief for patients can be fulfilled. Documenting pain assessment as "generalized" or "severe" and describing pain relief as "good," "better," or "fair" is inadequate and fails to show that the standard of care was met. Holding back pain medication in the belief that the patient is addicted without proper assessment, evaluation, and medical diagnosis is considered "inhuman treatment" and leaves the nurse professionally liable. The nurse has a shared responsibility and independent duty to provide appropriate pain management for patients, and the patient must be part of the decision-making process (see Figure 16-1B).

The courts have set the precedent for healthcare provider duty (liability) to properly manage pain by best evidence guidelines. The sentinel case is a North Carolina court decision in 1991. Mr. James was terminally ill with prostate cancer that metastasized to the spine and femur. He had 6 months to live. The long-term care nurse independently determined that Mr. James was addicted to morphine and used alternative pain management with no diagnosis, assessment, or orders from the primary physician, who had ordered pain relief every 3 hours. The family sued, and the court held that the treatment of Mr. James was "inhumane," that the nurse and her employer had a duty to the patient to relieve his pain and not withhold the pain medication. The verdict of $15 million sent a message to the healthcare community (*Estate of Henry James v. Hillhaven Corp.*).

In *State v. McAfee*, the issue before the court was the quadriplegic patient's right to refuse ventilator support. In holding that Mr. McAfee had the right to refuse lifesaving medical treatment, the court made clear that in discontinuing ventilatory support in a patient who was incapable of spontaneous respirations, he was entitled to sedative administration. The right to discontinue medical treatment was inseparable from his right to do so pain free.

■ REFERENCES

Agency for Health Care Policy and Research (now Agency for Healthcare Research and Quality). (1992, February). *AHCPR acute pain management guidelines 92-0032.*

Agency for Health Care Policy and Research (now Agency for Healthcare Research and Quality). (1994, March). *AHCPR cancer pain management guidelines 94-0592.*

American Nurses Association. (2003, December 5). *ANA position statement: Pain management and control of distressing symptoms in dying patients.* Washington, DC: Author.

American Pain Society. Glenview, IL. www.ampainsoc.org

Estate of Henry James v. Hillhaven Corp., 89 CVS 64 (N.C. Super. Ct. 1991).

State v. McAfee, 385 S.E.2d 651 (Ga. 1989).

Pierce, S. F., Dalton, J. A., & Duffey, M. (2001). The nurse's ethical obligation to relieve pain: Actualizing the moral mandate. *Journal of Nursing Law, 7*(4), 19–29.

Chapter 17

Patient Teaching and Health Counseling

Susan J. Westrick

A   Patient Teaching

- Assess patient need (include cultural, ethnic, literacy).
- Include teaching aids—written instructions.
- Complete documentation.

Discharge Instructions

- Include who was taught in documentation.
- Written instruction is recommended.
- Include name and phone number to call if questions arise later when at home.

Emergency Department

- Written instruction is recommended.
- Ensure that patient and/or family receives information.

Inpatient Settings

- Require patient to demonstrate skills.
- Collaborate with other healthcare providers to integrate teaching into patient's plan of care.

B   Minimizing Risks of Liability

- Completely document content, skills, and materials provided.
- Document if patient refuses teaching.
- Use standard teaching protocols.
- Evaluate teaching; ensure that patient receives and understands teaching.
- Fully inform patients of risks and benefits if alternate therapies.

The nurse's role in patient teaching and health counseling/education is receiving greater emphasis in practice because of changes in the healthcare environment (e.g., shorter stays for patients in institutions, more patients being treated in outpatient settings, increased numbers of patients in home care settings, increasingly chronic and complex healthcare conditions). These factors, along with greater emphasis on preventative care and health counseling and education, contribute to the need for nurses to be highly skilled and accountable in patient teaching.

■ LEGAL AND ETHICAL FRAMEWORK

Legal, institutional, and professional standards formulate the basis for the nurse's duty to teach patients. Most state laws that define nursing practice include specific language that addresses the area of patient education or health counseling. Even if not expressly stated, this duty is implied in language stating that nurses carry out plans of care for patients and treat their responses to healthcare problems. National standards, such as the American Nurses Association (ANA) standards of practice and The Joint Commission, require that patient education be included and documented in individual plans of care. Furthermore, these educational mandates are linked to the institution's participation in Medicare and Medicaid programs. The ANA standards require that teaching–learning principles be included in these activities. In addition, providing ethnic and culturally sensitive care requires incorporating these aspects into patient teaching. Patients' bills of rights, as published by the American Hospital Association, include the right to healthcare information, and nurses share responsibility for ensuring this right. Many nurses will find that their job descriptions include duties related to patient teaching and health counseling/education. Teaching hospitals usually incorporate teaching as part of their mission statement, and this may include patient teaching as well.

■ PRINCIPLES OF PATIENT TEACHING

The first step to consider in patient teaching is to assess the teaching needs of the patient or the teaching that is required in a particular situation (e.g., teaching related to a diagnostic or surgical procedure; see **Figure 17-1A**). The nurse should assess what the patient knows and begin from there. The nurse needs to consider language barriers, literacy, ethnic and cultural background, and age and emotional status of the patient; otherwise, teaching and learning can be impaired, placing the patient at risk.

For complex procedures that need to be taught (e.g., injection techniques), handouts, visual aids, and actual equipment should be used. The patient should demonstrate the learned procedure so the nurse can evaluate the effectiveness of the teaching. The taught content and skills should be documented in the appropriate health records that could include the use of flow charts and checklists. Using these principles ensures that the nurse

is meeting the standard of care as required for the situation.

■ TEACHING IN VARIOUS SETTINGS AND CIRCUMSTANCES

Discharge Instructions

Healthcare institutions are required by The Joint Commission to provide discharge instructions to patients as part of their discharge planning. These instructions should be in writing, with a copy retained for the healthcare record. In some situations, these instructions need to be given to a family member or other healthcare providers instead of the patient. If a patient is not provided with a copy of discharge instructions and harm results because of it, liability may result. Many healthcare organizations now require patients to sign discharge instructions indicating that they received and understood all components, including any follow-up instructions. It is most often the nurse who has the duty to provide the discharge instructions and to collaborate with the physician and other health team members for specific instructions.

In *Martin v. Abilene Regional Medical Center* (2006), a nurse documented that she instructed Mr. Martin about Plavix, an anticoagulant medication routinely given to postcardiac stent placement patients on discharge. The nurse had reviewed the discharge instructions with Mr. Martin, but there was no prescription written by the physician for this medication, so he did not receive the medication after discharge. The patient's coronary artery stent occluded 10 days following his discharge, and he was readmitted for further cardiac procedures. In his malpractice suit against the physician and the hospital, Martin alleged that the nurse should have questioned the physician as to why he did not write a prescription for the medication that the nurse had instructed him about. The nurse expert for the plaintiff agreed that the discharge orders should have been clarified and cited the Texas Nurse Practice Act, which requires a nurse to clarify any order that the nurse has reason to believe is inaccurate. The Court of Appeals of Texas allowed the case to go forward and overturned the lower court's ruling. This case illustrates that discharge instructions need to coordinate with the overall expected plan of care for the patient and that any inconsistencies must be clarified.

Sally Austin (2006) discusses a case of a patient discharged with a drainage tube in the rectal area who claimed she did not receive any instructions for follow up with her physician. Five years later, after complications occurred, the patient sued the facility and the nurse who was responsible for the discharge instructions. This case underscores the need for explicit and complete documentation of all instructions provided to the patient. Lawsuits such as this one can arise years later when memories of the incident are unclear. This makes permanent documentation in the medical record essential to defending a later claim of negligence.

Emergency Departments

When patients are discharged from the emergency department, specific instructions should be given to patients and caregivers. Written discharge instructions are a part of the standard of care for many conditions when patients are discharged from the emergency department and need to be incorporated into practice. Documentation should include that the patient or caregiver received the information.

Inpatient Setting

Even relatively simple patient procedures need careful teaching, as exemplified by *Chamberlain v. Deaconess Hospital, Inc.* (1975), a case that decided whether a patient was properly instructed on how to collect a 24-hour urine sample.

Health Counseling and Advice

The question of whether a nurse engaged in inappropriate teaching for a patient who requested information on an alternative treatment was raised in *Tuma v. Board of Nursing* (1979). A patient who received chemotherapy requested the nurse to return in the evening to discuss Laetrile treatments. The patient's physician heard about this from a family member, and the hospital later made a complaint about the nurse to the state board of nursing. After a hearing, her license was suspended for 6 months. She appealed this decision to the state supreme court, which overturned the suspension, reasoning that there was not adequate warning that this behavior would result in violating the statute for unprofessional conduct, and thus the statute was void for vagueness as applied to these facts. The issues discussed in the case raise valid concerns about how far patient teaching can go if it is viewed as interfering with the physician–patient relationship, as was alleged in this case. Teaching should always be collaborative with other healthcare practitioners.

Medications

Teaching patients about side effects and precautions while taking certain medications is a shared duty with other health professionals (see the *Martin* case as previously cited). Nurses in advanced practice with prescriptive authority need to be especially vigilant in this area. Physicians have been held liable in numerous cases where patients were not adequately warned of side effects and injury resulted. Liability can also extend to foreseeable third parties, such as those injured while patients under the influence of medications are operating a motor vehicle.

Alternative Therapies

The increasing popularity and use of herbal and complementary therapies has led to questions about the role and liability of nurses who are involved in teaching related to these therapeutic interventions. Although there is growing acceptance of many of these therapies, caution should be exercised when using or teaching about therapies that are not generally accepted by the nursing or medical communities. A particular concern arises when an allegation of malpractice is made by a patient, perhaps as a result of alleged negligent teaching about an alternative therapy. As in all negligence and malpractice cases, the "standard of care" required in the situation in question will be examined by the court. If the intervention used was not generally accepted by the nursing or medical community at the time, it becomes difficult to prove what the proper standard of care should have been. Courts that take a strict view may see this type of teaching or intervention as not falling within the acceptable standard of care. It is recommended that to protect oneself, the patient should be given explicit information about any risks as well as any benefits of the therapy. The nurse should also obtain consent and documentation that the patient fully understands this information. If the nurse has any question about whether this therapy in any way interferes with the medical regimen, the patient's physician should be notified and informed (see the *Tuma* case previously cited). In all cases there should be ongoing communication with other healthcare providers so that the patient has an integrated plan of care to ensure optimal outcomes.

Non-English Speaking Clients/Patients

Federal laws require hospitals to provide non-English speaking patients with meaningful access to health-related information. This includes the use of interpreters to assure that informed consent, discharge instructions, and other information meets legal requirements. Failure to do so can be a violation of federal regulations where fines and lawsuits could result. The Centers for Medicare and Medic-

aid (CMS) requires compliance by healthcare organizations to participate in these federal programs. It is not recommended that family members be used as interpreters because there is uncertainty as to what information is transmitted to the patient or stated back to the healthcare practitioner. If a family member is used at the request of the patient, there should be a written waiver for a staff interpreter signed by the patient, as verified by an impartial interpreter.

■ MINIMIZING RISKS OF LIABILITY FROM PATIENT TEACHING

Complete documentation related to patient teaching can help avoid claims that teaching was not done (see Figure 17-1B). Written materials should supplement teaching, and copies of these should be in patient records or easily accessible if a question arises. Family members or other caregivers should be included in the teaching, with the patient's permission. When a patient refuses to accept teaching, a note to this effect should be recorded. This documentation becomes important if the patient later makes a claim of negligence. "Contributory negligence" on the part of the patient will reduce or bar his recovery for damages.

Standard teaching protocols should be available for common conditions, and these should be reviewed and updated periodically. Continuing education classes on teaching strategies that incorporate cultural and literacy concepts can be especially helpful for nurses.

Focusing on the evaluation aspect of teaching can help ensure that the standard of care is met. Taking time to evaluate whether the patient and family *understand* the teaching is the best way to ensure this. In areas such as 1-day surgery, where there is limited contact with the patient, there should always be someone who can be contacted if questions later arise related to the discharge instructions. In fact, it is good practice for nurses to make follow-up phone calls to patients to evaluate their status after discharge.

■ REFERENCES

Austin, S. (2006). Ladies and gentleman of the jury, I present ... the nursing documentation. *Nursing, 36*(1), 56–62.

Brooke, P. (1998, May). Legal risks of alternative therapies. *RN,* 53–58.

Chamberlain v. Deaconess Hospital, Inc., 324 N.W.2d 172 (Ind. Ct. App. 1975).

Crawford v. Earl Long Memorial Hospital, et al., 431 S.2d 40 (LA 1983).

Dill, S., & Iyer, P. (2007, March). When patients don't speak English, what is the risk? *ED Nursing,* 53–54.

Martin v. Abilene Regional Medical Center, 2006 WL 241509 (Tex. App., February 2, 2006).

Tuma v. Board of Nursing, 100 Idaho 74, 593 P.2d 711 (1979).

■ ADDITIONAL RESOURCE

The Joint Commission. (2007). "What did the doctor say?": Improving health literacy to protect patient safety. Retrieved September 22, 2008, from http://www.jointcommission.org/NewsRoom/PressKits/Health_Literacy

Chapter 18

Medication Administration

Susan J. Westrick

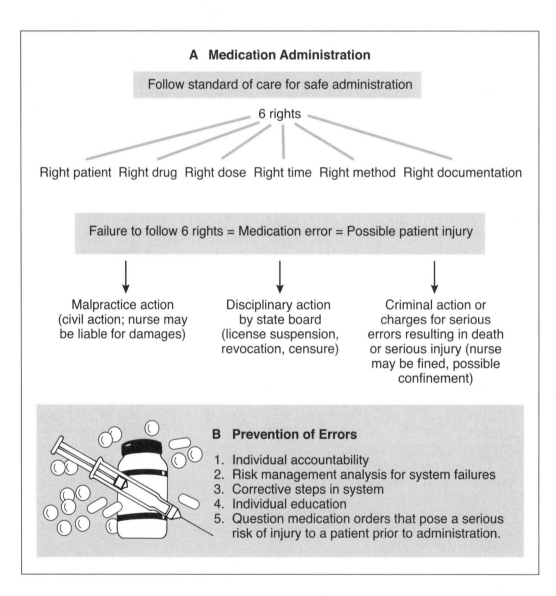

A Medication Administration

Follow standard of care for safe administration

6 rights

Right patient Right drug Right dose Right time Right method Right documentation

Failure to follow 6 rights = Medication error = Possible patient injury

Malpractice action
(civil action; nurse may
be liable for damages)

Disciplinary action
by state board
(license suspension,
revocation, censure)

Criminal action or
charges for serious
errors resulting in death
or serious injury (nurse
may be fined, possible
confinement)

B Prevention of Errors

1. Individual accountability
2. Risk management analysis for system failures
3. Corrective steps in system
4. Individual education
5. Question medication orders that pose a serious
   risk of injury to a patient prior to administration.

Nurses are responsible for administering almost all medications to patients, and they may spend an estimated 40%–60% of their time performing this task. Negligence in the area of medication administration has become one of the greatest areas of liability for nurses and their employers, sometimes resulting in multimillion dollar awards. Many times these errors result from failure to follow the basic rules of safe administration. Other reasons cited for the rise in errors include the vast numbers of medications a nurse is responsible for, the increasing complexity of drug administration methods, multiple medications dosing for individual patients, failure to update knowledge of drugs and their implications, poor product labeling, understaffing, distraction while preparing medications, poor communication, underlying system failures, and increased nurse–patient ratios. Researchers have validated that safe administration of medications is a highly skilled and complex process, involving much more than just the act of administering the medication to the patient. In fact, each patient situation is unique and involves judgment about dosing, timing, and selection of medications. Central to the process is the use of critical thinking skills to observe, verify and interpret data, predict consequences, problem solve, and communicate with others while considering the specific patient, context, and circumstances (Eisenhauer, Hurley, & Dolan, 2007).

■ STANDARDS RELATED TO MEDICATION SAFETY AND ERROR REPORTING

Government, professional, and public organizations have responded to the need to improve the safety of health care and in particular to prevent medical errors. The Institute of Medicine's (IOM) 2000 report identified preventable medical errors as accounting for 44,000 to 98,000 deaths per year in hospitals nationwide that cost between $17 billion to $29 billion per year. With this data widely in the public media, patients and healthcare organizations have sought ways to improve rates of medication errors and to create a "culture of safety" where workforce systems, such as electronic medication order entry systems, are used. The US Department of Health and Human Services Agency for Healthcare Research and Quality (AHRQ) has produced a 2008 Comparative Database Report with results for hospitals to use as benchmarks to establish a culture of safety and to reduce medical errors.

The Joint Commission is also committed to improving patient safety and publishes yearly safety goals and standards. The 2008 National Patient Safety Goals Hospital Program includes new goals for reducing the likelihood of patient harm from administration of anticoagulants and improved recognition and response to changes in patients' conditions. Other commission goals that are already in place and must be met include using two patient identifiers for patients when providing treatment, "read-back" verbal or telephone orders, standardized lists of abbreviations and dose designations that are not to be used in the organization, improving the timeliness of reporting, and implementing standardized "hand off" communication approaches when care transitions from one person to another or from one area of care to another. Specific medication goals include to identify, at least annually, a list of look-alike/sound-alike drugs and take action to prevent errors involving interchange of these drugs, label all medications and medication containers even on sterile fields, and accurately and completely reconcile all medications across the continuum of care. There must also be a process to compare the patient's current medications (when admitted) with those ordered for the patient while receiving care in the organization (referred to as reconciling the medications). Additionally, a complete list of medications must be communicated to the next provider of service when the patient is transferred, and a complete list must be given to the patient upon discharge. Other goal standards relate to patients' and families' active involvement in reporting safety concerns.

The Food and Drug Administration (FDA) reviews medication errors that come to MedWatch, the agency's adverse event reporting program. Since 2000 the FDA has received more than 95,000 reports, but because it is also a voluntary system, the actual number of medication errors is estimated to be much higher. The FDA reviews drug names, labels, packaging, and other processes to provide guidance to the public and industry. Error analysis may result in changes in the industry. For example, an FDA rule went into effect in 2004 to require bar codes on product labels for certain drugs and biologics, such as blood. Reporting adverse experiences to the FDA can be completed at www.fda.gov/medwatch.

The Institute for Safe Medication Practices (ISMP), a nonprofit research group that advocates for patient safety, has developed a list of high-alert drugs that are defined as drugs that have a heightened risk of causing significant patient harm when used in error. The list contains medications that continue to result in a large number of medication errors. As few as 20 drugs have been identified in 80% of deaths due to medication errors, and even when the errors aren't fatal, the ISMP has identified them with poor patient outcomes. Nurses also intercept many "near misses," and this data is invaluable to collect and trend as a risk management strategy.

In 2002 The Joint Commission adopted the ISMP's list of error-prone abbreviations, symbols, and dose designations for use in its National Patient Safety Goals. The ISMP develops a list of "Error-Prone Abbreviations, Symbols, and Dose Designations" (updated periodically) that have been reported as frequently misinterpreted and involved in harmful medication errors. The current list is available at its Web site.

The ISMP partners with the United States Pharmacopeia (USP) to operate a confidential national voluntary Medication Errors Reporting Program (MERP) to provide system analysis of the causes of medication errors. Healthcare professionals and consumers can report to this program, and information is also forwarded to the Food and Drug Administration (FDA) and the manufacturers or others to inform them of problems with labeling or packaging. An error report (including near errors) can be submitted online by accessing the secured Web page at www.ismp.org/order Forms/reporterrortoISMP.asp.

Examples of the impact of the USP-ISMP MERP include electronically distributed timely, nationwide hazard alerts to providers with recommendation for error reduction and press releases to the public when warranted. Organization and system changes, such as creating processes for near misses, have resulted in more complete data collection. Another example of a system change to prevent errors was The Joint Commission's 2003 adoption of ISMP's prohibition of the use of free-flowing infusion pumps without protection for accidental free-flow use. The commission retired this goal in 2006 after full compliance nationwide among accredited organizations.

Nursing organizations, including the American Nurses Association (ANA), continue to advocate for improved working conditions and reasonable nurse–patient ratios to improve safety and contribute to better outcomes for patients. The ANA position statement on "Assuring Patient Safety; Registered Nurses' Responsibility in All Roles and Settings to Guard Against Working While Fatigued" (2006) recognizes that working while fatigued threatens patient safety. Underscoring this position statement is the Institute of Medicine's (IOM) 2004 report, which found that when nurses work excessive hours, especially in excess of 12 hours in direct patient care, there is an increase in patient care errors. In another study, it was found that the likelihood of making an error was three times higher when nurses worked shifts lasting 12.5 hours or longer (Rogers et al., 2004).

■ LIABILITY ISSUES

Nurses are most often found liable for medication errors on the basis of negligence or malpractice, but criminal charges may also result from errors involving serious injury.

Negligence

Traditionally the area of negligence or mal-practice law has governed a nurse's actions in medication administration (see **Figure 18-1A**). This means that a nurse has a duty to follow correctly written physicians' orders (or advanced-practice nurses' orders if permitted by state statute) for medication administration to patients. This duty includes implementation of the six rights of medication administration: right patient, right drug, right dosage, right time, right method, and right documentation. Failure to follow any of these steps can result in a successful malpractice claim against a nurse. However, not all medication errors result in liability and a finding of professional negligence or malpractice. The plaintiff (or patient) who brings the lawsuit still must prove: (1) a duty, (2) a breach of the duty, (3) proximate causation between the breach of the duty and the injury, and (4) injury to the patient. Many medication errors do not result in injury to the patient and would not support a civil action for negligence.

Criminal Charges

A more recent, yet not widely reported, trend is to treat egregious errors, or those resulting in serious patient injury or death, as a criminal act. These rare but tragic cases are often the subject of widespread media attention, and the medication errors of nurses are often highlighted in the case. The criminalization of unintended medical errors has become a subject of heated professional and public debate. Professional nursing organizations continue to question whether these criminal charges will prevent errors by others. They advocate for analysis of the systems that led to the errors so that positive change and prevention can occur. Experts also point to the unintended negative effects of such actions in deterring others from entering the medical or nursing professions and the reluctance of

practitioners to report errors if criminal charges may result from human error.

Criminal charges were considered against nurses and a pharmacy technician after three premature infants died as a result of receiving an adult dose (10 times overdose) of heparin at Methodist Hospital in Indianapolis, Indiana. The pharmacy technician had accidentally stocked the unit with adult dose vials rather than infant dose vials. However, the nurses did not accurately read the labels before administration, and the vials for adults and infants both look alike, which contributed to the errors (Shalo, 2007). Another error of this same type has resulted in a lawsuit against the manufacturer of the drug in an attempt to force changes in packaging these medications.

Another widely publicized 2006 case involved an experienced obstetrics nurse, Julie Thao, who mistakenly administered an epidural medication IV instead of the ordered antibiotic, resulting in the death of a 16-year-old patient who was in labor. Nurse Thao had worked two eight-hour shifts the day before and stayed all night at the hospital to return for another shift the next morning. The mistake occurred at the end of her shift, and fatigue likely contributed to her error. The hospital had a bar code and patient identifier system that she did not implement properly. In addition, the IV bag with the epidural anesthetic had not been ordered, but she removed it from the medication system anticipating that it would be used. There were many errors in the administration process, including taking shortcuts with safety checks and bypassing protocols and procedures, but nurse Thao did not intend to cause harm to the patient. However, criminal charges can be supported when conduct becomes so careless and reckless that it places another in great danger. Nurse Thao was originally charged with a felony, criminal neglect, but she later pleaded guilty to two misdemeanor charges and was placed on two years probation, with work restrictions. The original criminal charge, a class H felony, could have resulted in a $25,000 fine and up to 6 years in jail. The plea agreement included that Thao could not work more than 12 hours in a 24-hour period and no more than 60 hours per week. Other conditions were that nurse Thao must take classes on preventing medication and health-care errors and make three presentations to nurses or nursing students on the topic. The Wisconsin nursing license board also suspended her license for 9 months and restricted the number of hours she could work for the following 2 years (Shalo, 2007; *State of Wisconsin v. Julie Thao*, 2006).

A Colorado case involving negligent administration of a drug to an infant also resulted in criminal charges against nurses. This tragic case in which the error resulted in the death of an infant involved multiple individual and system failures. The events occurred in 1996 when a physician prescribed "penicillin G benzathine, 150,000 U, IM" but had not written the order clearly. The order was handwritten and barely legible. The pharmacist misread the order and prepared two syringes with a dose of 1,500,000 U (having read the "U" to be an extra "O"). Because the volume of the drug was in 2.5 mL, the nurses determined that five separate injections would need to be administered. Not wanting to subject the infant to this, the nurses consulted with a neonatal nurse practitioner (NNP), who decided the drug could be given IV. They checked drug reference books but did not find the information to be clear and made incorrect assumptions about the name of the drug and its administration. This particular drug was to be given IM only. The NNP then changed the route of administration for the order, and the drug was given by IV push by herself and another advanced-practice nurse. After part of the medication was administered, the infant became unresponsive, resuscitation efforts were unsuccessful, and the infant died. It was determined that the infant died as a result of the drug (a 10-fold overdose) being injected IV, which caused a massive pulmonary embolism. After these events and following disciplinary action by the Colorado state board of nursing, the district attorney charged the nurses with "criminally negligent homicide." This was the first time criminal charges had been filed against nurses for a medication error (Smetzer, 1998a).

The outcome of the case was that two of the nurses (the nurses who actually administered the drug) pleaded guilty and accepted plea bargains rather than face a possible guilty verdict by a jury and potential permanent loss of their licenses. These nurses received a 2-year deferred sentence, probation, and an order for community service that included education of student nurses about their errors in this case. They could then return to court after the 2-year period and request that their cases be dismissed. The third nurse who was not directly involved in the administration stood trial and was acquitted of these charges by the jury. This case served as a signal to professionals as to the potential consequences of errors in their professional roles. The district attorney who brought the charges contends that the case was not about a simple medication error but rather a case of nurses changing the route of administration ordered by the physician, thus providing a "gross deviation from the standard of care" that unjustifiably placed the patient at extreme risk of danger.

The response of the nursing community to the criminalization of medical errors has largely centered around the need to treat this type of error as a system failure and address it as a risk management issue. Commentators have also stated that disciplining nurses involved with negligence resulting from human error should remain with the state board of nursing, the agency delegated to regulate the profession and to protect the public. An analysis of the Colorado case by the Institute for Safe Medication Practices (ISMP) identified over 50 system flaws that led to the medication error.

■ CASE LAW INVOLVING ADMINISTRATION OF MEDICATIONS

1. *Patient-controlled analgesia (PCA) pumps:* Prior to the requirement that PCA pumps must use tubing that prevents the free flow of medication, a patient who received an overdose of narcotic following surgery resulting in mild brain damage sued the defendant hospital and pump manufacturer, Baxter, for damages. In 1995 plaintiff Chavez received an overdose of Demerol when it escaped from the syringe in the PCA pump. Chavez claimed that a nurse incorrectly loaded the syringe and that the hospital negligently failed to use an extension set with an antisiphon valve. The jury found for the plaintiff and apportioned 55% fault to Baxter and 45% to the hospital, which was upheld on appeal. The hospital had argued unsuccessfully on appeal that syringe failure was the cause of the error (*Chavez v. Parkview Episcopal Hospital*, 2001).

In *Donna Ellis v. Bard, Inc. and Baxter Healthcare Corporation*, et al. (2002), the plaintiff, as her mother's guardian, claimed that the manufacturers were liable for her mother's brain damage due to their failure to adequately warn of the danger of having a person other than the patient activate the PCA morphine drip pump. In 1997 nurse Hamilton was caring for the plaintiff postoperatively after bilateral knee replacements at Georgia Baptist Medical Center (GBMC). She programmed the pump according to the physician's order with the prescribed amount of morphine, maximum hourly dosage, and lockout time between patient-activated doses. Nurses at GBMC were not authorized to permit a third party to activate the PCA pump without a doctor's order. However, nurse Hamilton instructed one of the patient's daughters to press the PCA button for her mother while she was sleeping so that she would not wake up in pain. The nurse said she made this exception to the rule because the patient appeared to be in great pain. She did not tell the daughter that this third-party activation could be dangerous. Later that same day, her daughter (after following nurse Hamilton's instructions) relayed the instruction about the pump to another of the patient's daughters, who also pressed the button while the patient was sleeping during the night. Around 7:00 a.m. when the doctor visited, the patient was having difficulty breathing, went into cardiac arrest, and suffered anoxic brain injury. Evidence presented at trial included that neither the pump itself nor the user's manual contained a label warning that third parties should not activate the pump. However, the defendant sales and medical distributor staff had educated GBMC hospital staff about the risk of third-party activation and provided patient brochures advising that only patients should press the PCA button. Additionally, another nurse at GBMC, Rhodes, testified that in preop teaching she had instructed the patient that only she should activate the pump. Nurse Hamilton, who provided the instruction for third-party activation, testified that she "was keeping an eye on Brown [the patient] to make sure she was OK."

The district court found for the defendant manufacturer and granted summary judgment, which was affirmed on appeal. However, prior to filing this lawsuit, Ellis sued GBMC for medical malpractice and settled the case for structured payments having a present value of $8 million.

A jury verdict was entered in favor of the plaintiff in another case where the patient's death was determined to be from the hospital's failure to monitor his condition while he was administered an opiate by use of a PCA pump (*McAllen Hospitals v. Carmen Garza Muniz et al.*, 2007). The appeals court affirmed the judgment. The patient, Muniz, had experienced pain after a leg amputation in 2002 and was prescribed postop Dilaudid IV by PCA pump. At 8:00 p.m. nurse Cesar Duque, a licensed vocational nurse, initiated the PCA. Following the initiation of the PCA, the amounts of Dilaudid administered or received by the patient were never recorded. At 9:00 p.m. a nurse took a blood sample from the patient for a glucose check. At about 11:00 p.m. nurse Duque found Mr. Muniz with no pulse or respirations and called a code, but the patient was later pronounced dead. Plaintiff's expert witness concluded that failure to monitor was the cause of his death and that the patient was known to be opiate sensitive due to a previous reaction to this medication. The expert opined that his respirations should have been monitored and if slowed, the infusion should be discontinued and possibly drugs should have been used to reverse the effects of the narcotic. Other testimony pointed out that the patient's mental status is also important to assess.

The failure to meet standards for documentation of medication and to monitor and record the patient's respiratory and mental status are clearly within the nurse's role. Also the hospital should have had a well-written policy and protocol for nurses to follow when patients receive PCA.

2. *Intravenous medications:* Appellants were heirs of a patient who claimed medical malpractice by a hospital in treating the patient Kapadia. The family alleged negligent nursing care in administering IV medications through a site in the patient's hand that caused tissue damage requiring later amputation. Kapadia, a diabetic, was admitted in 1984 to the emergency room in critical condition unconscious and with repeated seizures. A doctor had attempted to insert a central line but was unable to do so because of the seizures. Thereafter, nurse Bridgewater administered 1000 mg of Dilantin, as prescribed, through an IV in the patient's left hand. About an hour and a half later, nurse Bridgewater noticed that Kapadia's hand was blue or purple and cool to touch, so she moved the IV to the right arm, but the condition of the patient's hand worsened. There was conflicting evidence as to whether the eventual amputation of her hand was due to extravasation of Dilantin from the IV or from her diabetic condition. The jury found that the hospital was not negligent in its care and treatment of the patient, and the appeals court upheld the decision. Specific allegations against the nurses were failure to establish proper procedures for use of restraints above an IV site, use of a hand vein for giving Dilantin and other caustic drugs, dosage limits for Dilantin, and requirements for a nurse to question the amount of the drug or its method of delivery. However, nurse Bridgewater had verified the dose with the doctor and also called the pharmacist. She testified that she gave the dose slowly by IV push 50 mg at a time to dilute the drug with the saline that was infusing, and she demonstrated the procedure for the jury. Some experts at trial disagreed with this method of administration as meet-

ing the standard of care. Dilantin levels showed the patient received the medication. In finding no error, the appeals court commented that in light of the conflicting evidence, the jury was allowed to believe the substantial evidence that supported their conclusion (*Kamalaben L. Kapadia et al. v. Alief General Hospital*, 1996).

3. *Incorrect route of administration:* In 1988 a patient at defendant hospital received an intramuscular injection (IM) of Vibramycin from nurse Roe that should have been administered intravenously (IV). The patient, Gassen, had a mass in the area of the injection, pain, swelling, and disability as a result of the injection. The physician had incorrectly ordered the IM route, and the pharmacist changed the route of administration to IV on the patient's medication administration record (MAR). The Vibramycin is manufactured only for IV administration and was supplied by the pharmacist to the nursing unit with a label for "IV administration." Despite the labeled package, nurse Roe administered the medication IM as stated in the order because the MAR was not available to her until after she gave the injection. The appeals court reversed the district court and denied the summary judgment in favor of the pharmacist, holding that the pharmacist had a duty to check with the prescribing doctor to clarify the order for the clearly incorrect prescription. The case was remanded for further proceedings (*Lynn B. Gassen v. East Jefferson General Hospital*, 1993).

   The nurse in this case should also have questioned the fact that the drug was supplied specifying a different route of administration (IV) than the order (IM). This illustrates that even though the error started with an incorrect physician order that the pharmacist knew was

wrong and corrected (but only as to the route of administration), the nurse could have prevented the error as the last check for safety before administration. The nurse should have questioned the doctor's order at the point of preparing the medication because there was a clear discrepancy with what was supplied by the pharmacy.

4. *Improper treatment of pain and duty to clearly communicate nature and immediacy of patient problem:* In *Mobile Infirmary Association v. Robert E. Tyler* (2007), a jury verdict for wrongful death and medical malpractice was appealed by defendant hospital. The jury found that the hospital's nurses failed to exercise reasonable skill, care, and diligence as other similarly situated healthcare providers. The defendant's mother was admitted for an expected couple of days to the cardiac care unit in 1999 to monitor her condition and receive medications to prepare her for a later "cardioversion." The next day, Saturday, after her condition was normal in the morning, she complained in the afternoon to nurse Greene that she was having abdominal pain and then was given Darvocet and Phenergan. The nurse determined after examining her abdomen that it was normal, despite her complaints of severe pain. Nurse Greene's "focus note" for 1:15 p.m. indicated that the patient was having abdominal pain "the worse she had ever had," and at the same time her blood pressure and heart rate increased significantly. The nurse called the physician answering service and reported the pain and other symptoms related to her cardiac condition. The answering service did not perceive the call to be any type of emergency. The physician ordered some cardiac medications. At 2:00 p.m. the patient continued to have the pain and nausea, and the pain was "worse than usual." The family

requested that a doctor examine the patient (the second such request according to the family), so nurse Greene again called the answering service to report her symptoms but again did not indicate any emergency. The family claimed that the patient had been "doubled over" and was "screaming in pain."

Eventually there was a consult and examination that day by a gastroenterologist who found tenderness in the abdomen but bowel sounds and complaint of pain out of proportion with physical findings. On Sunday morning, nurse Greene returned for another shift and found the patient "moaning" and "only responsive to pain" with her abdomen hard and distended, and she was transferred to the intensive care unit. After doctors there examined her it was determined she needed emergency surgery. The surgery revealed her large intestine was necrotic and infected, the necrosis being caused by a mesenteric blood clot. Her condition was fatal, according to the doctor, and he recommended that the family authorize a "do not resuscitate" order. The patient died the next day. In the lawsuit the family claimed, among other allegations, that the nurses were negligent in administering pain medication before knowing the cause of her acute abdominal pain and that they failed to act on a significant decline/change in the patient early Saturday morning. The jury returned a verdict against the hospital finding that if the nurses had accurately communicated the patient's symptoms of pain (and not just treated it with pain medications), it was more probable than not that proper medical care could have prevented her death. The hospital appealed the $5.5 million damage award against them. The appeals court affirmed the trial court on the condition that the

punitive damage award be reduced in the amount of $2.5 million, leaving the plaintiff an award of $3 million.

This case underscores the need to clearly communicate patient symptoms and the immediacy of a required response. Additionally, treating the patient's pain without recognizing critical underlying reasons may lead to large damage awards, as in this case. Continuation of the patient's symptoms with inadequate pain relief should signal a need for further intervention.

5. *Overdose of medication and medication reconciliation error:* In 1999 a patient was admitted to the hospital after he fainted and hit his head. A neurologist prescribed an anticonvulsant medication, Dilantin, with an initial loading dose of 1 gram (1000 milligrams) to be followed by 300 milligrams every night thereafter during his hospital stay. The MAR was correctly transcribed as "Dilantin 300 mg po QHS." Four days later he was transferred to the rehabilitation unit requiring a new set of physician's orders, and the Dilantin was ordered as before: "300 mg po QHS." The new MAR generated by the pharmacy listed the Dilantin as "100 mg cap (Dilantin) oral, give = 3 capsules 300 mg TID." For the following 6 days, nurses administered and the patient received 900 mg per day while in the hospital, according to the instructions on the MAR. The error was also carried over to the discharge medication instructions, written by the nurse, but also verified by a doctor. The patient's community pharmacist questioned the order as being high and called the rehabilitation unit to verify it and was told that was what the MAR stated, so he filled the prescription. The patient never took any more of the medication after his daughter called his physician to report her father was having difficulty

swallowing and verbalizing, so the doctor advised that the patient should be taken to the emergency room. There it was discovered his Dilantin level was "54.4 mcg/ml," indicating Dilantin toxicity—the therapeutic level is 10–20 mcg/ml. The patient required further treatment for a month in the hospital. A jury entered a verdict for the patient, and the appeals court granted a new trial on the negligence claim but denied the claim against the hospital for punitive damages (*Robert Ferguson v. Baptist Health System, Inc.*, 2005).

Part of the evidence at the trial was that the overdose was not detected by a reconciliation process, wherein the first nurse who administers the drug is to compare the doctor's order with the MAR order and "reconcile" the two. The hospital acknowledged that one of its pharmacists had made an error in changing the dosage interval, but that error was compounded when the MAR was not properly reconciled by a nurse. The hospital had argued that those were the result of human error and should not be the basis of a punitive damage award based on "consciousness" that an act or omission would likely cause harm.

6. *Failure to question medication known to be contraindicated in patient's condition:* The jury found that hospital personnel, including an emergency room nurse, who did not question an inappropriate order for a medication that they knew was contraindicated in his condition, led to and was the proximate cause of the patient's injury (*Columbia Medical Center of Las Colinas Medical Center and Lisa Crain, R.N. v. Norma Bush*, 2003). Scott Bush, the 46–year-old patient who had been previously diagnosed with ventricular tachycardia, or rapid heartbeat, came to defendant hospital's emergency room in 2000 after "feeling funny." An

EKG confirmed that he was having ventricular tachycardia. Nurse Crain, a named defendant in the lawsuit, took Bush's initial information on the intake form and was the nurse working with him. Bush indicated that he did not want to be "shocked," that is, cardioverted. The ER doctor, Zeh, prescribed two different medications but neither was effective. Dr. Zeh then contacted the on call cardiologist, Dr. Osborne, and as a result of her conversation with him, she ordered that 5 milligrams of verapamil be administered to Bush. Eric Johanson, a paramedic working in the ER as an employee, administered the drug to the patient Bush. Within 2 minutes, his blood pressure "crashed," he had a convulsion, and he went into cardiac arrest, suffering brain damage as a result. Thereafter he became a resident in a nursing home, unable to speak, with no motor function.

Verapamil is a drug contraindicated for treatment of ventricular tachycardia. The Advanced Cardiac Life Support (ACLS) manual repeatedly warns against giving this drug to patients with ventricular tachycardia in the text, algorithm, and "critical points to remember." The package insert for the drug from the manufacturer similarly warns against this use. Nurse Crain and nurse Heskes, the house supervisor, were both present in the patient's treatment room when Dr. Zeh ordered that the verapamil be given to the patient. Nurse Crain, who is ACLS certified, testified that she immediately had a serious question about whether verapamil was an appropriate medication for him. She said, "Verapamil, are you sure?" and Dr. Zeh said "yes." Nonetheless, even after Dr. Zeh said "yes," nurse Crain still had a question about the order and knew it could be an extreme risk to the patient. She also agreed that the nursing standard of care required her to exercise her own judgment if she felt a doctor ordered a medicine with adverse consequences to a patient. In fact there was a specific policy entitled "Protocol to Follow When a Nurse Questions a Physician Order" outlining the process and the policy to ensure patient safety. Part of this protocol states that nurses are responsible for the "knowledge of the rationale for and the effects thereof, in the administration of medications and/or treatments as prescribed by a licensed physician or dentist. *Therefore, nurses are responsible for questioning medications ordered prior to administering the drug*" [emphasis added in text]. This policy imposed a separate duty on nurse Crain to intervene before the patient received the verapamil. Nurse Heskes also knew of the potential harm and testified that she may have breached a duty to intervene as a nursing supervisor.

The interaction between the paramedic, Johanson, who actually administered the drug, and nurse Crain was also part of the evidence at trial. Johanson had been hired 8 months earlier but did not yet have a written job description. However, the hospital's "Procedures Performed by Non Physicians" prohibited a paramedic like Johanson from administering cardiac medications. Johanson also testified that he had a serious question about giving this drug to Bush but that he and nurse Crain looked at each other "still, like unsure, like are we giving verapamil." Nurse Crain then nodded her head to Johanson, and he interpreted this nod as an indication that he was to go ahead and inject the verapamil. Also, Dr. Zeh, who ordered the medication, testified she felt verapamil was okay because she had con-

sulted about it with the cardiologist, and the patient had not responded to the other medications, thus she concluded that his situation was outside the ACLS guidelines. Dr. Zeh further said that she expected that the nurses or paramedic in attendance would bring it to her attention if they had a serious question about an order and to refuse to participate in carrying it out. None of them had done this. Dr. Osborne, the cardiologist who spoke with Dr. Zeh, testified that he did not order the verapamil but discussed various reasons that Bush had not responded to the previous medications "to enlighten her." Osborne said he told Dr. Zeh to "sit tight and I'll be there shortly."

A registered nurse paramedic expert witness for the plaintiff testified that both nurse Crain and Johanson's conduct fell below the standard of care and rose to the level of "malice" because they did not delay or prevent the administration, and they basically ignored the chain of command and went ahead and gave it knowing it posed great risk to the patient. The hospital argued unsuccessfully on appeal that the nurses and paramedic all relied upon "doctors we trusted" in administering the verapamil and that there should be no finding of malice as determined by the jury. The appeals court found the evidence to be sufficient for the jury's finding in that each professional, nurses Crain and Heskes, as the supervisor, and Johanson, as a paramedic, had an independent duty to intervene to stop the medication administration and not to just blindly follow a doctor's order, but they did not do so. The appeals court also supported the jury's failure to find that "the negligence, if any, of Dr. Zeh and Dr. Osborne proximately caused the occurrence in question." There was sufficient evidence to support a theory that it was the negligence of nurse Crain and Johanson in not refusing to administer verapamil, and the negligence of the nurse supervisor, Heskes, to intervene that was the proximate (legal) cause of the patient's injury. The appeals court also upheld the jury award of $10 million in future medical expenses and $3 million in punitive damages.

This case presents significant issues related to nurses questioning doctors' orders in appropriate circumstances when the nurse knows (or should know) that there is serious risk of harm to a patient. Although this may not be easy to do, many hospitals have implemented policies and protocols to clarify roles and responsibilities and to support nurses in this situation. Nursing judgment must be used to know when to question orders. Nurse supervisors are also reminded of their duty to intervene if the situation calls for it.

■ DISCIPLINARY ACTION BY THE STATE BOARD OF NURSING

The state board of nursing would normally be involved if a medication error resulted in a serious injury or death of a patient. Sometimes the state board will require a nurse to complete a continuing education course or will restrict his or her practice in some other way. Any of the sanctions available to the state board could be used, including revoking the license, which would mean the nurse could no longer work as an RN.

■ RISK MANAGEMENT CONSIDERATIONS

Nurses remain individually accountable for their own errors even if someone else started the chain of events, as illustrated in the preceding cases. For example, if a medication is ordered incorrectly, it is the responsibility of the nurse to clarify the order. The nurse administers the drug to the patient and becomes the last checkpoint for the patient's safety (see Figure 18-1B).

It is important for nurses to acknowledge mistakes and to document them accordingly on incident or adverse event reports and patient records. A nurse should never falsify any patient record, but doing so as related to medication errors (especially with narcotics) will usually violate the NPA. Nurses must follow all institutional protocols, but they may be required to go beyond protocols to provide for patient safety. Nurses are also encouraged to voluntarily and confidentially report medication errors online to the USP-ISMP Medication Error Reporting Program (MERP) or FDA MedWatch as previously noted.

When incidents related to medication errors (including near misses) are tracked and trended, patterns can be identified. This helps to positively identify system errors that can be dealt with effectively by the agency or institution. Another outcome of tracking errors is to identify medications with a high risk of injury to patients and to pay particular attention to these as high-alert drugs. Some of the medications that have resulted in significant patient injury and high awards for damages following litigation are insulin, potassium chloride, heparin, digoxin and other potent cardiac drugs, chemotherapeutic agents, narcotics, and anesthetics. It is recommended that extra checkpoints be included when administering these drugs, such as having two nurses check dosage, calculation, and administration methods.

Government and agency error reporting systems that use a nonpunitive approach are most effective, and confidential reporting has led to positive system changes to improve patient safety. Many experts agree that when egregious errors occur, it almost always involves system failure in more than one department and level of the organization. Others point to the fact that any activity involving human conduct will sometimes result in error, and individual blame is an ineffective strategy to prevent future occurrences. Along with this thinking, healthcare professions and the public are urged to accept errors as inevitable but manageable and not to expect perfection in practice. This, however, is at odds with the legal system, which is a fault-based system, and this can be a source of conflict in a particular situation (see **Figure 18-2**).

National studies and programs that track data related to medication errors estimate that nearly one-half of these errors are preventable. It is clear from the preceding legal cases that nurses are expected to assume an increased role and duty to question inappropriate medication orders in promoting patient safety while advocating for patients. In light of these considerations, nurses must be vigilant in their practice in fulfilling their responsibility to patients in terms of safe administration of medications.

■ REFERENCES AND BIBLIOGRAPHY

American Nurses Association. (2006). *ANA position statement: Assuring patient safety; registered nurses' responsibility in all roles and settings to guard against working while fatigued.* Washington, DC: Author.

Brooke, P. (2007). Program update: Promoting patient safety and preventing medical errors. *Journal of Nursing Law, 11*(3), 124–128.

Chavez v. Parkview Episcopal Hospital, 32 P.3d 609; 2001 Colo. App. LEXIS 996; 2001 Colo. J.C.A.R. 3250 (2001).

Columbia Medical Center of Las Colinas Medical Center and Lisa Crain, R.N. v. Norma Bush, 122 S.W.3d 835; 2003 Tex. App. LEXIS 9914 (2003).

Dennison, R. (2006, November). High-alert drugs: Strategies for safe I.V. infusions. *American Nurse Today,* 28–33.

Dennison, R. (2007). A medication safety education program to reduce the risk of harm caused by medication errors. *The Journal of Continuing Education in Nursing, 38*(4), 176–184.

Donna Ellis v. Bard, Inc. and Baxter Healthcare Corporation, et al., 311 F.3d 1272; 2002 U.S. App. LEXIS 23421; CCH Prod. Liab. Rep. P16,442; Fla. L. Weekly Fed. C 38 (2002).

Patient Safety Is Always Paramount

- Follow all recommended manufacturer instructions and agency protocols.
- Question inappropriate orders that pose a serious risk of injury to a patient.
- Document according to the organization's "do not use" list, and avoid using any ISMP's list of "Error-Prone Abbreviations, Symbols, and Dose Designations."
- Use extra caution and safety checks when administering "high-alert" drugs.
- Submit confidential and voluntary reports of medication errors or "near misses" to the ISMP and FDA Web sites to improve medication safety.
- Support nonpunitive approaches to reporting medication errors.
- Work to promote a culture of safety in the workplace for medication administration.

Figure 18-2   Additional practice tips for safe medication administration.

Eisenhauer, L., Hurley, A., & Dolan, N. (2007). Nurses' reported thinking during medication administration. *Journal of Nursing Scholarship*, *39*(1), 82–87.

Hughes, K. (2007, July 2). Wave of the future. *Advance for Nurses—New England*, 16–20.

Institute of Medicine. (2000). To err is human: Building a safer health system. Washington, DC: National Academy Press.

Kamalaben L. Kapadia et al. v. Alief General Hospital, 1996 Tex. App. LEXIS 4116 (1996).

Lynn B. Gassen v. East Jefferson General Hospital, 628 So. 2d 256; 1993 La. App. LEXIS 3985 (1993).

McAllen Hospitals v. Carmen Garza Muniz, et al., 2007 Tex. App. LEXIS 9683 (2007).

Mobile Infirmary Association v. Robert E. Tyler, 2007 Ala. LEXIS 192 (2007).

Plum, S. (1997). Nurses indicted. *Nursing 97, 27*(7), 34–35.

Robert Ferguson v. Baptist Health System, Inc., 910 So. 2d 85; 2005 Ala. LEXIS 19 (2005).

Rogers, A., et al. (2004). The working hours of hospital staff nurses and patient safety. *Health Affairs, 23*(4), 202–212.

Shalo, S. (2007). To err is human—But for some nurses, a crime. *AJN, 107*(3), 20–21.

Smetzer, J. (1998a). Lessons from Colorado—Beyond blaming individuals. *Nursing Management, 29*(6): 49–51.

Smetzer, J. (1998b). Voices from Colorado. *Nursing Management, 29*(6): 52–53.

State of Wisconsin v. Julie Thao, 2006 CF2512, Wisconsin Cir., Dane County, November 2, 2006.

The Joint Commission. (2008). *2008 national patient safety goals*. Retrieved September 22, 2008, from http://www.jointcommission.org/PatientSafety

US Food and Drug Administration. (2008, March 14). *FDA 101: Medication errors*. Retrieved September 22, 2008, from http://www.fda.gov/consumer/updates/medicationerrors031408.html

■ ADDITIONAL RESOURCES

Institute for Safe Medication Practices: www.ismp.org

United States Pharmacopeia: www.usp.org

Centers for Medicare and Medicaid Services (CMS): www.cms.hhs.gov

Agency for Healthcare Research and Quality: www.ahrq.gov

Chapter 19

Clients with AIDS and HIV Testing

Katherine Dempski

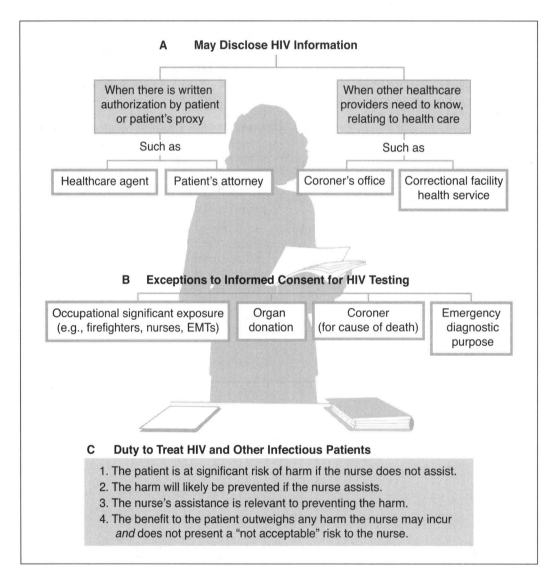

A   May Disclose HIV Information

When there is written authorization by patient or patient's proxy

When other healthcare providers need to know, relating to health care

Such as

Such as

Healthcare agent

Patient's attorney

Coroner's office

Correctional facility health service

B   Exceptions to Informed Consent for HIV Testing

Occupational significant exposure (e.g., firefighters, nurses, EMTs)

Organ donation

Coroner (for cause of death)

Emergency diagnostic purpose

C   Duty to Treat HIV and Other Infectious Patients

1. The patient is at significant risk of harm if the nurse does not assist.
2. The harm will likely be prevented if the nurse assists.
3. The nurse's assistance is relevant to preventing the harm.
4. The benefit to the patient outweighs any harm the nurse may incur *and* does not present a "not acceptable" risk to the nurse.

The Centers for Disease Control and Prevention (CDC) recommendations changed from HIV testing of those with high risk factors to HIV screening of all patients between the ages of 13 and 64 years (CDC, 2006). With these recommendations, the CDC sought to address the two major barriers cited by healthcare providers to HIV testing: the pretest counseling requirement and the need for a separate written informed consent for HIV testing. To encourage widespread testing, federal and state statutes ensure confidentiality surrounding the testing process and diagnosis of HIV and AIDS. The federal statute sets the minimum amount of confidentiality that must be in place for each state. Each state has its own rules governing AIDS and HIV testing (see **Figure 19-2**).

■ CONFIDENTIALITY

In general, healthcare providers who obtain HIV information must keep that information confidential. There are usually a few exceptions to the rule of strict confidentiality (see **Figure 19-1A**). Whenever disclosure is made, it must include a written statement warning the individual receiving the information that it is confidential and protected by law. A violation of the confidentiality law makes the individual liable in a private cause of action by the patient. The ANA Position Statement on HIV Testing (1991b) supports voluntary, anonymous, and confidential testing and not mandatory testing.

■ WARNING KNOWN PARTNERS

Specific rules govern warning third parties of a patient's HIV status. Physicians and nurses have a duty to their patients to keep HIV information confidential. This is an ethical duty and in most states a legal duty defined by statute. Most statutes do not authorize nurses to pass this information to known partners. However, the ANA has a position statement on warning known third parties who are at risk (1991a). The ANA supports the ethical responsibility of disclosing HIV information to an identified partner who is at risk by the nurse's patient when certain conditions apply. The nurse must be the primary care provider, the patient must have received counseling on the benefits of warning partners, and the nurse must reasonably believe the patient will not warn the partner. Any nurse in the position of disclosing HIV information to warn a third party should consult an attorney who is familiar with both the state statute defining the legal duty and professional organizations' position statements defining any ethical duty. When the two are at odds, the nurse will need to know how to reconcile them.

■ INFORMED CONSENT FOR HIV TESTING

Healthcare providers may not order HIV testing without written or oral consent documented in the medical record. Each state will have its own HIV informed consent statute with which healthcare providers need to be familiar. Some states have followed the CDC recommendations to encourage widespread testing by dropping the specific written HIV testing informed consent and the pretest counseling on issues such as the reliability and confidentiality of the test. Other states

- Testing is voluntary with patient consent. Consent no longer needs to be on a specific HIV Testing Informed Consent Form.
- Consent can be verbal with written documentation by the provider.
- Oral or written information on HIV testing and the test results must be given to the patient.
- Posttest counseling is required only if the test is positive. The counseling must be done in person and include reliability of test results, preventative practices in spreading HIV, and referrals for health care and support.

Figure 19-2   Sample state HIV testing statute.

still require that the HIV informed consent be very specific. First, the person obtaining the informed consent must explain the purpose of the test and the benefits of early diagnosis and treatment. The patient must be informed of the confidentiality in the testing process and that HIV testing is not a prerequisite to medical treatment. The patient must also be aware that recording HIV information in the medical records when it relates to medical treatment is permissible and that disclosure to known individuals who are at risk may be statutorily required. Documentation must show that all of the criteria were met. To avoid liability, healthcare providers who order the test must make a good faith effort to comply with all requirements and convey that informed consent was given.

Posttest counseling remains an important element in all HIV informed-consent statutes. Positive test results must be given with personal contact between the caregiver and patient. Counseling must be offered about discrimination, emotional issues, prevention of transmission, and the possible need of notifying others who are at risk. Documentation of all counseling provided is an essential element of the informed-consent statutes. Laboratories need to verify that informed consent is in the record before running the test. The results must go directly to the healthcare provider who ordered the test to protect confidentiality.

■ EXCEPTIONS TO INFORMED CONSENT

There are specific exceptions to obtaining informed consent for HIV testing (see Figure 19-1B). In urgent care situations when the patient is unconscious or otherwise unable to consent and no one authorized to consent is available, testing may be done if needed for immediate diagnostic purposes. Testing may be done when healthcare providers or other occupations (firefighters or emergency medical technicians) have a significant exposure

in the course of their occupational duty and the patient refuses testing. This means that nurses who have a needle stick injury should be able to have the patient tested even if he or she refuses. Agency policies need to be followed strictly in reporting the injury. The deceased may be tested if the diagnosis is necessary for the cause of death. Testing may also be done prior to organ donation. In each situation the specific statute and agency policies must be followed carefully.

State statutes are very specific on when one may be compelled to submit to HIV testing. First there must be a bona fide exposure (generally defined as blood or body fluids with visible blood coming in contact with an open wound, broken skin, or mucus membrane). A Minnesota court held that the state could not compel an offender who bit and spit in the eye of a police officer because no visible blood came in contact with the officer's mucus membrane (eye), and although his skin was broken there was no visible blood in the offender's saliva (*In Matter of Welfare of ESC,* 2007).

■ MANDATORY TESTING

States that have enacted mandatory HIV testing for pregnant women require counseling of HIV testing as part of routine prenatal care of all women including early treatment benefit to the newborn. The woman may "opt out" with documentation of such in her medical records. At time of delivery the woman would be counseled again as to the benefit of early treatment, and unless she provides specific written refusal, the test will be performed.

■ AMERICANS WITH DISABILITIES ACT

The ignorance and fear surrounding the AIDS virus leaves HIV-positive individuals vulnerable to discrimination. Federal courts have recognized HIV as a disability because the stigma attached to it interferes with one's ability to perform "activities of daily living." Therefore,

HIV has become a protected disability under the Americans with Disabilities Act (ADA).

An HIV-positive patient made a successful discrimination claim against his surgeon for an unnecessary 2-day delay in surgery while the operating team waited for HIV "safe suits" to arrive. The federal court ruled that the delay was unreasonable because the CDC guidelines for universal precautions do not require safe suits, and therefore the patient was treated differently from others based on his HIV status.

■ DUTY TO TREAT HIV PATIENTS

Both the American Medical Association and ANA have issued ethical statements on the duty to care for HIV-infected patients. Both agree that it is professionally unethical to deny medical and nursing treatment to a patient based solely on the patient's HIV status. This includes denying care to a patient who refuses to undergo HIV testing. HIV patients may be transferred to another healthcare provider or facility that is better equipped to provide care to the patient, but the transfer must be to benefit the patient's care rather than the personal preference of the healthcare provider. However, the ANA recognized that nurses are not legally or ethically required to put their personal health at risk. For example, an immunosuppressed nurse is justified in requesting to not care for infectious patients just as a pregnant nurse should not care for a patient with cytomegalovirus (which is harmful to the fetus).

Guidelines issued by professional organizations are often used to show the standard of care in these situations and should be followed (see Figure 19-1C). The ANA position statement supports needle exchange programs with infection control, referral for treatment, and HIV education (1993b). The ANA also supports those at risk for HIV by providing HIV testing and prophylactic treatment to patients who were raped (1993a).

■ REFERENCES

American Nurses Association. (1991a). *ANA position statement: Guidelines for disclosure to known third parties about possible HIV infection.* Washington, DC: Author.

American Nurses Association. (1991b). *ANA position statement: HIV testing.* Washington, DC: Author.

American Nurses Association. (1993a). *ANA position statement: HIV exposure from rape/sexual assault.* Washington, DC: Author.

American Nurses Association. (1993b). *ANA position statement: Needle exchange and HIV.* Washington, DC: Author.

American Nurses Association. (2006, June 21). *ANA position statement: Risk versus responsibility in providing nursing care.* Washington, DC: Author.

Centers for Disease Control and Prevention. (2006). *Revised recommendations for HIV testing of adults, adolescents, and pregnant women in healthcare settings.* Retrieved September 22, 2008, from http://www.cdc.gov/mmwr/preview/mmwrhtml /rr5514a1.htm

In Matter of Welfare of ESC, J6-06-551059 (Minn. May 2007).

Chapter 20

Abusive Situations

Katherine Dempski

- **Physical Abuse:**
  - Infliction of injury or punishment that results in harm, unreasonable confinement, beating, slapping, kicking, rough handling, or other abuse causing welts, cuts, burns, abrasions, sprains, bruises, dislocations, fractures, or broken bones.
- **Neglect by Caregiver/Others:**
  - Deprivation of essential needs such as adequate shelter, lack of supervision, failure to give medicine, food, or personal care, not attending physical impairments such as pressure ulcers.
- **Self-Neglect:**
  - Reportable when adult is incompetent. Manifested by failure to provide self-care in ADLs, overmedication/undermedication, untreated medical or mental conditions, danger to self.
- **Psychological/Emotional Abuse:**
  - Denying visits with family/friends, verbal threats or insults, cursing, belittling, or isolation.
- **Sexual Abuse:**
  - Sexually transmitted diseases (STDs), pregnancy, bruises, bleeding, pain or itching in genital or anal areas, difficulty in walking or sitting.
- **Financial Abuse/Exploitation:**
  - Using the adult's money for personal use, mismanaging money or stealing property, savings, credit cards, unusual activity in bank accounts, misuse of assets, forcing change in will.

Nurses are often at the entry point for patients faced with family violence. *Family violence* is defined as inappropriate and damaging interpersonal harm among individuals with interpersonal relations regardless of their actual biological or legal relationships. Such harm includes child physical abuse and neglect; child sexual abuse; domestic partner abuse; and elder or vulnerable adult mistreatment, abuse, and exploitation. The general types of abuse are defined in **Figure 20-1**.

■ CHILD ABUSE

It is critical that nurses, as well as other healthcare providers, be able to identify children in abusive situations. A discrepancy between the physical findings and the explanations of how an incident occurred is a valid reason for a nurse to suspect abuse. A classic example is evidence of healed fractures that have no plausible explanation. The effects of child abuse on younger children can include aggressive behavior, social withdrawal, depression, lying, stealing, thumb sucking, as well as behaviors that are inappropriate for the child's age. Older children and adolescents are more likely to be involved in substance abuse, exhibit problems at school, engage in risky behavior (high-risk sexual encounters, high-speed driving, etc.), or suicidal behavior.

All states have mandated child abuse reporting laws. Mandated reporting laws require that suspected abuse of a child be communicated to the appropriate authorities. Each state has specified social services or law enforcement agencies to which an incident of suspected child abuse must be reported. In addition to healthcare professionals, a number of other professionals are considered to be "mandated reporters." It is important to note that the usual confidential nature of medical treatment usually is waived in the child abuse situation. Therefore, health professionals are expected to report suspected child abuse even if their knowledge comes from the patient. Moreover, most states have provisions that protect individual healthcare professions (including nursing) from legal liability as long as the reporting was done in good faith. Finally, many states have laws that expose a healthcare provider to legal action, criminal and/or civil, for failing to report suspected abuse to the appropriate authorities.

■ ELDER AND VULNERABLE ADULTS

All 50 states have mandatory reporting statutes for healthcare providers who have a reasonable belief that a vulnerable adult (physical or mental impairment limiting self-care) or elder (an adult older than the age set by the statute, such as 60) is being abused or exploited.

- *Elderly:* An elderly person is usually about 60 years of age. It is important to be familiar with individual state adult reporting statutes because all are not uniform. Some states define all adults over a certain age to be elderly and thus fall within the scope of adult protective services regardless of independent living and competency to make their own informed decisions. Others require an elderly person to also be a vulnerable adult before adult protective services mandates reporting of abuse.
- *Vulnerable adult:* A vulnerable adult is over 18 years of age, with impaired ability to complete ADLs due to mental, emotional, or physical impairment (including the infirmity of age). Most states specifically include all residents of a care facility regardless of age.

All 50 states have adult protective services to support vulnerable adults and elderly to live free of abuse and exploitation. A significant majority of states have named nurses as mandated reporters. As such nurses need to understand the relevant definitions. *Elder or vulnerable adult abuse* refers to: (1) neglect; (2) abuse, both physical and psychological; (3) financial exploitation; and (4) neglect by self or caregiver.

Mandated reporters extends to those professions that may come in contact with elderly or vulnerable adults, such as attorneys, financial planners, insurance brokers, residential care staff, accountants, as well as healthcare workers.

The most easily recognizable abuse is physical abuse. Recognition, assessment, and treatment of abuse in the elderly are complicated by a number of factors. An abused elder may be fearful of the abuser, be ashamed to acknowledge dependency on the abuser (especially his or her own adult children), or be loyal to the abuser. The complexities of identifying abuse benefits from a multidisciplinary approach. The physician determines competency of the patient. The nurse assists in the injury assessment, documentation, and the health history, while the social worker assesses the psychosocial situation and identifies community support services the patient may benefit from.

When a healthcare provider suspects that an elderly patient is a victim of physical abuse, there are often clues to assist in assessment of the situation. Explanations inconsistent with noted injuries and delay in seeking treatment of the injuries are examples of signs and symptoms of abuse. The behavior of the family members or caretakers also can suggest a pattern of abuse. For example, behaviors include excessively detailed accounts of the injuries, undue concern with the cost of treatment, and refusing to let the elderly person be interviewed or treated without their presence. Interventions for abused elders and vulnerable adults should focus on maintaining safety and evaluating the patient's capacity to protect himself or herself.

Some elders may lack the mental capacity to make informed choices about their situation. Therefore, the nurse as a mandated reporter who recognizes elder abuse will need to make the state report with the assistance of the healthcare institution or agency's legal counsel so adult protective services may begin the process for conservatorship or guardianship. Elders who are competent to make informed choices may choose to not report that they are the victim of some form of abuse. The nurse will need to educate the patient in his or her options to seek support services from adult protective agencies or other community services.

Immunity is provided to healthcare providers (such as a civil libel suit) when the report is done in good faith. This immunity extends from the initial reporter (to encourage reporting) to the nurse who is asked postreport to provide corroborative evidence as part of the abuse investigation (*Casbohm v. MetroHealth Med. Ctr.*, 2000). The Casbohm court affirmed immunity for the nurses who

were sued for a negligent physical exam that determined sexual abuse based on a skin rash and a perianal wart that later was diagnosed as a skin tag. However, most statutes provide that a mandated reporter who intentionally and with malicious intent either fails to report abuse or makes a false report may face a criminal charge under the statute and disciplinary action by the licensing board. The statute will specify the reporting process (see **Figure 20-2**). In addition, the agency may have a specific policy to follow and require specific documentation and, more importantly, there may be an internal notice requirement of the report (such as legal counsel or risk management). Under most state statutes, an institution may have a protocol to notify legal counsel and seek guidance in making the report, but the policy may not hinder the mandatory reporter.

The person with the power of attorney can be the abuser (*Boyce v. Fernandez*, 1996). The abuser is not always a person but can be an entity. A long-term care facility was reported and found liable for neglect and abuse of a vulnerable adult who suffered stage IV pressure ulcers, frequent falls, and dehydration (*Denton v. Superior Court of Arizona, American Family Care Corp., Olster Certified Healthcare Corp., Todd Koceja and Jane Koceja*, 1997).

■ PARTNER ABUSE

Unless the abused partner is a vulnerable adult, there is no mandatory reporting requirement. However, the emotional impact a violent environment has on children is well documented. In situations in which there may be child abuse, mandated reporting laws, which require reporting, may assist in providing the vehicle for family treatment. Again, the signs and symptoms of partner abuse can be clouded by the patient's fear in disclosing information that he or she has been a victim of abuse by a partner. In many abusive situations, the battered partners will try to remedy the situation themselves by trying to change

```
┌─────────────────────────────────────────────────────────┐
│                                                           │
│                    Reporting Process                      │
│                                                           │
│         Suspected abuse/neglect of:                       │
│             Child or vulnerable adult (physical/mental    │
│             condition limiting self care OR elderly, age  │
│             defined in statute)                           │
│                                                           │
│         Report to:                                        │
│             Child Protective Services                     │
│             Adult Protective Services                     │
│                                                           │
│             Long-term care ombudsman (usually when an     │
│             agency or healthcare provider is involved)    │
│                                                           │
│             State licensing board (when healthcare        │
│             provider is involved)                         │
│                                                           │
│             Law enforcement (if required under statute)   │
│                                                           │
│         When:                                             │
│             Written or verbal report within 24 hours of   │
│             incident                                      │
│                                                           │
└─────────────────────────────────────────────────────────┘
```

Figure 20-2 Sample state HIV testing statute.

their behavior. For example, "I shouldn't argue so much, he gets so angry."

Nursing assessment and interventions include asking the right questions and referrals to appropriate social service or law enforcement agencies.

■ REFERENCES

Boyce v. Fernandez, 77 F.3d 946 (1996).

Capezuti, E., et al. (1995). Meeting the challenge of elder abuse. *Nursing Dynamics, 4*(1), 5–9.

Casbohm v. MetroHealth Med. Ctr., 746 N.E.2d 661 (Ohio Ct. App. 2000).

Denton v. Superior Court of Arizona, American Family Care Corp., Olster Certified Healthcare Corp., Todd Koceja and Jane Koceja, 94f5 P.2d 1283 (1997).

Greenberg, S. A., Ramsey, G. C., Mitty, E. L., & Fulmer, T. (1999). Elder mistreatment: Case law and ethical issues in assessment, reporting, and management. *Journal of Nursing Law, 6*(3), 7–20.

Kearney, K. (2007). Nurse's duty to report child abuse versus the attorney's duty of confidentiality: The nurse attorney's dilemma. *Journal of Nursing Law, 11*(1), 13–25.

National Clearinghouse on Child Abuse and Neglect Information. 330 C Street, SW, Washington, DC, 20447. (800) FYI-3366 or (703) 385-7565. E-mail: nccanch@calib.com.

Chapter 21

Reproductive Services

Katherine Dempski

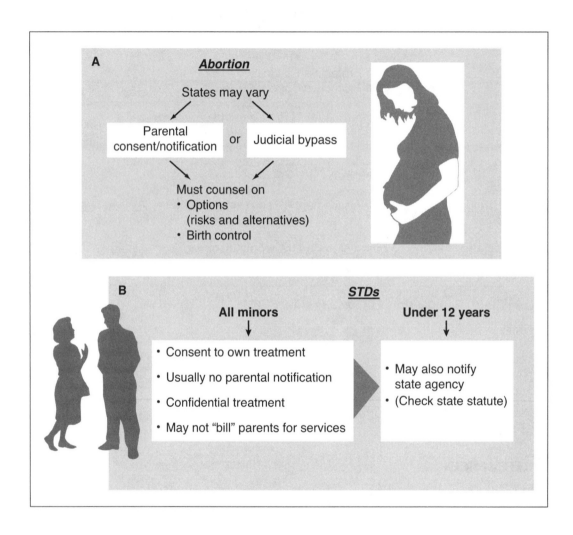

Patients have a right to privacy and a right to make informed heathcare decisions based on full disclosure of information. Healthcare providers have an obligation to inform the patient of all healthcare choices that are legal. Healthcare providers can objectively discuss reproductive services such as abortion, contraception, and treatment of sexually trans-mitted diseases and be aware of the informed consent and notifications issues involving the treatment of minors.

■ ABORTION

Termination of pregnancy is not absolute, with each state setting limitations for adults and minors.

Adults

A woman's right to privacy includes her decision to continue with or terminate a pregnancy up to the point of fetal viability. When the point of fetal viability is reached (somewhere in the second trimester), the state has some interest in preserving life and can put some limits on abortion. However, these limitations cannot cause an undue burden on the woman. Undue burden has not been completely defined and has been determined on a case-by-case analysis. The court has upheld a restriction on federal and state funding for abortions (*Maher v. Roe*) but struck down provisions requiring a woman to obtain her husband's written consent (*Planned Parenthood of Missouri v. Danforth*). Husbands may not compel a wife to complete or terminate a pregnancy.

The court has also struck down a state provision requiring physicians to follow a specified informed-consent form prior to completing abortions. The court found it too intrusive on the physician–patient relationship because the consent form disregarded the physician's judgment on what was relevant to each individual's case. Recently, the court upheld a statute requiring physicians to test fetal viability when the pregnancy is around the 20th week. Technology has changed in the 20 years since the *Roe v. Wade* decision, enabling younger fetuses to survive longer. Some states have a medical emergency exception that permits dispensing with the informed-consent requirement when the physician makes a good faith conclusion that medical complications of pregnancy necessitate a therapeutic abortion. This exception sometimes includes serious mental health issues. Each state specifically enumerates what constitutes a medical emergency (such as loss of life or major bodily function).

Minors

Each state has statutes governing abortions on minors (see **Figure 21-1A**). Nurses who practice in areas providing abortion to minors must be concerned with parental notification and counseling. There are variations in each state on whether a minor may receive an abortion without parental consent. The US Supreme Court answered the question of whether the right to privacy included a minor's right to an abortion in *Planned Parenthood v. Danforth* and *Bellotti v. Baird*. An unemancipated minor's right to reproductive choice is not equal with that of an adult, even in the early stages of pregnancy. No state provision may categorically deny a minor the right to an abortion, and parents may not have absolute veto power over the minor's decision. Although states and parents may not exercise absolute veto power over a minor's reproductive choice, a minor has no absolute right to exercise that choice without authorization from a parent, guardian, or judge. Therefore, states may involve parents by requiring parental notification without giving parents the power of consent. States must be consistent in ensuring that third parties do not have absolute power over another's decision to terminate a pregnancy. Constitutionally, states may require parental consent (usually only one parent will meet statutory requirements), but the state must also include an alternative to parental consent. This alternative has become known as a bypass provision. The bypass provision grants courts the power to determine if a minor is mature enough to consent to an abortion without parental consent or notification. This alternative recognizes that parental consent is not always in the best interest of the minor. Abusive or strained relationships may only worsen when parental consent or notification is required.

All minors must be counseled on options such as adoption and keeping the baby. The minor must sign a form stating she was not coerced and she understands the risks and alternatives. Birth control options also must be discussed. States also may require the healthcare providers to counsel minors on available clinics for birth control services as part of abortion informed consent.

Treating a minor without parental consent for a morning after pill to prevent pregnancy was not a violation of the parents' constitutional rights to parental liberty or the minor's due process rights because the minor sought treatment. The parents brought suit against the city clinic when the minor became sick from the treatment. The court held the conduct the parents complained of was devoid of any compulsion or constraint, and under these circumstances, neither the due process clause nor other constitutional provisions required the parent to be notified (*Anspach, et al., v. City of Philadelphia et al.*, 2007).

■ MINORS AND TREATMENT FOR SEXUALLY TRANSMITTED DISEASES

Minors have the highest sexually transmitted disease (STD) rate of any age group, yet they seek treatment the least because they fear parental notification by healthcare providers. Healthcare providers in the position of treating minors must be aware of the specific state legislation on minors. Most healthcare providers treating minors for STDs are concerned with parental consent even though litigation against providers in their area is uncommon. State statutes will enumerate the age of minority for consenting to reproductive services, which include testing for HIV and STDs (see Figure 21-1B). Some states may require that the state public health or family advocate services be notified that a minor under a certain age (usually 12 years) is seeking reproductive services. This is not the same as parental notification.

When a minor is diagnosed and treated for an STD, the confidentiality statutes require that all information related to the treatment be given only to the young patient. State statutes may require parental notification

that a minor has been hospitalized for STD-related treatment if the minor will be hospitalized for greater than a set amount of time (such as 12 or 16 hours).

The state, however, may compel a clinic that provides treatment to minors for sexually transmitted diseases to notify the state when the clinic become aware of sexual contact between a minor and an adult or other of disparate age when the conduct is in violation of the state statutory rape laws. In *The People ex. Re. Eichenberger v. Stockton Pregnancy Control Medical Clinic, Inc.* (Ca. 1988), the appeals court held the state had a compelling interest in the sexual conduct of a minor 14-year-old and another of disparate age, which constituted a felony sexual assault. The violation of the minor's privacy was justified.

Communicable disease reporting and public health notification requirements are the exception to this. Confidential treatment includes the billing process. The minor is responsible to pay for services, and the parents may not be billed.

Healthcare providers must obtain the minor's informed consent to treatment and determine whether the minor understands the nature, risks, and benefits of the procedure as well as any alternative treatments.

■ SEXUAL ASSAULT

Several states have statutes that authorize providers to treat minors for sexual assault with the minor's consent to treatment and education on sexually transmitted diseases. Parental notification is required unless the parent is the suspected abuser. Absent a specific state statute to treat, the institution should have a guideline for treating minors in this situation under the mature minor exception or emergency exception.

■ EMERGENCY CONTRACEPTION

Emergency contraception reduces the likelihood of pregnancy by 81%–90% if taken within 72 hours of intercourse. Although emergency contraception has been available in the United States for several years, less than half of the states have legislation regarding emergency contraception. States laws either mandate emergency departments to offer sexual assault victims the contraception or allow pharmacists to dispense directly to women without a physician's prescription. Currently very few states provide for both.

■ REFERENCES

American Nurses Association. (1989). *ANA position statement: Reproductive health*. Washington, DC: Author.

Anspach, et al., v. City of Philadelphia et al., 503 F.3d 256 (Circ. 3d 2007).

Bellotti v. Baird, 443 U.S. 622 (1979).

Maher v. Roe, 432 U.S. 464 (1977).

Planned Parenthood of Missouri v. Danforth, 428 U.S. 52 (1976).

Robertson, A. J. (2007). Adolescent informed consent: Ethics, law, and theory to guide policy and nursing research. *Journal of Nursing Law, 11*(4), 191–196.

Roe v. Wade, 410 U.S. 113 (1973).

The People ex. Re. Eichenberger v. Stockton Pregnancy Control Medical Clinic, Inc., 203 Cal. App. 3d 225; 249 Cal. Rptr. 762: 1988 Cal. LEXIS 724 (Ca. 1988).

Chapter 22

Restraints

Katherine Dempski

CMS Definitions

Restraints: Restraints are physical or mechanical devices, equipment, or materials that immobilize or restrict movement of arms, legs, body, or head. Drugs used to manage behavior or restrict freedom of movement and are not standard doses of treatment for the patient's condition are forms of restraint. Examples are jackets, vests, leg and arm restraints, arm boards, hand mitts, and lap cushions or lap trays that the patient cannot easily remove. Restraints also include sheets tightly tucked in or wrapped across the patient to prevent movement from the bed. Placing a wheelchair against a barrier that prevents a patient from moving is a form of restraint. Side rails can be a form of restraint when used on a patient for the purpose of restricting movement of someone who is unable to put the side rail down to get out of the bed.

Not restraints: Orthopedic devices, surgical dressings, protective helmets, and devices that hold a patient in a position for a physical exam or test are not restraints. Devices, materials, or equipment that protect the patient from falling out of bed or are age-appropriate devices, such as cribs or strollers, are also not restraints.

Seclusion: Seclusion is involuntary confinement where the patient is alone in a room or area and the patient is prevented from leaving. Seclusion may only be used for management of violent or self-destructive behavior.

Licensed independent practitioner (LIP): Licensed independent practitioners are practitioners who are permitted by state law and hospital policy to order restraints for patients independently within the scope of practice of the individual's license and when the order is consistent with clinical privileges. Examples are physician's assistants or nurse practitioners.

The current medical trend is for a restraint-free environment. Restraint and seclusion use are inherently dangerous. Increased scrutiny has made this a highly regulated intervention. The Patients' Bill of Rights (1999) states that patients shall be free from restraints and seclusion for punishment, retaliation, coercion, discipline, or convenience of staff. Restraint and seclusion are to be used only in emergent situations for physical safety and if less restrictive interventions are ineffective. Under state and federal regulations, restraint and seclusion use requires that specific steps be taken in assessment, ordering, implementation, monitoring, and documentation, as well as training of staff members who are authorized to use these interventions. Furthermore, restraint and seclusion use have their own liability issues when implemented negligently with harm to the patient. A provider's disregard to follow state and federal regulation as well as professional standards could lead to manslaughter charges following a patient's death due to restraint or seclusion. Additionally, patients may bring an action under the Americans with Disabilities Act with an allegation that they were denied access or participation in an activity based on a disability that was not a direct threat of harm to the safety of others.

■ FEDERAL REGULATION

The Centers for Medicare and Medicaid Services' (CMS) final rule on restraints regulates the minimum requirements for restraint and seclusion use (Patients' Bill of Rights, 1999; final rule published December 8, 2006, effective February 6, 2007). States may have more stringent requirements. CMS no longer differentiates between clinical restraint use and restraints of behavioral management. The indication for restraint is only for the immediate physical safety of the patient, staff, and others (Patients' Bill of Rights, 482.13 (e); see **Figure 22-1**).

The FDA publishes safety alert notices that warn of the hazards associated with certain restraint devices. Therefore, nurses should be familiar with these notices. Continued use of a restraint that is a known hazard could be considered a violation of the standard of care.

The FDA requires the manufacturers to label the restraints. Nurses should verify that the vests, jackets, and other torso-restraining devices are labeled for size, weight limits, and device orientation (such as front/back and top/bottom). Labels should also include cautionary information (such as flammable), application steps, and warnings for incorrect application.

The Safe Medical Devices Act (1990) obligates facilities that use restraints to report to the FDA all restraint-related deaths or injuries within 10 working days.

■ INDICATIONS

Under the Patients' Bill of Rights (1999), patients shall be free from restraints and seclusion for punishment, retaliation, coercion, discipline, or convenience of staff. Restraints and seclusion are to be used only in emergent situations for physical safety of the patient, staff, and others and if less restrictive interventions are determined to be not effective. CMS recognizes that in some emergent situations there is no time to use less restrictive interventions, therefore a determination by the practitioners that less restrictive interventions will not be effective will meet this requirement. The use of restraints requires a comprehensive assessment of the patient and the environmental risks along with an individual patient care plan to determine interventions that will ensure patient safety.

■ INITIAL ORDER

Restraint or seclusion must be ordered by a physician or a licensed independent practitioner (LIP) where permitted by state laws. Restraint orders may not be "as needed" (PRN) or standing orders. Under the Patients' Bill of Rights, initial restraint and seclusion orders for management of violent or self-destructive behavior that jeopardizes the immediate safety of self or others are limited and must be reviewed at 4 hours for an adult, at 2 hours for a child age 9–12 years, and at 1 hour for a child under age 9 years. The initial order must then be renewed at 24 hours with an examination by a physician or LIP. Restraint or seclusion to ensure the physical safety of the patient may be renewed per institution policy.

■ EVALUATION AND MONITORING

Both CMS and The Joint Commission require that all patients placed in restraints or seclusion must have a face-to-face evaluation by a physician, LIP, or RN who is trained for assessing the physical and psychological effects of restraint and seclusion. Determination to continue or discontinue the restraint must be made in the face-to-face assessment. When a trained RN or LIP perform the face-to-face assessment, the attending physician must be consulted (see **Figure 22-2**).

■ DOCUMENTATION

States may have regulations that are more restrictive, but at a minimum, CMS requires specific documentation in medical records for restraint and seclusion intervention:

- Describe patient behavior, interventions used, and the patient's condition that warrants the restraint or seclusion
- Document the 1-hour face-to-face evaluation
- Document the patient's response to the intervention and the rationale for continued use
- A staff member's training must be documented in his or her personnel file as evidence of training/competency

- Document monitoring and continual assessment of the patient during restraint and seclusion use
- Report to CMS and document when a death in restraint or postrestraint occurs, including date and time of death
- Institution policies should also outline documentation requirements, such as assistance of patient in completing activities of daily living, notification to the patient's family, and their response

■ STAFF TRAINING

Patients have the right to have a restraint or seclusion intervention by trained staff only. As such, CMS has specific training requirements for staff members, which includes a demonstration of competency in applying restraints and implementing seclusion before performing each on a patient. This training must be part of initial orientation and be part of peri-

---

CMS (all restraints and seclusion):
1. A 1-hour face-to-face evaluation is required.
2. Patients must be assessed and monitored as determined by hospital policy to guide staff members to an appropriate interval based on patient needs and restraint type used. This could be continuously (moment by moment) or periodic (every 15 minutes).

The Joint Commission:
1. Behavioral restraints and seclusion
   a. A 1-hour face-to-face evaluation is required.
   b. Patients must be continuously observed by staff members who are present with the patient, including assessment every 15 minutes of vital signs and physical and psychological status. Patients must be assisted with nutrition, elimination, and hygiene.
   c. It is acceptable for staff members who are in close proximity to monitor a secluded patient who has been free of restraints for more than 1 hour via video and audio.
2. Nonbehavioral restraints
   a. An LIP examination within 24 hours is required.

Figure 22-2   Evaluation requirements.

odic training. The institution is responsible for setting the frequency. Evidence of individual staff training must be in personnel files.

■ DEATH REPORTING

Death under the following circumstances must be reported to CMS within the next business day and documented in the medical record:

- Death while in restraints or seclusion (regardless of cause)
- Death that occurs within 24 hours after removal of restraints or seclusion (regardless of cause)
- Death known to the institution that occurs within 1 week of restraint or seclusion removal when it is reasonable to assume the restraint or seclusion contributed to the death

■ INFORMED CONSENT

By the definition of restraint and seclusion, practical informed consent may be improbable, impractical, or even impossible. CMS recognizes that patients do not have a right to refuse, nor do family members have a right to demand that a loved one be restrained. The intervention is based on physician and trained staff assessment. It is recommended to always notify family members of the intervention.

■ LIABILITY

Timely intervention with a restraint or seclusion to prevent patient harm to self or others can avoid liability, but as these cases prove, the intervention must adhere to the regulations and laws.

When his daughter was found dead in seclusion from a ruptured ectopic pregnancy, a father brought suit claiming standards were not followed for monitoring. The court held that the father, as executor of his daughter's estate, stated a claim of action because significant facts showed there was a gap in the medical records showing vital signs and observation until she was found dead (*Hopper v. Callahan*, 1990). Another court determined that the plaintiff–patient did correctly state a claim of negligence when the facts showed the physician and emergency department personnel incorrectly identified the patient's need for drug-induced restraint and failed to obtain consent in a nonemergent situation. The patient was brought to the emergency department because she was upset and uncooperative with the police. She was assessed by the physician to not be a danger to self or others, but she was upset and crying, so the physician ordered Ativan (a sedative), which was administered without an explanation of its purpose or effects.

The Americans with Disabilities Act (ADA) was used to bring suit against a hospital for having a policy to seclude all patients who were brought in for a psychiatric evaluation and strip search them for harmful objects before assessing the patient's behavior for harm to self or others. A patient was left in seclusion for hours before a physician examined her and determined she was to be discharged. The court held she brought forth facts to state a claim under the ADA, such as denied access or participation in an activity based on a disability, and her acts did not fall under the exception to the ADA for being a direct threat to the safety of others (*Scherer v. Waterbury*, 2000).

■ REFERENCES

Hopper v. Callahan, 562 N.E.2d 822 (Mass. 1990).

Patients' Bill of Rights, 42 C.F.R. § 482.13 (1999).

Safe Medical Devices Act, Pub. L. No. 101-629, § 1(a), 104 Stat. 4511 (1990).

Scherer v. Waterbury, 2000 Conn. Super. LEXIS 481 (2000).

Substance Abuse and Mental Health Services Administration. (2008). *Homepage.* Retrieved September 27, 2008, from http://www.samhsa.gov

Chapter 23

Emergency Psychiatric Admissions

Katherine Dempski

A Preventing Liability
- Know and strictly follow the state law and the facility's policy.
- Always work in conjunction with a skilled interdisciplinary team that specializes in mental health assessment.
- Assess the patient in a safe and nonthreatening environment, with particular attention to the presence of weapons and the immediate opportunity for harm.
- Establish a checklist that readily identifies the criteria for involuntary admission.
- Precisely document all findings, conclusions, and bases for commitment.
- Encourage confidential peer review and case studies on all patients who have been civilly committed.

B Dangerous Individuals Are
- Suicidal or homicidal
- At risk of imposing serious bodily harm to self or others
- Unable to satisfy their own basic physical needs if allowed to remain at liberty

Categories of Patients Most Frequently Found to Be Dangerous
- Substance abusers
- Individuals who are noncompliant with medications
- Individuals with long histories of violent behavior

C Procedural Process
Clinical assessment (usually performed initially by the nurse, followed and confirmed by other members of the interdisciplinary team)
- Detailed patient history
- Mental status examination with emphasis on suicidal/homicidal and safety issues
- Physical evaluation pertaining to self-care, nutrition, and coping strategies

Careful documentation
- Subjective and objective data
- Detailed support for the decision to commit
- Comprehensive plan of treatment

Civil certificate
- Signed by physician
- Witnessed as required

Strict adherence to institution policy governing commitment
- Admission procedures
- Clinical and judicial review
- Time parameters
- Discharge procedures

Although most individuals who are mentally ill recognize and welcome the need for treatment, others, by virtue of their impaired judgment and sense of reality, may resist treatment. In many settings, the nurse is the frontline consultant who, in conjunction with an interdisciplinary team of mental health professionals, is charged with the duty of ensuring that an individual in psychiatric crisis receives proper treatment. At times, proper treatment includes involuntary admission, also known as *civil commitment*. To avoid legal liability, the nurse must exercise due diligence in assessing and identifying patients subject to emergency civil commitment (see **Figure 23-1A**).

■ PATIENT RIGHTS VERSUS RISK OF HARM

Under the federal constitution, all individuals have the right to free speech, liberty, privacy, and procedural due process. Likewise, societal values encourage individuals to maintain a sense of personal integrity by exercising these rights without fear of undue judgment or constraint. The manner by which these rights are to be protected within healthcare settings is outlined in state statutes, case law, and patients' bills of rights. Of primary concern is the delicate balance that exists between the patient's right to refuse medical treatment and the need to protect the patient and others from harm. The balancing of the two is greater in the mental health setting where legislation frequently recognizes a heightened sense of patient vulnerability.

The concept of emergency psychiatric admissions is akin to that of general emergency treatment. Specifically, patient consent is usually not required when lifesaving measures are necessary. Although nonconsensual treatment of mentally ill patients is almost never legally permissible, it is allowed when the individual demonstrates a danger to self or others.

■ CLINICAL CRITERIA FOR DETERMINING DANGER

Danger is generally defined as a serious mental condition that poses a risk of harm to the patient or others. Unfortunately, predicting which patients are dangerous is an imperfect science. However, several criteria have been established to identify patients who are dangerous (see Figure 23-1B). Approximately one-third of all psychiatric emergency service patients present with suicidal or homicidal ideation or both. The difficulty in predicting whether or not an individual is dangerous occurs when the patient presents without any history of having attempted suicide or having performed an assaultive act. Nurses have a tendency to overpredict individuals whom they believe to be dangerous, which is significant when considering legal liability and whether proper weight was given to the issue of patient rights versus risk of harm. On the other hand, liability has been imposed when nurses have failed to identify a dangerous patient who warrants emergency admission.

■ LEGAL BASIS

As noted, mental illness alone is not a sufficient legal basis for detaining a patient. Additionally, in *O'Connor v. Donaldson* (1975), the US Supreme Court held that a state cannot constitutionally confine a patient without providing the necessary treatment or rehabilitation to enable reintegration into society.

Civil commitment is permitted but not required under all state statutes. Although civil commitment statutes vary from state to state, most set forth the essential elements pertaining to the nature and extent of commitment including the length of time one may be detained, mandatory psychiatric and judicial review, and the procedure by which a patient may challenge the process.

Under no circumstances should civil commitment be automatically equated with incompetence because civil commitment does not negate the presumption of competence. Rather, even patients who have been admitted involuntarily to psychiatric service enjoy an absolute right to refuse medical treatment, including antipsychotics, unless or until they are deemed incompetent to make such decisions. Likewise, the nurse may not assume that involuntary admission results in the forfeiture of basic patient rights or allows for legally sanctioned imposition or expansion of treatment. Simply stated, civil commitment provides the patient a safe environment under which he or she may seek treatment. The typical process under which civil commitment evolves is shown in Figure 23-1C.

■ LEGAL CAUSES OF ACTION

Several legal causes of action are associated with civil commitment, four of which are outlined below. The first three are legal actions brought directly by the patient who alleges he or she has been wrongfully committed, and the fourth is typically commenced by a third party (i.e., someone other than the patient or mental healthcare worker) for damages allegedly sustained when the patient should have been committed but was not.

False Imprisonment

Although this cause of action is most commonly associated with improper civil commitment, it is the most difficult to sustain. The reason is that the claim implies that the mental health professionals deliberately and maliciously held the patient by ignoring the statutory requirements for commitment or by failing to evaluate the patient prior to commitment. The patient must prove the following to recover damages:

1. In the absence of his or her consent, the patient has been willfully restrained, restricted, or confined as a result of the defendant's actions.
2. The defendant intended to restrain, restrict, or confine the patient.
3. The defendant failed to adhere to the statutory requirements governing civil commitment.
4. The defendant's actions caused the patient injury.

A claim of false imprisonment following involuntary treatment will not stand when the detention was predicated on a valid process (*Ridgeview Institute, Inc., v. Wingate,* 1999). The plaintiff sought treatment for alcoholism and voluntarily committed him-

self, then he discharged himself against medical advice. A few months later he voluntarily committed himself again. When he sought to once again discharge himself before completing the program, his physician initiated involuntary commitment proceedings based on the plaintiff being unsafe to self or others. The proceedings followed the statutory requirements including an independent medical examination and a hearing at probate court. After completion of treatment, the plaintiff was treated as an outpatient. When Ridgeview sued for payment of services, the plaintiff countersued for false imprisonment. The court held the statutory requirements were met, and the defendants showed the plaintiff was a present danger to himself.

Wrongful Commitment

A cause of action for wrongful commitment is based on negligence as opposed to deliberate intent. To prove that he or she has been wrongfully committed, a patient must show that the mental health professional erroneously certified the patient for commitment by virtue of a negligent diagnosis. Thus, although the diagnosis was rendered in good faith and without malice, it was negligently determined. The malpractice claim for failure to follow the standards of care for committing a patient or failing to involuntarily commit a patient usually stems from a substandard psychiatric assessment for determining an immediate danger to self or others.

Plaintiffs brought a malpractice action against a medical center contending that the emergency room nurse breached the applicable standard by having security remove their paranoid brother instead of notifying the physician and having their brother detained. Mr. Marcantel came to the emergency department and appeared to be having delusions. Mr. Marcantel accused the nurse of plotting with the voices to control his thoughts. When the nurse told him the doctor would be in to see him, he left the building, then returned demanding his medical record. When he became loud and belligerent he was told if he did not want medical treatment he needed to leave. He drove away. Several hours later a crisis intervention team was called to Mr. Marcantel's home when shots were fired. When Mr. Marcantel approached the police officers brandishing a weapon, he was shot and killed. His siblings brought the suit against the medical center and nurse. The state medical review panel concluded the nurse breached the standard of care by not informing the doctor of the patient's presence and his condition. The family proceeded to court where the jury concluded there was no duty owed to Mr. Marcantel. The plaintiffs appealed. The emergency physician on duty the night Mr. Marcantel sought treatment for depression and anxiety testified that he was treating several patients at that time who were having chest pains, rectal bleeding, and stitches. He stated he would not have left a more serious patient to see Mr. Marcantel unless the nurse indicated the patient was dangerous. He could not have detained the patient until he first evaluated him and determined he was suicidal, homicidal, or gravely disabled. He also testified the nurse did not have authority to detain the patient. A sheriff in the emergency room that night testified that he ran Mr. Marcantel's plates, determined he had no criminal history, was posing no threat, and therefore he could not have taken Mr. Marcantel into custody. The appeals court affirmed the jury verdict that the medical center and the nurse did not breach the duty to Mr. Marcantel. The standard of care called for the nurse to notify the physician to examine the patient, but Mr. Marcantel's hasty departure prevented him from doing so. Furthermore, the nurse and the security officers did not perceive Mr. Marcantel as a threat to self and others and therefore had no authority to detain him (*Bellard v. Willis Kingston Medical Center*, 2001).

Infliction of Emotional Distress

Although relatively uncommon on their own, causes of action sounding infliction of emotional distress are frequently linked with claims of negligence. Most claims alleging causation between an act and an emotional injury require evidence that the alleged mental stress produced physical injury. However, courts in various states have loosened this requirement, and some have allowed recovery in the absence of actual physical injury. It is conceivable that a patient who has been falsely imprisoned or wrongfully committed may be awarded damages solely based on emotional distress.

Failure to Warn of Harm to Third Party

This cause of action allows a third party to recover for injuries related to a mental health provider's failure to commit a dangerous patient who makes a threat to harm an identifiable third person. The seminal case is *Tarasoff v. Regents* (1976) whereby the defendant was held liable for failure to warn an identified victim that the patient was dangerous and intended to harm her. The holding requires the physician who is made aware of a threat by a patient that poses serious danger of harm to an intended victim to take reasonable steps to warn the intended victim. This may include notifying the intended victim and police of the threat of harm. The underlying legal issue was whether the patient should have been civilly committed in light of his expressed violent ideations.

■ REFERENCES

Bellard v. Willis Kingston Medical Center, 797 So.2d 676; 2001 La. LEXIS 2699 (2001).

O'Connor v. Donaldson, 442 U.S. 563, 95 S. Ct. 2486, 45 L.Ed.2d 396 (1975).

Ridgeview Institute, Inc., v. Wingate, 520 S.E.2d 445: 271 Ga. 512 (1999 Ga. LEXIS 805).

Tarasoff v. Regents, 17 Cal.3d 425, 551P2d 334 (1976).

Chapter 24

Organ and Tissue Donation and Transplantation

Susan J. Westrick

The Matching Process

What Can Be Donated

Organs—kidneys, heart, lungs, liver, pancreas, intestine
- Organs must be used within hours of removal from donor's body.
- A living donor can donate a kidney or part of pancreas, intestine, lung, or liver.

Tissue—corneas, the middle ear, skin, heart valves, bone, veins, cartilage, tendons, ligaments
- Tissue can be stored in tissue banks.

Stem Cells—can be obtained from bone marrow, peripheral blood stem cells, or umbilical cord blood
- Healthy adults age 18–60 years may donate.
- The donor and recipient must have closely matched tissue type or HLA (human leukocyte antigen).

Blood and Platelets
- Donors can donate multiple times if they are a suitable donor because blood and platelets are replaced in the body.
- Blood and platelets are stored in a blood bank according to blood type (A, B, AB, O) and Rh factor.

When Does Donation Occur?

Donation after Brain Death
- Most organs are from those who have suffered brain death or total cessation of brain function including the brain stem.
- After the organs are removed, the patient is taken off artificial support.
- Organs in good condition are removed surgically and used between 6 and 72 hours after removal from the donor.
- Tissues can be stored in tissue banks for later use.

Donation after Cardiac Death (DCD)
- Some patients after traumatic brain injury cannot be declared dead based on the definition of brain death.
- A patient is declared dead after cessation of cardiac death, which is cessation of cardiac and respiratory function when the patient is withdrawn from life support.
- DCD occurs only after the patient or family has decided to withdraw life-sustaining therapies for reasons entirely separate from any potential for organ donation.

Living Donors
- Each living donor is evaluated for suitability to donate.
- Most donations occur between family members.
- The long-term effects to a donor of a living donation is not known.
- A living donation is a personal decision.

Waiting List

The United Network for Organ Sharing (UNOS) maintains a centralized computer network, UNet, that links all organ procurement organizations (OPOs) and transplant centers. Access to the list is available only to professionals who are members of the Organ Procurement and Transplantation Network (OPTN).

Factors considered to determine who is offered an organ include, but are not limited to:
- Age
- Blood and tissue type
- Medical urgency
- Waiting time
- Geographical distance between donor and recipient
- Size of the organ in relation to the size of the recipient
- Type of organ needed

Source: Adapted from OrganDonor.gov. (2008). *Access to U.S. government information on organ & tissue donation and transplantation.* Retrieved May 23, 2008, from http://www.organdonor.gov

■ LEGISLATION

Organ and tissue donation and transplantation are regulated by federal and state legislation. Current legislation in the United States prohibits the buying and selling of organs based on the belief that human organs and tissues are not products to be sold but rather are humanitarian gifts. The following key acts affect donation:

1. The *National Organ Transplant Act*, passed in 1984, provides for the establishment of a task force on organ transplantation, an organ procurement and transplantation network, and authorizes financial assistance for organ procurement organizations (OPOs).
2. The *Omnibus Reconciliation Act* of 1986 sets forth hospital protocols for organ procurement and standards for organ procurement agencies. Hospitals participating in Medicare and Medicaid programs are required to establish written protocols to identify potential organ donors. Under these protocols, a healthcare facility must:
   a. Ensure that families of potential organ and tissue donors are aware of their options to donate, or decline to donate, organs and/or tissues;
   b. Encourage discretion and sensitivity with respect to the circumstances, views, and beliefs of the families of potential donors; and
   c. Notify an OPO designated by the Secretary of Health and Human Services of potential organ donors.
3. The *Uniform Anatomical Gift Act* (UAGA) of 1968 (as amended in 1987 and 2006) was recommended by the National Conference of Commissioners on Uniform State Laws and the American Bar Association to serve as model legislation for states regarding organ donation. Every state has enacted some form of this legislation. Through this act, all states rec-

ognize the limited capacity of minors and mentally disabled individuals to make such decisions. The act also requires written documentation of one's intent to donate one's body after death. However, the physician usually seeks permission of surviving family members, even where such documentation exists. The 1987 version of the amended act included a controversial provision that authorized various personnel, including public health officials, coroners, and medical examiners, to remove body parts from cadavers in their custody for transplantation if the officials had no knowledge of the decedent's or qualifying relative's objection. Such provisions are referred to as "presumed consent" organ donation. In a Florida case, a surviving family challenged the removal of a family member's corneas under a presumed consent statute on constitutional grounds. The family was unsuccessful because the court determined that the family's interest in the disposition of the dead relative's corpse was not a protected liberty, due process, or property interest under the Constitution (*State v. Powell*, 1986). Some states have enacted other provisions of the 1987 UAGA authorizing routine inquiry about organ donation and require requests for adult patients admitted to a hospital. Some provisions permit designated hospital representatives to discuss organ donation with dying patients.

The 2006 UAGA attempts to make procedures even more uniform and to clarify areas of uncertainty resulting from previous enactments. It is limited to donations from deceased donors as a result of gifts before or after their deaths. One provision of the 2006 act strengthens prior language barring others from attempting to override the individual decision to make or refuse donation. If adopted by a state, the 2006 UAGA repeals the 1968 and 1987 versions.

■ DONATION NETWORK AND ORGAN PROCUREMENT ORGANIZATION (OPO)

The Organ Procurement and Transplantation Network (OPTN) maintains a computer system, known as the United Network for Organ Sharing (UNOS), that contains the names of individuals waiting for organs in this country. The OPTN establishes policies related to organ procurement and transplant that are followed by member organ procurement organizations (OPOs). All US transplant centers and organ procurement organizations must be members of the OPTN. The OPOs are authorized by the Centers for Medicare and Medicaid (CMS) to procure organs for transplant. CMS defines geographic procurement territory within which the OPO concentrates its efforts. Various provisions are required for the OPOs by the OPTN, including a plan for equitable organ distribution based on the ethical principles of utility and justice. The OPOs may have sharing agreements to increase the availability of organs in those regions. The organization must also define donor acceptance criteria consistent with standards of the OPTN. Another feature is the requirement that the OPO carry out studies and demonstration projects to improve procedures for organ donation to attempt to increase transplantation among populations with special needs, including children and members of racial and ethnic minority groups. There is a specific prohibition making it unlawful for any person to knowingly acquire, receive, or otherwise transfer a human organ for valuable consideration for use in human transplantation if the transfer affects interstate commerce (except for human organ paired donation). Thus, it is illegal to sell organs. This prohibition implements an important public policy that seeks to protect vulnerable persons from being subject to abuse for monetary gain. The definition of "human organ" has been expanded to mean human (including fetal tissue) kidney, liver, heart, lung, pancreas, bone marrow, cornea, eye, bone, skin, or any subpart thereof, and any subpart derived from a fetus.

■ AGENCY PROTOCOLS

Hospital policies and procedures must include criteria for identifying potential organ and tissue donors and a mechanism for notifying the family of each potential organ and tissue donor of the option to donate or to decline to donate organs or tissues after the death of the family member. The protocol must indicate who notifies family members of their options and how such notification is handled. The protocol must also provide for acceptance of a family's decision to decline the option to donate organs. Only staff members who have completed a training program designed to ensure discretion and sensitivity with respect to circumstances, views, and beliefs of the family are involved in the effort to identify potential donors and to make families of potential donors aware of their options. Additionally, hospitals must establish a training program consistent with these requirements in cooperation with the OPO to train and retrain staff members who are designated to notify the family of its options.

■ DONATION PROCESS

Organ donors usually die as a result of trauma, stroke, primary brain tumor, or cerebral anoxia (lack of oxygen to the brain). Homicide and suicide victims can donate organs with a medical examiner's permission. A person of any age may be a candidate for organ donation. Excluding criteria include transmissible disease (e.g., AIDS, hepatitis), sepsis, cancer (other than primary brain tumor or skin cancer), and organ-specific disease. The current organ donation system also faces liability issues related to donor and organ screening, similar to successful lawsuits for negligent transmission of bloodborne diseases from blood transfusions. Donors can be classified as a cadaveric organ donor (a person who died of an injury or illness that did not affect the major organs and who can be maintained on mechanical support); living related organ donor (a living person who donates a kidney or a part of the liver or a lung to an immediate blood relative); or living nonrelated organ donor (a nonblood relative or other person). A living person can make a donation to a specific individual, and this is known as a "paired donation."

Tissue donors do not require intact circulation, but timing is still a critical factor, and tissue donation surgery needs to take place within a maximum of 24 hours after death. A person who dies of cardiac (heart) failure is automatically disqualified from organ donation but may be a tissue donor. Even if an autopsy is required (e.g., for homicide and some accident victims), tissue donation is often possible. Organ donors can also donate tissue. Age limits vary for each type of tissue.

A healthcare team member or family member can alert the OPO of a potential organ or tissue donor. Prior to donation, donation coordinators begin donor evaluation by obtaining information about the time and cause of death, past medical history, and the immediate medical condition. Medical contraindications are ruled out and the family is approached and given the option of donation. The opportunity to donate is discussed with the family if the deceased has not consented previously. Consent for organ or tissue donation has to be given by the individual or by the legal next of kin.

CONSENT FOR DONATION

Becoming an organ or tissue donor is as simple as filling out a Uniform Donor Card, signing it in the presence of two witnesses, and obtaining their signatures. It is important for the donor to notify family members of the wish to be a donor because donation will be discussed with them at the time of death. Sometimes the donor card is lost or not available, in which case the family will be asked to make the decision on the patient's behalf.

If there is no donor card, current policy in the United States requires that the donor or the next of kin give permission to proceed with organ and tissue donation (informed consent). In some states, "presumed consent" (as in Florida with cornea donations) allows organs and tissues to be removed at the time of death without the permission of the donor or next of kin as long as there has been no indication that donation is against the wishes of the donor. Legislation and policy have been written to protect the rights of the patients who have indicated, by signing a donor card, their desire to donate organs and tissue.

LIABILITY RELATED TO CONSENT

The following two cases both involve nurses' interactions with families who consented to organ and tissue donation for a deceased family member. In both cases it was disputed what was consented to, and the communication was viewed as different as based on the nurse's and families' testimony.

In *Schembre v. American Transplant Association, Jefferson Memorial Hospital, and Chris Guelbert* (2003), the decedent suffered a fatal heart attack. Nurse Guelbert approached the family while in the "quiet room" as to whether they would consider donating organs, bone, or tissue from the decedent's body. He told the family that the decedent did not meet criteria for donating organs but suggested that they donate eyes, bone, or tissue if they wished. Initially, the decedent's wife, Schembre, declined to give any consent, but after discussing with her children the decedent's wish to help others, she agreed to donate his corneas. Schembre stated she was adamant against using any donated organs for research purposes. Guelbert then inquired about consenting to donate the bone in his legs. According to the plaintiff wife, nurse Guelbert indicated with his hands the amount of bone would be approximately 2 inches, and he told her it would be 2 to 4 inches. Because she still had questions about the donation, another nurse came to clarify the process, explaining that the eyeball would be slit to facilitate harvesting the corneas but that the eye would not be removed from the body. The other nurse also affirmed nurse Guelbert's statement that 2 to 4 inches of bone would be removed from the decedent's leg. The plaintiff and her son also stated that the other nurse was writing on a clipboard, and they thought she was noting the limitations on the consent form.

In contrast, nurse Guelbert testified that he explained the donation process in detail to the plaintiff and her family. He testified that he told the family the entire eyeball would be removed and that the long bones of the leg would be removed if they chose to donate bone. He said he would have noted any limitations on the consent form. Nurse Guelbert assisted the decedent's wife in completing the consent form. The form indicated "yes" in boxes for donation of "eyes" and "bone." Guelbert said he read the completed form to the plaintiff, which she then signed. The plaintiff said she did not read the form because she was too distraught. Nurse Guelbert then made arrangements for defendant Mid-American Transplant Services (MTS) to harvest the corneas, bone, and tissue. The compliance manager for MTS testified that "bone" is a term of art used in the organ donation community that generally encompasses the removal of the lower bones of the leg, including the iliac crest, femur, tibia, fibula, and fascia lata. Moreover, he stated that the entire eye is removed for cornea donation. MTS removed and procured all of decedent's organs according to the consent document. The decedent's wife and children learned of the removal of all of his lower leg bones and eyes at the time of funeral preparation. This was a case of first impression in Missouri, and the court examined decisions

from other districts. Because MTS removed the decedent's corneas, bone, and tissue according to the consent form, the court held they acted without negligence. However, the court reversed the summary judgment for the nurse and hospital defendants. The court found there were issues of fact related as to whether the conduct of nurse Guelbert was without negligence and was in good faith in procuring consent from the decedent's wife. Thus the case was remanded to determine these facts.

In a similar case, the court found that a reasonable person could have determined that defendant's conduct in obtaining consent for tissue donation with false information exploited a position of trust (*Mary Ann Perry et al. v. St. Francis Hospital and Medical Center and American Red Cross,* 1995). Shortly following decedent's death, nurse McDonald approached the plaintiff's spouse and children in the waiting room to discuss the matter of tissue donations. Saying they were opposed to disfiguring his body, they initially said "no" to nurse McDonald's question about donations of bone, skin, or corneas. Nurse McDonald then explained the procedure for donating corneas in which they were just "peeled off" without removing the eyes from the body. The plaintiffs then decided that they would find donating the corneas acceptable to the decedent because it would just be "peeling them off." Later the nurse then asked the family about skin or bone donation, but family members were adamant that they did not want the decedent's body to be taken apart. Nurse McDonald then started discussing bone marrow donation, which she explained as involving a needle and syringe without any disfigurement. When she came back with the consent form, the family expressed their wish to donate only the corneas and bone marrow. Both boxes on the consent form for bone and eyes were written with "yes" beside them. Plaintiff Mary Ann Perry, the decedent's wife, said she asked nurse McDonald why bone was marked when they only wanted bone marrow, but nurse McDonald assured them that those doing the surgical procedure would understand that bone marrow and not bones were to be removed. Plaintiff then signed the form. Nurse McDonald testified in her deposition that she fully explained to the family that the long bones would be removed and replaced with rods and that the entire eye would be removed and replaced with a form, and that the changes would not be noticeable during an open casket funeral. She also stated that this was the first family she had approached about organ donation, but she was comfortable doing so at the time due to her recent in-service training concerning organ and tissue donation.

Plaintiff Perry testified in her deposition that she did not know if nurse McDonald intentionally misled them, and that "I feel that once she got us to say okay to one thing, she pushed on to another. I mean, now, I feel like she was taking advantage of our situation and pushing the issue. . . . She wasn't yelling. She wasn't rude." Other family members said that nurse McDonald was sympathetic and displayed empathy and a demeanor consistent with what one would expect when discussing organ donation. Also noted was that St. Francis had a team of tissue donor coordinators who were on call to handle inquiries and answer questions. Nurses are told during orientation to call this coordinator if they have questions. The American Red Cross team that removed the tissues removed sections of the upper arm, femurs, tibia, fibulas, and iliac crests. The decedent's wife and family first learned of this when they were told to bring heavy clothing to cover where the bones had been removed. The defendant St. Francis argued that they acted with "good faith" and there was no evidence of wrongdoing, and that they were therefore immune from liability under the UAGA organ donation statute. The court, however, did find that under the family's version of the facts related to the consent process, there were issues of fact that could support a conscious or intentional wrongdoing carried out for a dishonest purpose or furtive design. The court found no intent in the UAGA to cut off liability when hospitals act knowingly or recklessly mislead family donors and denied St. Francis's motion for summary judgment on its defense of good faith immunity pursuant to the statute. The court also rejected the plaintiff's attempts to construct an enforceable contract from the facts and said that the signed consent is not a contract but simply memorializes their consent to donate.

Both of these cases underscore the need to balance the sensitive nature of obtaining consent during a time of great emotional distress for families, with the need to increase organs available for transplant. While the nurse may think that the communication has been clear regarding the specifics of consent and that the family was not "pressured," the family may think otherwise. It is suggested that organ donation coordinators be used when possible to ensure consistency and reliability in providing information. Any consent forms should clearly indicate specific restrictions and limitations for organ or tissue donations. Training programs must be ongoing to ensure that new information is incorporated and that only well-trained staff participate in the donation process.

◼ MATCHING DONORS AND RECIPIENTS

The United Network for Organ Sharing (UNOS), an organization under contract with the US Department of Health and Human Services Health Resources and Services Administration (HRSA), maintains a centralized computer network that links all organ procurement organizations (OPOs) and transplant centers. This computer network is available at all times, and organ placement specialists are available to answer questions.

After being referred by a doctor, a transplant center evaluates a patient's mental and physical health and social support system to determine if the patient is a suitable transplant candidate. If the person is a suitable candidate, the name is added to a "pool" of patients waiting for transplants.

When a deceased donor is identified, a transplant coordinator from an OPO accesses the UNOS computer network where each patient in the pool is matched by the computer against donor characteristics. The computer then generates a list of donors who are ranked according to organ allocation policies. Factors affecting the rank include tissue match, blood type, length of time on waiting list, immune status, and the distance between the potential recipient and the donor. For heart, liver, and intestines, the degree of urgency is also considered. The organ is then offered to the first person on the list, but the person must be available, healthy, and willing to be transplanted immediately. Further laboratory tests may be required resulting in the candidate not being suitable, such as from high antibody levels that can prove to be incompatible.

■ PROCURING THE ORGAN

When the organ donor has been evaluated completely and consent has been obtained, the donor will be taken to the operating room to have the organs removed. Matching of tissue donors with recipients is performed after the tissues are removed (see Figure 24-1). Unlike organs, which must be transplanted within hours, tissue can be stored for a longer time, up to several years for bone tissue. Because most cadaver tissue is processed, genetic matching is not required.

■ REFERENCES

Mary Ann Perry et al. v. St. Francis Hospital and Medical Center and American Red Cross, 886 F.Supp. 1551; 1995 U.S. Dist. LEXIS 7089 (1995).

OrganDonor.gov, U.S. Department of Health and Human Services. (n.d.). *Homepage.* Retrieved September 29, 2008, from http://www.organdonor.gov

Organ Procurement and Transplant Network. (2003). *Homepage.* Retrieved September 29, 2008, from http://www.optn.org

Schembre v. American Transplant Association, Jefferson Memorial Hospital, and Chris Guelbert, 2003 Mo. App. LEXIS 1125 (2003).

State v. Powell, 497 So.2d 1188 (Fla. 1986), *cert. denied* 481 U.S. 1059 (1997).

Chapter 25

Discharge Against Medical Advice

Katherine Dempski

A Discharge Against Medical Advice–Competent Adult
1. Offer services and treatment.
2. Explain risks and benefits for refusal of care.
3. Is this a competent adult?
4. Document item 2.
5. Attempt to have patient sign a waiver of treatment.
6. Continue to offer support, transportation, discharge instructions, supplies, and medications.
7. Document item 6.

B Discharge Against Medical Advice–Other Than Competent Adult
1. Offer services and treatment.
2. Explain risks and benefits for refusal of care.
3. Is this adult not competent, i.e., a minor, adult with questionable behavior, adult with evidence of alcohol or drugs?
4. Document item 3.
5. Seek surrogate for consent, i.e., parent, court-appointed conservator, healthcare agent.
6. If surrogate not available, seek guidance through risk management, social services, and administration.

C A Nursing Checklist for Patients Requesting to Leave Against Medical Advice

 Try to ascertain why the patient wishes to leave and take necessary steps to correct the situation, if possible.

 Inform the patient and family of the risks and alternatives of refusing care and document this conversation and their understanding.

 Depending on the situation, notify the appropriate members of the healthcare staff–the physician, the nursing supervisor, social services, and if necessary, risk management, security, or the police.

If all efforts to convince a patient to stay and receive necessary care have failed, provide the patient with a waiver to sign which states that the patient has been advised of the risks, benefits, and alternatives of refusing treatment and the potential consequence of such refusal. If the patient refuses to sign the waiver, document on the form that the information was given to the patient, provide the date, and sign your name after your comments and place in the patient's medical record.

Patients who leave an environment where medical care is available and either refusing initial treatment or continuing treatment is a cause for concern from a medical, legal, and ethical viewpoint. Issues surrounding the rights of the patient, the accountability and liability of the provider, and the various settings where discharge against medical advice (AMA) may occur frequently cause uncertainty on the part of medical and nursing staff alike.

When a patient wishes to leave the hospital against medical advice, the goal is to provide the standard of medical care in less than ideal circumstances. Institutions must provide standardized protocols to guide staff because AMA often occurs on nights and weekends when resources are minimal.

■ PATIENTS' RIGHTS

Under both common law and various constitutional rights, competent adults have the right to make decisions regarding their medical care and any invasions into the privacy of their body. *Competency* is defined as having the ability to understand the nature and effects of one's acts (see **Figure 25-1A** and **B**).

■ PREDICTORS

Patients at risk to leave AMA tend to be young men who are admitted emergently with a history of substance abuse, personality disorders, and who exhibit anger. People who have a previous history of leaving against medical advice are more likely than not to repeat this behavior. Patients who do not have a primary care physician and those who have to wait an extended period for clinic appointments or emergency department visits have a higher incidence of choosing to leave without being seen. Other factors are religious beliefs and personal or financial obligation including lack of insurance.

■ NURSES' ROLE

Nurses are often the first to become aware of the patient's desire and insistence to leave AMA. The nurse has the pivotal role in coordinating communication among the providers to identify the patient's capacity to understand the diagnosis, treatment proposed, and consequences of refusing and leaving against medical advice. While it is a physician's responsibility to explain the risks, benefits, and alternatives to patients to enable them to make an informed decision or to give

informed consent, the nurse may be the key player in getting patients to consider the alternatives or consequences of accepting or refusing care.

The nurse should document all efforts to provide the patient with the information necessary to make a decision to accept or refuse care. Documentation should be objective and include the date, time, who spoke with the patient, what the patient was told, comments made by the patient, and the final disposition. The nurse should also document names, telephone numbers, and referrals given to the patient on discharge as well as a description or listing of any preprinted instructions or verbal instructions on discharge and medications. Most AMA patients do not turn in prescriptions, so it is reasonable to make an effort to dispense necessary medications through the hospital pharmacy if possible.

A waiver, or refusal of care form, should be presented to the patient for signature and inclusion in the record. A refusal to sign the form should be noted on the document, which the person who proffered the information should sign. Continuing efforts to help the patient who refuses care or chooses discharge against medical advice should also be documented. For patients who do not fall into the designation of competent adult, attempts should be made to seek a surrogate decision maker, such as a parent, court-appointed conservator, or healthcare agent, while maintaining the patient in a safe environment (see Figure 25-1C).

■ PROVIDER LIABILITY

Various legal consequences should be considered when patients choose discharge against medical advice. If there is any question of the competency of the patient, and the patient leaves, sustains an injury from failure to provide medical care, and sues, an action could be brought against the provider for abandonment or negligence.

The nurse has a duty to take appropriate action when there is a question of patient competency. The question should be raised with the examining physician and a psychiatric evaluation should be performed, if necessary, prior to allowing the patient to leave. The nurse as well as the provider could be held liable if a patient is allowed to leave against medical advice and there was any question as to the patient's ability to make a decision in his or her best interest.

If the assessing physician disregards the nurse's question of competency, the nurse should notify the supervisor of the concern and follow the chain of command. All efforts to protect the patient from future harm based on decisions made when the patient was incapacitated should be documented in chronological order, as should any follow-up efforts to check on the patient's safety after discharge.

The nurse might be in the dilemma of trying to balance the duty to protect the confidentiality of the patient against the duty to warn others of potential harm by the patient (to self or others). At times the nurse may have to make a decision to notify the police to either detain the patient, help find the patient who left without treatment, or notify relatives or friends if the patient verbalized threats against them. The nurse should be familiar with the employer's policy on police notification and involve the appropriate supervisory personnel in the decision to notify the authorities. Any decisions that would lead to a breach of confidentiality should be discussed and approved by the physician and appropriate management personnel.

Conversely, if a competent adult chooses discharge against medical advice and attempts are made to detain the patient, a legal action could be brought against the provider for assault, battery, or both and for false imprisonment.

Providers mistakenly believe that documenting that the patient consented to leaving

AMA and getting a signature on an AMA form offers immunity from professional liability. Successful defenses to negligence in AMA cases are based on the provider's ability to show no negligence in delivering care (see **Figure 25-2**). Documentation should show not just a signed "AMA form" but rather a process:

- Well performed capacity assessment
- Benefits and risks of proposed treatments and continued hospitalization
- Risks and consequences of early discharge against medical advice and patient understanding

Competent adults with decision-making capacity must take responsibility for their own healthcare decisions when the consequences have been explained to them. A nurse and her employer were sued for alleged failure of her duty to not discharge a sedated patient without an adult driver present. Nurse Brown was responsible for the care and discharge of patients from an endoscopy center after recovery from sedation. The patient was told pre-procedure that he would not be able to drive home and must be accompanied by an adult driver on the day of the procedure. Mr. Young presented without a driver but told Nurse Brown his friend "Trundle" would pick him up. When the friend did not show, the nurse called the patient's wife, who informed the nurse that no one was available to drive the patient. Mr. Young signed himself out AMA. He was in a one car motor vehicle accident and died several months later. His wife sued alleging failure to not sedate the patient without an adult driver and failure to not discharge the patient without a driver. After hearing expert testimony, the court held that a provider must rely on the information a patient tells them and must be responsible for his own care. It would be an onerous burden to require the nurse to assume the patient provided incorrect information. She was within

Capacity to make decisions:
- A responsible physician assesses the patient's ability to understand necessary treatment and justifies continued hospitalization.
- Assess if the patient understands the consequences of refusing treatment and discharging AMA.

Communication:
- Provide the patient with information on diagnosis, treatment needed, and medications.
- If the responsible physician who makes the capacity assessment is not the primary care physician, then notify primary care physician of the AMA and the discussions with the patient, including discussed follow-up care plan.

Follow-up care plan:
- When consented by the patient, notify the family or next of kin of AMA and the necessary follow-up.
- Follow hospital policy on arranging follow-up outpatient appointments and obtaining contact information.

Figure 25-2   The AMA process.

her duty to sedate the patient for the procedure based on the patient's statement that his friend would drive him home. The court further dismissed the plaintiff's contention that the nurse had a duty to prevent the patient from being discharged by calling the police, taking his clothes, involuntarily admitting him to the hospital, or restrain him until the sedation wore off. The court instead held that the nurse had no duty nor a right to call the police, restrain the patient, or otherwise hold him against his will. Furthermore, the court noted that Mr. Young was not "discharged" by the nurse but left against medical advice (*Young v. Gastro-Intestinal Center and Diane Brown, RN,* 2005).

■ EMERGENCY MEDICAL TREATMENT AND LABOR ACT

Nurses should be cognizant of the Emergency Medical Treatment and Labor Act (EMTLA). The federal government enacted this "anti-

dumping" law in 1986, and after several years of amendments, the Health Care Financing Administration (HCFA) adopted new regulations that expanded its scope in 1994 with amendments again in 2000 and 2003. Under EMTLA, emergency department physicians and nursing staff are required to perform an appropriate medical screening examination and stabilize the patient prior to transfer if an emergency medical condition is identified (Regulations for Necessary Stabilizing Treatment for Emergency Medical Conditions, 2003). Patients may not be discharged or transferred unless they *refuse* treatment or request a transfer. Nurses working in an emergency department should be familiar with the federal mandates, hospital's policies, procedures, and forms to comply with this law in case a patient refuses a medical screening examination and stabilization or transfer. Nurses should ensure that documentation is appropriate and that the patient has a full understanding of the risks and alternatives of accepting or refusing care. Federal regulations specifically require that when a patient presenting for an emergency treatment then refuses further medical screening and treatment, the staff must document the exam and treatment offered and refused, the risks and benefits of each, and the patient's refusal to consent. Reasonable steps must be taken to obtain the patient's refusal in writing.

Nurses in the hospital emergency department may encounter particular problems when a pregnant patient has an actual or potential emergency medical condition, refuses care, and attempts to leave against medical advice. The risks to the unborn child must be weighed in relation to the rights of the mother to refuse care. In these instances, the nurse must immediately involve the supervisor, social services, and potentially outside agencies, such as the department of children and families, to protect the life of the unborn child.

■ REFERENCES

Devitt, P., Devitt, A., & Dewan, M. (2000). An examination of whether discharging patients against medical advice protects physicians from malpractice charges. *Psychiatry Services, 51,* 899–902.

Emergency Medical Treatment and Labor Act, 42 U.S.C. § 1395dd(b)(2), 1985.

Regulations for Necessary Stabilizing Treatment for Emergency Medical Conditions, 42 C.F.R. § 489.24(d)(B), 2003.

Young v. Gastro-Intestinal Center and Diane Brown, RN, 205 S.W.3d 741; 361 Ark. 209 (2005 Ark. LEXIS 171).

Part II Review Questions

1. A Medicaid patient has confided in the nurse that he took an illegal drug prior to being admitted because he was nervous about the elective standard procedure he is to undergo. He is not acting inappropriately, but the nurse is concerned about the effects of the drug when mixed with the anesthetic. The patient's nurse should first:

   (A) Keep the information quiet for the sake of protecting his privacy
   (B) Recognize that Medicaid patients have little or no understanding of the ramifications of such actions and ignore it
   (C) Tell the charge nurse and attending physician
   (D) Speak with the patient about his fears and concerns

2. A man in a white lab coat is seen perusing a patient's charts. Although the nurse assumes he is a physician or on staff at the hospital, the nurse has never seen him before. The nurse should:

   (A) Ignore him because the nurse is too busy to stop and ask him who he is
   (B) Look for some kind of identification on his person that would indicate a connection to the hospital
   (C) Identify himself or herself as the patient's nurse and ask him his name
   (D) Ask other staff members if they have ever seen him before, and if someone recognizes him, let it go

3. The nurse has just learned some information of a sensitive nature from a patient. To fulfill an ethical duty to the patient and maintain confidentiality, the nurse should:

   (A) Determine if the information has any bearing on the patient's healthcare needs before it is charted
   (B) Document the information in the healthcare record before it is forgotten
   (C) Maintain the confidentiality of the information and not chart or report it regardless of what it is about
   (D) Communicate the information only if the nurse feels it is in the best interest of the patient

4. The nurse should be vigilant in protecting private patient information. Which of the following indicates the nurse is following proper legal and ethical duties in this regard?

   (A) Visitors are informed of the patient's progress if they are close relatives
   (B) Spouses are automatically informed of their spouse's medical procedures if reproductive information is involved
   (C) Work papers with patient-identifying information are kept behind the desk where only staff are allowed
   (D) A newspaper reporter calls for information on a patient and the nurse reveals only favorable information of the patient's status

5. A nurse is caring for a patient who is heavily sedated. The patient previously told the nurse that he does not want chemotherapy. However, the family now wants to begin treatment. The best course of action for the nurse is to:

(A) Start the chemotherapy because the physician has provided orders for it

(B) Refuse to begin the chemotherapy because the patient now lacks the capacity to consent to therapy and has given clear notice that he does not want it

(C) Request the social worker to initiate guardianship proceedings because the family cannot give valid consent without a court order

(D) Consult the hospital ethics committee

6. A home care nurse notices that an elderly patient is having trouble managing her affairs. There is evidence that she is not eating properly and does not follow through on taking medications. There are no immediate family members to monitor her. The nurse should:

(A) Consider this to be a problem for the social worker and make a referral before her next appointment, which is scheduled next month

(B) Continue to observe the patient but take no further action until after a few more visits

(C) Document the observations in the healthcare record, initiate a social worker referral, and make some temporary arrangements (with the patient's permission) for assistance through the agency

(D) Initiate guardianship proceedings because the elder is not competent to care for herself

7. Informed consent is obtained prior to:

(A) All nursing procedures that involve touching the patient

(B) Only surgical procedures

(C) Invasive medical procedures that involve risks

(D) All emergency treatment

8. Informed consent requires which three elements?

(A) Confidential communications, patient competence, and consent standard

(B) Information, patient competence, and voluntary consent

(C) Voluntary consent, patient competence, and patient's signature

(D) Voluntary consent, information, and patient's signature

9. A 78-year-old widow presents to the emergency department after a reported fall down the stairs at her home. She appears slightly confused and frail. She is complaining of back and hip pain. The physicians have recommended hip surgery. She tells the nurse how her late husband died on the operating room table several years ago, and she has sworn never to have surgery. The nurse should:

(A) Contact the legal department immediately

(B) Tell the patient she is being silly and she needs to have the surgery or she will never walk again

(C) Discuss your concerns with the charge nurse or the social worker or both

(D) Assess the patient's understanding and ability to comprehend the information further before taking any other action

10. A 27-year-old woman with strong religious beliefs against blood transfusions presented to the emergency department following a severe motor vehicle accident. Given the large lacerations and significant blood loss, the physicians wish to order several blood transfusions. She

refuses, indicating that according to her religious beliefs she may not receive blood transfusions. The medical staff believes that if she does not receive blood transfusions in the next several hours, she will go into shock and possibly die. The nurse should:

(A) Call the risk management department immediately

(B) Seek intervention or consultation with the patient's spiritual adviser

(C) Assess whether the patient appears to be fully competent and aware

(D) Do all of the above

11. The nurse is caring for a 40-year-old woman who underwent a colon resection under general anesthesia 12 hours earlier. Upon arrival to her room, she is holding her abdomen, is not moving in bed, and is clenching her teeth. She complains of pain that has been present in the incisional area for the last hour. She is also complaining of nausea. She requested pain medication earlier. However, it was approximately 30 minutes too early for her as-needed dose of meperidine (Demerol), 75 mg intramuscularly every 4 hours. Her vital signs are as follows: temperature by mouth 100°F, blood pressure 140/90 mm Hg, respiratory rate 20, and heart rate 100 beats/min. All of these values are increased over her last set of vital signs. What should the nurse do first?

(A) Administer the meperidine

(B) Ask the patient additional questions about her pain to determine the nature, source, and intensity of the pain

(C) Notify the physician for an increase in the dosage of meperidine

(D) Medicate the patient for nausea

12. A home care nurse is caring for a 62-year-old man who is terminally ill with lung cancer, with metastases to the kidneys and cervical spine. Upon the nurse's arrival to his home, the bedridden patient is semiconscious and moaning. His blood pressure is 104/66 mm Hg, heart rate 88 beats/min, and respiratory rate 10. His wife and son are present and express concern about his pain and the ineffectiveness of the previous dose. The nurse checks the physician's orders and notes an order for morphine sulfate, 5 mg subcutaneously every 4 hours as needed. The nurse checks the medication records and notes the patient's last dose was administered approximately 4 hours earlier. The nurse knows from the medical records that the patient does not want to be in pain but is concerned about the respiratory depression associated with the administration of morphine sulfate and the respiratory rate of 10. Under the ANA's position on the administration of opioids to terminally ill patients in pain, an appropriate intervention would be to:

(A) Withhold the medication because of the diminished respiratory rate

(B) Offer alternative comfort measures

(C) Reassure the family that this pain is expected

(D) Administer morphine sulfate now

13. To ensure that the standard of care is met when the nurse is providing discharge instructions, the nurse should do all of the following *except:*

(A) Provide written instructions

(B) Assess the patient's literacy level

(C) Request the patient to demonstrate any skill needed for home care (such as dressing change)

(D) Take no further action if the patient refuses to participate in discharge teaching

14. A patient requests the nurse to teach him about an experimental drug that is not available at the hospital where he is

receiving treatment. In fact, his physician does not approve of this treatment, but the nurse has some knowledge of it. Before the nurse decides how much teaching would be appropriate in the situation, she should consider that:

(A) She can teach the patient anything and refer him for treatment elsewhere

(B) No matter what the patient wants to know and how it is affecting his present treatment, it will not interfere with his present relationship with his physician

(C) She should not inform the physician about this or make a note in the chart because it may be contrary to the present treatment

(D) It may be best to explain to the patient that if he chooses this alternate therapy, the physician needs to be informed so the physician can consider this in light of his present treatment

15. A colleague who is busy asks a nurse to help administer her medications. The nurse is not familiar with one of the IV drugs to be given. The most *reasonable* action for the nurse to take is to:

(A) Give the medication following steps she has used with other IV drugs

(B) Refuse to give the medication because she is unfamiliar with it, and take no further action

(C) Look up the medication in authoritative drug references or check with a pharmacist regarding administration

(D) Consult with another nurse about how to administer the drug

16. A nurse has given the wrong medication to a patient. The nurse should do all of the following *except:*

(A) Chart the medication in the patient's medical record

(B) Take no action if there is no apparent patient injury

(C) Fill out an incident report

(D) Monitor the patient and document observations and assessment data

17. Nurses may disclose a patient's HIV information:

(A) When a known sexual partner is also a patient of the nurse

(B) To a family member who requests the information

(C) Never

(D) To other healthcare providers for the purpose of medical treatment when the information is in the medical record

18. The purpose of the HIV statutes related to public health and safety is to:

(A) Provide confidentiality

(B) Encourage early detection and treatment and prevent further transmission

(C) Disclose information to protect third parties

(D) Make HIV a protected disability

19. A 78-year-old widow presents to the emergency department after a reported fall down the stairs at her home. She is disoriented and frail, and her clothing appears to be somewhat disheveled and wrinkled. She is complaining of back and neck pain. Upon removing her clothing, the nurse notices several bruised areas on her arms. She is unable to tell what happened. Her adult son, however, is quick to point out how clumsy his mother is and how she won't change her clothing from day to day. He also will not leave the examining room while the nurse attempts to assist her in putting on a hospital gown. The nurse should:

(A) Contact protective services immediately

(B) Order the adult son to leave the room

(C) Discuss concerns with the charge nurse or the social worker

(D) Ask the patient directly if her son has harmed her

20. A 6-year-old first grader presented to the school nurse for the 10th time with a headache at 11:00 a.m. The child does not have a temperature or chills but appears to be a bit shaky. Orange juice and crackers usually relieve the headache and the shakiness. The child is not very talkative about her home life and is evasive when asked about breakfast each time she is in the nurse's office. This time she has several large welts on her arm as well. When asked about the welts, she says she was "very bad." The nurse should:

(A) Contact the parents by letter
(B) Call the police
(C) Send her back to class after the juice and crackers
(D) Speak to the principal about reporting concerns to the local child protective agency, and if the principal wants to wait, follow her advice
(E) Speak to the principal, and if she doesn't want to contact the child protective agencies, do so anyway because the nurse is that concerned

21. An 11-year-old seeking STD treatment and birth control goes to the nurse practitioner in a family health clinic. The nurse knows that in most states the nurse:

(A) Must notify the girl's parents, but this can be done after she is treated because the nurse doesn't need their consent for treatment
(B) Must notify her parents and get their consent prior to treating her
(C) May have to notify the state family services agency because she is under 12 years old
(D) Can treat her without parental consent and charge her parents for services rendered

22. A surgical nurse who is religiously opposed to abortion for any reason is assigned to the operating room where an abortion is scheduled to save the mother's life. The nurse may:

(A) Not refuse an assignment for moral reasons
(B) Refuse an assignment for moral reasons but not under these facts because the goal of the abortion is to save the mother's life
(C) Refuse the assignment by notifying the supervisor and immediately leave the room to show the refusal
(D) Notify the supervisor and stay in the room until adequate relief is provided

23. The first line of defense in preventing falls is to:

(A) Properly restrain the patient
(B) Use side rails
(C) Assess the patient's risk factors
(D) Provide continuous monitoring

24. Proper use of restraints is indicated when:

(A) The family requests that the patient be restrained
(B) It is medically necessary for diagnostic or treatment purposes
(C) The patient is at risk and the staff is shorthanded and cannot provide monitoring
(D) The patient is noncompliant with a bed rest order

25. When predicting whether a patient is dangerous, all of the following factors should be considered *except*:

(A) Suicidal or homicidal ideation
(B) The risk of imposing bodily harm
(C) Whether the patient is taking antipsychotic medications
(D) Whether the patient can satisfactorily care for his or her own basic needs

26. Civil commitment or involuntary emergency admission is:
    (A) Mandated by all states
    (B) Analogous with a determination of incompetency
    (C) A means by which treatment can be imposed even in the absence of patient consent
    (D) A method of protecting the patient and others during psychiatric crisis

27. Hospital protocols for organ procurement (required for hospitals that participate in Medicare and Medicaid programs) must incorporate all of the following *except:*
    (A) Notifying family members of their options to donate or to decline donation
    (B) Use of only trained hospital personnel to work with families to discuss these options
    (C) Use of patients who have donor cards without consideration of other potential donors
    (D) Criteria for identifying potential organ and tissue donors

28. To ensure that their wishes are carried out at the time of consideration of organ donation, the nurse should inform patients or potential donors that:
    (A) Persons should have made out a donor card and carry it with them at all times
    (B) Family members should be informed of the patient's wishes
    (C) Registration with an organ donation agency must have taken place for donation to occur
    (D) Both A and B

29. A pregnant patient is admitted to the emergency department for a fever and respiratory illness. After being screened and examined, the physician finds that the patient is stable but recommends inpatient treatment with IV antibiotics. The patient refuses this plan and wants to be discharged against medical advice (AMA). The nurse determines that:
    (A) The patient cannot be discharged AMA because she is pregnant
    (B) The Emergency Medical Treatment and Labor Act (EMTLA) prevents her from leaving because the hospital can institute treatment, even in a non-emergency situation
    (C) Because the patient has been determined to be stable, she can most likely be discharged as long as there is an alternate treatment plan that does not present harm to the fetus
    (D) The patient should be allowed to leave as soon as the risks of nontreatment are explained to her, without considering the risks to the fetus

30. A patient tells the nurse that she is leaving against medical advice despite the fact that she is seriously ill and in need of treatment. An acceptable action to take when someone chooses discharge against medical advice is to:
    (A) Threaten to call security if the patient tries to leave the facility
    (B) Put the patient in four-point restraints
    (C) Medicate the patient so he or she is unable to leave without assistance
    (D) In a nonthreatening manner, explain the risks and alternatives of refusal of treatment; ask the patient to sign a release; offer assistance in discharge, transport, and medications/supplies; and give the patient written discharge instructions and names and numbers to call if the condition worsens.

Part II Answers

1. *The answer is D.*

   Although telling the charge nurse and attending physician is warranted, speaking with the patient *first* to obtain an understanding of his concerns may facilitate a means to educate and inform the patient of his rights. A direct explanation of the procedure and the possible drug interaction gives him some of the information he needs to make a choice about whether to proceed or not. One cannot protect a patient's privacy if the possibility of medical complications is present. The patient needs to know that as well.

2. *The answer is C.*

   As a professional, the nurse cannot be timid or cavalier about protecting a patient's confidentiality. Although another staff member may have seen the man before, that does not ensure that he has a right to read a patient's chart or has a role in the patient's care. The nurse should confront the stranger, in the spirit of trust and cooperation, and ask enough questions to resolve concerns about his status.

3. *The answer is A.*

   The nurse needs to first determine if the information is relevant and necessary to patient care. Patients may confide private information related to financial difficulties, marital infidelity, or other informa-

   tion that has no bearing on medical treatment. Answer B is not correct because the information may not necessarily need to be documented in the medical record. Answers C and D are not correct because the nurse may need to reveal the information to an official agency as required by law or regulation, and it may not necessarily be in the best interest of the patient to do so. Sometimes confidential information must be revealed because it will protect others.

4. *The answer is C.*

   Keeping work papers behind the desk keeps them from public view and protects the patient's right to privacy. Answer A is incorrect because permission must be received from the patient before information is disclosed to any relatives. Answer B is incorrect because even though it is tempting to give spouses this information, it may be something that the patient wishes to keep confidential. Answer D is incorrect because any information, even if favorable, cannot be revealed without the patient's permission.

5. *The answer is B.*

   The nurse should not begin the treatment when there is a conflict with the patient's expressed wishes when he was competent. Answer A is incorrect because there is a question of patient consent, so the order should not be initiated. Answers C and D are not necessary until other interventions have been implemented. These actions are used as a last resort.

6. *The answer is C.*

The nurse needs to document properly the observations, but action should be taken as well. The support of a home health aide may be all that is needed, and the least restrictive alternative to the patient's autonomy should be sought. Answer A is incorrect because this problem should be dealt with in an interdisciplinary manner. Answer B does not include an intervention that would protect the patient's health and welfare. Answer D is incorrect because it is too drastic and makes assumptions that are beyond the facts presented.

7. *The answer is C.*

All invasive medical procedures that carry risk require informed consent. B is incorrect; although surgical procedures are invasive and usually carry some risk, there are also medical procedures that require consent. A and D are incorrect because informed consent is necessary before all invasive procedures that carry a risk. Not all emergency treatment is invasive and risky, and touching a patient requires consent (usually implied by the patient's action) but not informed consent.

8. *The answer is B.*

It states all three of the elements. A is incorrect because confidential communication is always a necessary requirement of patient care but not a specific element of informed consent. C and D are incorrect. While consent, patient competence, and information are all elements of informed consent, the patient's signature is not necessary in some states as long as there is documentation on the informed consent in the medical record.

9. *The answer is D.*

Patients can refuse any type of medical intervention if they are competent to do so. Being slightly disoriented and frail does not necessarily assume incompetence. Certainly the patient's fears of surgery are based on her own experience with the loss of a life partner. While answer C may also be appropriate, a further assessment of her understanding is warranted before any other action is taken.

10. *The answer is D.*

This is an example of the difficult decision nurses and other healthcare providers may face. Hospitals usually have policies concerning the appropriate steps a healthcare provider must take in a nonemergent situation. However, borderline cases occur all the time. The spiritual advisor may help clarify the patient's choice, but maybe not. The risk manager will assist the staff with following agency policy for this situation. When a patient refuses lifesaving treatment, it is important to determine the patient's competency through appropriate medical channels and to document it. It may become necessary to obtain a court order when third parties are involved. For example, the patient may be the mother of a breastfeeding infant with no other family to care for the baby or may be pregnant. There are state statutes limiting a pregnant woman's right to refuse lifesaving treatment. Healthcare providers must be aware of the statutes in their state. The bottom line is that each case must be evaluated individually. While laws and guidelines give healthcare providers rules to follow, no one case can define this area completely.

11. *The answer is B.*

    The nurse must determine whether the patient is in acute pain associated with the surgical procedure and not from a new source, such as a pulmonary embolus or deep vein thrombosis. A, C, and D are appropriate interventions, but they are secondary to B.

12. *The answer is D.*

    According to the ANA's position, the medication should be administered for pain management even if it hastens death. It is the nurse's ethical and moral obligation. (It must be consistent with the patient's wishes.) A is wrong because the patient wishes to be pain free. B and C are appropriate but secondary to the administration of pain medication.

13. *The answer is D.*

    The nurse needs to document the fact that the patient refuses to take part in discharge teaching. This protects the nurse and the institution if a problem arises later from this lack of follow up by the patient. Answers A, B, and C state principles or guidelines that should be followed to ensure that the proper standard of care is met.

14. *The answer is D.*

    Although the nurse does have the right to teach patients about alternative treatments, this needs to be done in consideration of the patient's present plan of care. Because the physician is implementing a treatment at present, the physician should be informed if the patient seeks alternative treatment. Answers A and B are incorrect because the nurse cannot just refer the patient elsewhere—this could be considered interfering with the physician–patient relationship. Answer C is incorrect because the nurse may need to make a note in the chart so that others

on the healthcare team can consider this in their care of the patient.

15. *The answer is C.*

    The nurse should always seek information from the most authoritative references available. Nurses are not expected to know all information about drugs and their administration but are expected to use resources. This is a reasonable action under the circumstances. Answers A and D do not reflect safe practice because all IV medications are not given in the same way and another nurse could give incorrect information. Answer B is not the best answer because the nurse has not attempted to find out how to give the medication safely. If she did lack the skill to do so after obtaining this information, then she should refuse to give the medication.

16. *The answer is B.*

    All answers except B reflect reasonable and expected actions to follow in this situation. Accountability requires the nurse to document the medication in the patient's medical record, take steps to monitor the patient for any untoward effects, and file an incident report according to institutional policy. These actions will ensure that the proper standard of care has been followed. This does not mean, however, that the nurse may not be liable for a malpractice claim, disciplinary action by the state nursing board, or even criminal charges if a serious error has occurred.

17. *The answer is D.*

    Most states allow disclosure to other healthcare providers when the information is in the record. Disclosure should be made for the purpose of medical diagnosis and treatment, and each provider who has the information has a duty to guard it confidentially. A is incorrect because some states only permit *physicians* to tell known partners. B is incorrect because the information is confidential even to family members unless the patient has authorized otherwise. C is incorrect because nurses may disclose information in the medical record when it relates to health care.

18. *The answer is B.*

The purpose of the statutes is to encourage patients to seek testing and medical care for HIV infection. Providing confidentiality is a means to achieve this (answers A and C). D is true under the Americans with Disabilities Act.

19. *The answer is C.*

Many times patients have been abused by their adult children; however, direct confrontations (as in B and D) probably will not facilitate a solution quickly. Contacting protective services may be helpful but would not be available immediately. The social service department of many hospitals is equipped to intervene and assist with interviews and arrange appropriate referrals if necessary.

20. *The answer is E.*

There may be policies and protocols for the school nurse to follow in any institution when it comes to reporting suspected child abuse. However, the bottom line is that not only does the nurse have a legal responsibility to report suspected child abuse in virtually every state but also ethical codes for nurses mandate this action as well.

21. *The answer is C.*

Most states require notice to the family service agency when a minor under a specified age (usually 12) seeks STD treatment or birth control (check the state statute). A is incorrect because notifica-

tion requirements relate to abortion services. B is incorrect because most states encourage minors to seek STD treatment by dispensing with the usual parental consent requirement (check state statute). D is incorrect because most STD confidentiality statutes require that all information go only to the minor, and this includes billing for services.

22. *The answer is D.*

A, B, and C are incorrect because nurses may refuse assignments for moral reasons but within the legal constraints of refusal, such as assuring that proper and appropriate nursing care will be given to the patient by another nurse and that the patient will not be harmed by the nurse's refusal.

23. *The answer is C.*

Risk factors must be identified to prevent falls, and this certainly must be done before restraints are used. A, B, and D are second lines of defense.

24. *The answer is B.*

Restraints are only indicated for diagnostic or treatment purposes. A is incorrect because a family may not order restraint use, although their concerns should be addressed and the patient assessed for the need for restraints. C is incorrect because restraints are never used for staff convenience, and their use requires more monitoring, not less. D is incorrect because restraints are not used for punishment or noncompliance.

25. *The answer is C.*

That a patient is taking antipsychotic medications is not a factor to consider because the patient may qualify as dangerous even when taking medication. The remaining factors must be considered to identify whether a patient is a danger to self or others.

26. *The answer is D.*

    Civil commitment is allowed but not mandated by states. Although it recognizes that a patient is dangerous, it does not equate to incompetency, nor does it take away the patient's right to refuse treatment. The goal of civil commitment is to afford protection while encouraging the patient to undergo treatment that will enable a safe return to the community.

27. *The answer is C.*

    Donors who do not have donor cards can be considered. Families of potential donors may know of the patient's wishes to be an organ donor whether or not the patient has an organ donor card. Answers A, B, and C state features required in the protocols.

28. *The answer is D.*

    Potential donors should have a card and inform family members of their wishes. These suggestions ensure that donors' rights are upheld, but donation can occur without either of them present. Families can still be asked at the time of death to donate their loved one's organs. Answer C is incorrect because one does not have to register with an agency for organ donation.

29. *The answer is C.*

    The risks of the discharge to the mother and the fetus must be considered before a pregnant patient can be discharged AMA. It is likely that if there is a safe alternative plan (e.g., home care with IV antibiotics), and all risks and alternatives have been explained, the patient should be allowed to determine her course of treatment. Answer A is incorrect because the patient does not lose all her rights to self-determination just because she is pregnant. Answer B is incorrect because the patient does not need to be stabilized, and it is not an emergency situation. Answer D is incorrect because the needs of the fetus need to be considered as well, not just the patient.

30. *The answer is D.*

    Answers A, B, and C would constitute assault, battery, and false imprisonment. Answer D provides for respect for the patient's autonomy while offering alternatives and ongoing support, as well as explaining the risks associated with the patient's choice in an objective and nonjudgmental manner. Documentation of these actions will protect the provider from future allegations of abandonment or neglect.

PART III

Documentation Issues

Chapter 26

The Medical Record

Katherine Dempski

A

Objective Documentation
- Give all facts necessary to communicate the patient's status.
- State facts as you witnessed them — never making assumptions.
- Give supporting facts for assessments and objective findings.
- Document patient's condition, the nursing interventions, and outcomes.
- Document that you are safety conscious.
- Document the standard of care — keep in mind complications and your steps to avoid them.
- Never add subjective comments about the patient, family members, or colleagues.

B

Make Accurate Corrections
- Draw a single line through incorrect entry; date, time, and sign the correction; never use correction fluid or scribble out incorrect entries.
- Use addendums when important data are left uncorrected; date, time, and sign the addendum; indicate date and time the addendum refers to.
- Use late entries; document date and time.
- Never rewrite a note.

Documentation in medical records serves several functions. It serves as the main source of information regarding the patient's treatment and progress. It facilitates communication to all members of the healthcare team, which ensures continuity of care for the patient. Additionally, record reviews are done by state licensing and accrediting bodies to determine if federal regulations, standards of care, and agency policies are followed. Proving providers delivered appropriate care is difficult when a medical record is incomplete.

◼ REVIEW OF MEDICAL RECORDS

Peer review committees access records to determine whether quality patient care is rendered. Infection control and utilization review committees determine if agency policy and procedures are followed. Healthcare records also are used by those who are not members of the healthcare team but may have the authority to do so, including state licensing boards, an attorney with authorization, and insurance companies. Patients and their representatives have the right to information in the medical records including a copy of records or a review of the medical records, but this should be done with a healthcare provider to educate and prevent misinformation.

■ A COMPLETE RECORD

Under CMS regulations the medical record must contain information to justify the admission and continued hospitalization, support the diagnosis, and describe patient progress and response to medications and interventions (42 C.F.R. § 482.24). CMS regulations require that a complete medical record contain:

- Admission conditions and admitting diagnosis
- Health history dated not more than 30 days prior to admission and no later than 24 hours after admission
- Consults, results, and evaluations
- Informed consents for procedures determined by medical staff bylaws
- Physicians' orders and progress notes on patient's condition and treatments
- Nursing notes and medication records
- Lab reports
- Discharge summary with follow-up treatment needed and final diagnosis

The Joint Commission regulations are similar to the CMS broad overview requiring all medical records to contain documentation to justify admission, hospital course, and response to treatment, but it also has specific documentation requirements:

- Patient identification including authorized representative
- Special language/communication needs
- Advance directives
- Allergies
- Discharge medications
- Preadmission emergency care
- Treatment goals, reassessments, responses to interventions

- Communications with patient regarding care and treatment
- Documentation on receiving and verifying verbal orders

■ NURSING CONSIDERATIONS

A complete record gives a detailed and accurate description of the patient's condition, nursing assessment, nursing interventions, and outcomes. The nurse should document objectively all the facts necessary to communicate the patient's status to other members of the healthcare team (see **Figure 26-1A**). A clear and concise description of a patient's condition will assist nurses in noting changes.

When documenting nursing assessments and interventions, nurses should keep the standard of care for that particular patient in mind. Nurses need to show their awareness of a patient's potential complications and show that steps are being taken to avoid them. Nurses also should document precautions being taken to safeguard the patient (see **Figure 26-2**).

A complete record always includes the following:

1. Timeliness: Nurses' notes are best written while events are fresh in their memory. It is difficult to remember an incident years later when most liability cases come to trial. An accurate and complete record can be used to refresh the nurse's memory. During legal proceedings, the medical record is often called the "witness that never dies." Complete and timely documentation works in the nurse's favor.

2. Date and time notes: A nurse's note is never complete without documentation of the date and time the note was written. Often the note is actually written after a nursing assessment. The correct time of the note should be written, but the note can include when the assessment actually took place. Providing the

Initial nursing assessment: Physical and psychological assessment and risk assessments (restraints, falls, etc.)

Nursing admission notes: Advance directives, primary language, communication issues (use of interpreter, hearing impaired)

Integrated interdisciplinary assessments on one form: Minimizes contradictory assessments, required by CMS

Nursing care plan: Nursing assessments, nursing interventions, and patient response

Nursing progress notes: Nursing factual observations, patient education

Figure 26-2   Documenting precautions taken to safeguard the patient.

chronological order of events is important to ensure the patient receives the correct progression of medical care. For example, the healthcare team needs to know exactly when a patient's condition began to respond well to treatment or deteriorated.

3. Name and title: A nurse's name and title in every note is part of a complete record. When a multidisciplinary team approach is being used, RNs, physicians, dietitians, physical therapists, occupational therapists, or nurse's aides are all documenting on the same progress reports. Documentation of titles explains which discipline has taken part in the medical care and who the team members are. It also shows which members of the team have performed their part in patient care. It is acceptable for the nurse to place initials on a data flow sheet, but full name and title should appear somewhere on the sheet to coincide with the initials.

4. Patient's name: The patient's name must appear on each page of the medical records. It is too easy to place a loose flow sheet from one patient's record or bedside into the record of another. That flow sheet will inaccurately become a permanent part of another patient's medical history. Often specific sections of medical records are photocopied and sent to consulting healthcare providers. It is difficult to prove which patient these nameless records belong to. Poor record keeping could be construed as poor nursing care.

5. Neatness counts: Nurses don't have to win penmanship contests, but they do have to meet the professional standard of care in documentation. Communication between healthcare providers is the primary purpose of healthcare records. A nurse's note that is difficult to read or understand will fail to meet this standard. Sloppy records often equate with sloppy nursing care.

■ OBJECTIVE DOCUMENTATION

Nursing assessments are stated objectively and based on facts and observation. Whenever possible, the nurse should use measurable terms. For example, a wound should be described as "the size of a dime" or "2 cm wide" instead of just referred to as "small."

When describing a patient's demeanor, the nurse should give an objective reason for the assessment. An example would be, "Patient's affect was flat as evidenced by his monotonous tone." The only subjective data in a nurse's note should be the patient's own statements placed in quotes. Generally, the nurse should not state conclusions without supporting facts.

When at all possible, the nurse should document facts that are personally witnessed rather than what someone else states. The exception to this would be the patient's own words in quotes or paraphrased. The nurse should be cautious about assuming anything, even what may be obvious.

■ MEDICAL ABBREVIATIONS

The Joint Commission National Patient Safety Goals prohibits the use of unapproved abbreviations. Providers must document using only hospital-approved medical abbreviations. Patients are safer when providers communicate the same meaning to all other providers. Abbreviations that are not standard or agency approved through its policy and procedure manuals will only hinder communication.

■ CORRECTING MISTAKES IN DOCUMENTATION

All mistakes made in documentation must be corrected according to the agency policy. Failure to properly correct a mistake could be construed as altering a record and is indefensible. Figure 26-1B lists general tips on proper corrections, but the nurse should always check policy first. Inappropriate corrections or alteration of the record damages the credibility of the record.

■ MAINTAIN PROFESSIONALISM IN DOCUMENTATION

A nurse's subjective comments concerning a patient or patient's family members do not belong in a medical record and will only cause legal problems for the nurse. When a patient

is being uncooperative to medical care, the nurse should document the patient's behavior and subjective comments in quotes. This gives the reader notice of the uncooperative behavior in matter-of-fact terms without the nurse's subjective opinion.

Likewise, nurses and other healthcare providers should be careful not to express opinions concerning colleagues in a patient's medical record. Unprofessional documentation can equate unprofessional nursing judgment and care in the eyes of the patient or anyone else reviewing the medical record. Problems with coworkers should be addressed through other more appropriate channels.

■ CHARTING BY EXCEPTION

Charting by exception is being practiced in some healthcare agencies to decrease the amount of documentation. Under a charting-by-exception policy, nurses do not document expected outcomes; they only document changes in a patient's condition outside the expected norm for that disease process and hospital course. However, nurses should document data such as daily vital signs.

Nurses need to be aware of any state or local regulation on documentation. No matter what form of documentation is used, nurses must document the standard of care for each specific patient. Hospital documentation policy must be cross referenced with any local regulation. The department of public health and the local chapter of the ANA may be a source on state regulations.

A court reviewing a malpractice claim for a postoperative wound infection commented that a more accurate account of the patient's hospital course could not be recreated because the nurses were negligent in the charting by exception method of documentation. Court held that a jury could find that substandard record keeping by the nurses was the proximate cause of the delay in diagnosing the patient's wound infection thereby causing the patient's harm. The hospital and the surgeon's motion for judgment in their favor was denied (*Lama v. Borras*, 1994).

■ AUTHORIZED ACCESS TO MEDICAL RECORDS

Federal and state statutes define who has authority to medical records and the information contained within. Institutions must have policies outlining authorized access and a process for monitoring staff access to records. In general, providers involved in direct care and treatment of the patient are authorized, as are those in quality improvement. Providers who are not in direct care do not have authority to access medical records and will be subjected to professional discipline.

■ RETENTION REQUIREMENTS

CMS requires medical records to be retained or reproduced for 5 years (42 C.F.R. § 482.24).

State statutes will vary due to different statutes of limitation on various legal claims, but 10 years or longer is a usual retention rule before records may be destroyed. Even when records are destroyed, institutions must keep specific information, and records may be kept longer upon requests of attorneys, physicians, or the patient or representative.

■ REFERENCES

CMS Regulations for Medical Record Services, 42 C.F.R. § 482.24.

Lama v. Borras, 16 F.3d 473 (P.R. 1994).

The Joint Commission. (2007). *2007 national patient safety goals (NPSG 2B)*. Oakbrook Terrace, IL: Author.

The Joint Commission. (2007). *Comprehensive accreditation manual for hospitals*. Oakbrook Terrace, IL: Author.

Chapter 27

Electronic Health Information and Communication

Susan J. Westrick

A   Computerized Patient Records: Key Issues for Nurses

Authentication of entries to patient records

Protection of confidentiality of the information

Prevention of unauthorized access

B   Electronic Signatures Deemed Acceptable

1. Unique to person using it
2. Capable of verification
3. Under the sole control of the person using it
4. Linked to data in such a manner that if data are changed, signature is invalidated
5. Conforms to regulations adopted by the Secretary of State

C   Keys to Computer System and Patient Record Security

Password protection

System education and training

Control and limit user access

Monitor access and detect breaches

Be alert

Overprotection is the best approach

As movement toward electronic health records (EHR) for patients advances, concerns grow with respect to protecting privacy and maintaining confidentiality of medical information that is stored in computers, other devices, or is maintained in electronic databases. Advantages of such systems include availability of patient records at the time and place when needed, availability of large volumes of data that can assist in medical research, quick retrieval of data, and stream-lined billing practices due to recording treatment in a uniform manner. Additionally, data are likely to be more accurate, organized, legible, and subject to less error than handwritten records. One important impetus for the use of electronic health records (EHRs) is the desire to minimize and prevent medical errors as cited by the Institute of Medicine (IOM) 1999 report. Many institutions are using computerized physician order entry (CPOE), computerized medication administration records

(MARs), and bar code systems to reduce medication errors. Risks associated with such systems include access by unauthorized users, potential alteration of vital medical information, improper disclosure or use of private information, and infection by computer viruses or other system failures that could impair or shut down a system entirely.

The expanding needs for healthcare information must be balanced against the requirement to ensure the security and personal privacy of each individual's electronic health record and information. Those responsible for management and maintenance of the system may be liable for harm caused by improper intrusions into the system. As with traditional paper records, the nurse has a responsibility to ensure that EHRs remain confidential, accurate, legible, secure, and free from unauthorized access. All recommended standards, policies, and procedures related to documentation remain in effect when using electronic technology for computerized charting. Key issues for nurses are listed in **Figure 27-1A**.

■ LEGAL FRAMEWORK—FEDERAL AND STATE PROTECTIONS

Privacy protects an individual's control with regard to use and disclosure of personal information. Courts are generally in agreement that patient records are protected by a privacy right grounded in the 14th amendment of the US Constitution. The Privacy Act of 1974 protects health information collected by federal agencies and includes regulations concerned with alcohol and substance abuse records. The Computer Fraud and Abuse Act of 1986 makes it a federal offense to alter, damage, or destroy information contained in a computer used by or for the US government. It also defines that tampering with medical records warrants punishment without needing to show incorrect or harmful treatment as a result of the tampering.

The Health Insurance Portability and Accountability Act of 1996 (HIPAA) involves standardizing the electronic data interchange of certain administrative and financial transactions while protecting the security and privacy of the transmitted information. The law is intended to improve portability and continuity of health insurance coverage and regulates covered entities such as health plans, clearinghouses, and healthcare providers. This also includes all of their employees and business associates, making the impact of the law far reaching. The HIPAA privacy rule standard includes mandated adoption of federal privacy protections for any protected health information (PHI). These rules apply to all healthcare information including electronic protected health information (EPHI) and records. Furthermore, Congress provided civil and criminal penalties for covered entities that misuse PHI. Current state laws and regulations vary from state to state and are inadequate and inconsistent. Accordingly, nurses should familiarize themselves with the laws of the state in which they practice to know what effect they might have on management of electronic health records or information and nurses' responsibility.

■ LIABILITY FOR UNAUTHORIZED DISCLOSURE OF MEDICAL INFORMATION

A common-law fiduciary duty is an obligation imposed between parties who have a relationship of special trust and confidence. Nurses occupy this trusted position with respect to their patients and with regard to maintaining the privacy of information derived from the course of that relationship. Use or disclosure of this private information without consent or authorization may result in liability for damages. In addition, all healthcare providers have an ethical duty to maintain confidentiality of patient information.

Nurses also have a legal duty to maintain the confidentiality of a patient's medical information, a duty that arises from the obligation to perform according to the appropriate professional standard. A nurse who breaches this duty to perform according to the proper professional standard (negligence) may be liable for any resulting harm.

In *Pribble v. Edina Care Center* (2003), a licensed practical nurse copied confidential medical information from patient charts to help assert her claim that she was entitled to unemployment benefits. She photocopied the records and sent them electronically by fax to her attorney to show that her charting was not deficient, as her defendant employer had maintained when she was terminated. The court held that she was not entitled to unemployment benefits because she was discharged for cause. They further found that she had violated the confidentiality of patient medical records in sending these copies to her attorney. Although she denied that she had done this, her acts were witnessed by other nurses.

■ AUTHENTICATING ENTRIES—ELECTRONIC SIGNATURES

Entries made to a record, whether paper or electronic, must be signed. There are two categories of signatures associated with electronic transmission—electronic signatures and digital signatures—and their purpose is to guarantee a level of validity, authenticity, and security in electronic transactions that are not conducted in person. *Electronic signatures* are any form of electronic mark on a message or document. It is typically defined by any combination of letters, characters, or symbols entered directly into a computer or by some other electronic means. It is executed or adopted by a party to authenticate a document or entry. The electronic signature must meet the criteria of message integrity (confirming that the document has not been altered), nonrepudiation (the signer must not be able to deny signing the document), and user authentication (the recipient must be able to confirm that the signature was in fact "signed" by the real person). A *digital signature* is an electronic encoded message containing a unique alphanumerical notation. A "key pair," a private and a public key, is used to scramble or encrypt a message and then

unscramble or decrypt the information. A computer software program results in a unique digital signature that can then be linked back to the sender by using the appropriate public key. This system assures each party that the other is who they say they are and that the message received is valid and unchanged.

Several states have imposed criteria that must be met to determine whether a particular electronic signature is legally sufficient to have the same force and effect as the use of a manual signature (see Figure 27-1B). Rules and regulations for electronic authentication are contained within the federal HIPAA privacy rule.

■ MAINTAINING SECURITY OF ELECTRONIC HEALTH INFORMATION

Nurses are key users of the electronic record systems and must be alert to issues associated with control of access to the system (see Figure 27-1C). Electronic documentation systems are rapidly becoming commonplace in nursing practice and will become increasingly prevalent in the future. Accordingly, nursing input at the outset can help design system controls that will minimize risks associated with implementation and use. Persons or entities using electronic technologies must adopt policies and procedures that reflect reasonable efforts to protect patient confidentiality. Security standards include administrative safeguards, physical safeguards such as restricting access and retaining off-site computer backups, and technical safeguards to control access and transmission of electronic protected health information (EPHI).

The major means to control direct access at this time is usually an individual's password. Passwords should *never* be revealed to another person and should be changed periodically. The password should contain multiple letters, characters, and symbols to increase its difficulty of duplication. In addition, a user should not leave the computer workstation without logging out or signing out according to proper procedures.

At this time, the greatest threat to the integrity of an electronic health record and charting system is inappropriate entry by someone from within the organization who has stolen passwords by observing users' keystroke entries or who has copied private files on to portable disks or storage devices and carried them out of a facility or office. Maintaining alertness with regard to use of the computer itself and enforcing explicit policies against such practices may prevent these acts. It is also suggested that employees periodically be reminded of these policies and sign written agreements as a condition of using these systems and of continued employment. These policies should also address use of e-mail and data storage devices including personal data assistants (PDAs), smart phones, CD-ROMs, cell phones with picture taking or Internet access, and other devices used for electronic transmission of information in the workplace. Computer disk drives may be disabled to prevent copying information. If remote access to electronic health information is permitted, appropriate safeguards must also be in place to protect the information. The ease of access and transmission of sensitive information is a continuing and immediate challenge in any healthcare setting.

All staff using electronic systems must have proper, adequate training prior to their actual use of the system. Access to data should be permitted only according to limits based on a person's "need to know." This includes nursing faculty or students who may be using these systems as part of clinical experiences at an institution. By signing on with a unique password, users are permitted access only to the areas of the system necessary for their work.

■ PREVENTING UNAUTHORIZED ACCESS/AUDIT TRAILS

The system must also monitor and record all users to track access to the system. If a breach is detected, the "audit trail" that maintains a log of who accesses each computer and when can provide valuable help in investigating the breach and permit corrective action and any necessary changes to the system. Any alleged breach of the system can be tracked through an audit trail by internal information technology personnel or forensic computer analysts. Nurses must intervene if they do not know who is at a terminal or if they observe a person accessing a screen that he or she should not have access to or that appears improper. The alertness of nurses in the patient care workplace has prevented many problems in the past and will no doubt be critical to preventing the type of problem that can occur when there is improper access to this highly confidential information (see **Figure 27-2**).

■ LITIGATION INVOLVING ELECTRONIC RECORDING OR TRANSMISSION OF HEALTH OR WORKPLACE INFORMATION

1. *Improper use of e-mail.* In *Wanda Kay Woodson v. Scott and White Memorial Hospital*

Administrative: Person responsible for security, training, and policies

Physical: Design, restrict access, privacy screens, protect from public view

Technical: Authentication controls, key pairs for messages, computer analysts

---

Figure 27-2   Workplace safeguards.

(2007), nurse Woodson brought a claim for retaliatory discharge in violation of the Family Medical Leave Act (FMLA). Woodson had received a "final warning" before she requested the leave. The final warning alleged that she had used the computer of a coworker without consent, had looked at the coworker's e-mail, and printed at least one of them. Woodson showed the e-mail to two other employees and told them she thought her supervisor and a coworker had an affair. The appeals court ruled in favor of the employer and found there was a legitimate reason to terminate Woodson based on these acts and other unprofessional conduct, thus her retaliatory discharge claim failed.

2. *Audit trail of internal memo.* A memorandum containing allegedly libelous statements against nurse Bannert was copied to a diskette by an employee under her supervision. The employee gave her the copies of the memo stating that managers were trying to gain Bannert's resignation by creating rumors of her unprofessionalism and drug use. The employee later testified that the "file" for the memorandum document was copied on a diskette (which he later produced at the lawyers' request) from the shared drive of the hospital's computer system, and the author appeared to be Bannert's supervisor, LaMont. However, LaMont denied writing it and asked the director of information services to find the source of the memo. Bannert was fired for dishonesty after the investigation concluded that the source of the memo was actually Bannert's computer. Bannert then sued her former employer and supervisor LaMont for defamation and other causes of action. The trial court awarded Bannert $1.5 million dollars in actual and punitive damages on the defamation claim. However, this verdict was overturned and reversed on appeal with the court finding that there was no evidence to support the conclusion that one of the managers wrote the memo. At trial, computer analyst experts for the defendant hospital had found that the chronology of the memo was first from the employee's computer, then copied to the diskette, then to Bannert's computer, and then last to the hospital shared drive. Thus the claimed source and trail of the memo was not verified by analysis of the computers (*Columbia Valley Regional Medical Center v. Bannert* (2003)).

This case illustrates how "forensic electronic evidence" is increasingly used to prove the source and integrity of written material. Computers can be examined to determine the chronology of source material and also whether it has been changed or manipulated.

3. *Billing charges for nurse practitioners— forensic electronic evidence.* In *United States of America ex rel. Kelly Woodruff and Robert Wilkinson v. Hawaii Pacific Health et al.*, (2008), plaintiffs filed a motion to compel defendants to comply with discovery requests, including electronically stored data, in their lawsuit alleging violations of the federal False Claims Act. Defendants allegedly submitted false UB-92 forms for reimbursement of charges for medical procedures. Some of these claims for reimbursement from the government involved procedures allegedly performed by nurse practitioners who were not licensed to perform them. Cost reports related to these charges were also sought, which the court found that the plaintiffs were entitled to. Plaintiffs also requested raw data, stored electronically and on microfiche, from the UB-92 forms, which the court did not grant at this time pending more information on the electronic discovery request.

Increasingly, billing data and information to back up charges for procedures will be requested as part of litigation. It is imperative that documentation of who performed procedures, coding, and billing records all match and comply with standards for reimbursement. The plaintiffs in this case also requested that the defendants pay for forensic analysis of their computer systems because of their failure to comply with previous court orders. Defending litigation to prove compliance with standards can be extremely time consuming and expensive for organizations.

4. *Computerized medication administration records.* Nurse Dufault was discharged by her employer for "failure to adhere to the standards of narcotic/controlled substance administration-suspected drug diversion" (*The Mercy Hospital, Inc. v. Massachusetts Nurses Association*, 2005). The medication administration machine in the ICU was a computerized dispensing system requiring an electronic keypad for entering personal codes. The defendant employer found that on several occasions nurse Dufault had withdrawn narcotic medication from the machine without offsetting entry for administration in the separate documentation system. The nursing supervisor found other inconsistencies, one of which involved withdrawing an unusually large dose of a narcotic drug. Nurse Dufault stated that this was done to prepare an intravenous drip bag of the medication rather than having to return periodically to the system to withdraw smaller doses prescribed in the physician's orders. She also explained other discrepancies as resulting from working with a nurse orientee that resulted in incomplete documentation because some patients were under their joint control. In directing the hospital to reinstate nurse Dufault, the court found that although it was not good practice,

the arbitrator found that there was evidence that such practice of taking out larger doses for intravenous administration was common practice in the ICU as a time-saving measure. The district court agreed with the arbitral award of reinstatement for the nurse.

Nurses are cautioned that medication dispensing and administration records should always be in compliance with physician orders and patient administration records. Bypassing standards for correct administration may lead to the inference that there is drug diversion as in the Dufault case.

■ REFERENCES AND BIBLIOGRAPHY

Christiansen, A., & Frank-Stromborg, M. (2001). The protection of patient privacy in a high tech era. *Journal of Nursing Law, 8*(1), 17–26.

Columbia Valley Regional Medical Center v. Bannert, 112 S.W.3d 193; 2003 Tex. App. LEXIS 5857 (2003).

Computer Fraud and Abuse Act of 1986, 42 U.S.C. § 290dd-3 (1988).

Gartee, R. (2007). *Electronic health records.* Upper Saddle River, NJ: Pearson Prentice Hall.

Health Care Portability and Accountability Act of 1996 (HIPAA), Pub. L. No. 104-191, 110 Stat. 1998 (1996).

Institute of Medicine. (1999). *To err is human: Building a safer health system.* Author.

Nelson, R. (2007). Electronic health records: Useful tool or high-tech headache? *AJN, 107*(3), 25–26.

Pribble v. Edina Care Center, 2003 Minn. App. LEXIS (2003).

Simpson, R. (2007, February). Easing the way for the electronic health record. *American Nurse Today,* 48–50.

The Mercy Hospital, Inc. v. Massachusetts Nurses Association, 429 F.3d 338; 2005 U.S. App. LEXIS 25073; 178 L.R.R.M. 2548; 151 Lab. Cas. (CCH) P10,583 (2005).

United States of America ex rel. Kelly Woodruff and Robert Wilkinson v. Hawaii Pacific Health et al., 2008 U.S. Dist. LEXIS 4933 (2008).

Wanda Kay Woodson v. Scott and White Memorial Hospital, 2007 U.S. App. LEXIS 24702 (2007).

Chapter 28

Interdependent Nursing Functions: Verbal Orders and Telenursing

Katherine Dempski

CMS and The Joint Commission verbal order use:

- Policy and procedures in place to minimize verbal order use
- Policy identifies practitioners authorized to receive verbal order under state and federal law
- Policy identifies practitioner authorized to give verbal orders under state and federal law
- Organizational method to identify practitioner giving verbal order by phone or fax
- Immediately document order and sign by the person who receives the order
- Record on order sheet or enter in CPOE
- Read back verification

Implementing verbal orders as well as triage telenursing are interdependent nursing functions because they rely on a physician's or other licensed independent practitioner's assessment, diagnosis, and judgment. As such, the nurse who implements the orders must exercise independent judgment and carry his or her own legal liability.

■ VERBAL ORDERS

Ideally, physicians' orders should be written or entered in the computerized order entry (CPOE) to decrease the potential for errors. However, in emergency situations, verbal orders are often a necessary method of communication between physicians and nurses (see **Figure 28-1**).

To minimize use of verbal orders, CMS requires authentication (date, time, and signature) of verbal orders within 48 hours by the prescribing practitioner. Absent a state law specifying a time frame for verbal order

authentication, verbal orders need to be signed within the 48 hours. To give organizations time to comply with the 48-hour rule, CMS allows a temporary exception (5 years from the date of publication: January 26, 2007), allowing responsible providers (authorized by state law and organization policy) to authenticate the verbal order even when the order did not originate with that provider.

To minimize the potential for human error and to comply with federal and accreditation standards, the nurse receiving a verbal order performs a read back verification, which includes writing down the order, reading back the order, and receiving back confirmation from the practitioner giving the order so any misunderstanding can be clarified immediately (The Joint Commission, 2008a, 2008b; see **Figure 28-2**). Organizations must have procedures in place to identify the practitioner giving verbal orders by phone or fax (CMS Regulations for Nursing Services, 2004). A nurse should not

> • Receiver of order *writes* complete order
> • Receiver *reads* back order to person who is ordering
> • Receiver *receives* back confirmation from person who is ordering

Figure 28-2 Read back verification: write—read—receive.
Source: The Joint Commission, 2008a, 2008b.

take a verbal order from a physician through third parties such as the physician's office staff.

■ CHAIN OF COMMAND: QUESTIONING A PHYSICIAN'S ORDERS

The nurse's duty to the patient does not end with documentation that the nurse disagrees with the physician's orders, assessment, or diagnosis. Nurses can be held liable to a patient for injuries received from a physician's negligence when the nurse recognized (or failed to recognize) the negligence and did nothing to prevent it by failing to exercise appropriate nursing standards and institute the organization's chain of command policy. The nurse should begin with discussing the situation with the physician. When a physician reacts negatively, the nurse has a duty to take the next step up the chain of command by following policy. The nurse should document on the appropriate form each level taken.

Failure to institute a notification up the chain of command to prevent the discharge of a pregnant woman with severe preeclampsia was the subject before the court in *Whittington v. Episcopal Hosp.* (2001). The patient was discharged and then returned for an emergency caesarean section and eventually died as a result of the untreated condition, and the family brought suit. Experts testified that the nurses knew vital lab data had not returned from the lab and the patient's high

blood pressure had not been assessed for hours, yet they followed the physician order to discharge the patient against standards of practice and without prophylactic medications. The experts testified the nursing standards required the nurse to go up the hospital chain of command to notify their supervisor, the nursing director, and the chairman of Obstetrics to institute the correct action (admission, delivery of the baby, and monitoring of her blood pressure). The court held the expert testimony did show a breach in the standard of care.

Failure to question or notify the physician of an omitted prescription led to the liability of the nurse, physician, and medical center for the readmission of the plaintiff for cardiac complications following a stent placement procedure. When the patient was being discharged following a stent placement, the nurse viewed the discharge instructions with the patient, which included information on anticoagulation therapy but did not include a prescription for the medication. The nurse did not communicate the missing script to the physician. Subsequently the patient suffered complications due to the lack of anticoagulation. The court held that expert testimony on the standards of care for the nurse showed a relationship between the nurse's act and the patient outcome (*Martin v. Abilene Regional Medical Center*, 2006).

While taking concerns up the chain of command, a nurse can still be liable for a patient's change in condition and has an independent duty to monitor and assess the patient while making proper notification to supervisors and responsible physicians.

■ TELENURSING

Telemedicine uses technology to communicate patient care information from one place (or institution) to another, including transmitting a patient's radiographic scan images (teleradiology) and telephone triage (telenursing). Telenursing offers efficient use of healthcare resources to provide a timely, appropriate level of care to patients who are often in remote areas.

Giving advice or triage over the telephone constitutes the practice of nursing under the NPAs of most states. Accordingly, triage advice given by a nurse must follow applicable standards of care and should not include a medical diagnosis. Nurses performing telephone triage should follow clearly defined protocols based on medical and nursing disciplines. Scripted protocols or software programs can guide the nurse in questioning the caller for an appropriate assessment, medical history, and the nature of the injury. The telenurse may then recommend the patient seek medical care at an emergency department or urgent care clinic. Protocols serve as evidence on whether the standard of care was followed should a lawsuit arise from the incident. Although the nurse is following protocols, triage nursing requires independent nursing judgment and skills.

■ LEGAL CONSIDERATION: NURSING LICENSE

Telenursing for regional or national HMOs or healthcare institutions may require nurses to speak to patients in another state. Telenursing is advancing faster than the law in this area. Nursing, as a licensed profession, is subject to the laws governing the practice and regulation of nursing in each state. Because the definition of telenursing would be included in most NPAs, the nurse may need a license to practice nursing in the state where patients are calling from as well as the state where the nurse is.

Recognizing the advantages to telenursing while maintaining public health and safety, the process for creating a nurse licensure compact among state nursing boards began. The National Council of State Boards of Nursing approved a "mutual recognition policy" to recognize the nursing license of one state allowing the nurse to practice in another state. The Nurse Licensure Compact was organized to protect public health by promoting compliance with laws governing nursing practice by mutual recognition of state licensure. The mutual recognition model requires adoption of the compact by each state and subjects the nurse to the laws and regulation in each state. The nurse with a license in one state would have reciprocity to practice in those states that adopt the compact. It requires that the licensing state and the state of practice cooperatively process complaints regarding the nurse's license. The practicing state may issue an order for the offending nurse to stop practicing in that state while the licensing state processes disciplinary action.

The nurse who triages across state lines should contact the state nursing boards to clarify the need for a license or check with the employer's risk management office for the protocol on multistate triaging.

Although telemedicine is a relatively new technology, several states have statutes regulating this practice. Some states require out-of-state physicians performing telemedicine to be licensed when making a diagnosis and ordering treatment in that state. Accordingly, nurses should be aware of this when implementing the orders of an out-of-state physician. Additionally, several states require the physician to inform the patient about the limitations of telemedicine and obtain *written* informed consent (usually informed consent can be written or oral).

■ REFERENCES

American Nurses Association. (1992). *ANA position statement: Nursing care and do not resuscitate decisions.* Washington, DC: Author.

CMS Regulations for Nursing Services, 42 C.F.R. § 482.23 (c)(2)(i-ii) (2004).

CMS Regulations for Medical Record Services, 42 C.F.R. § 482.24 (c)(1)(iii) (2004).

Greenberg, M. E. (2000, May/June). Telephone nursing: Evidence of client organizational benefits. *Nursing Economics, 18*(30), 117–123.

Martin v. Abilene Regional Medical Center, 2006 Tex. App. LEXIS 897 (Tex. 2006).

National Council of State Boards of Nursing (NCSBN). (2008). *Nurse Licensure Compact (NLC).* Retrieved September 27, 2008, from http://www.ncsbn.org/nlc.htm

The Joint Commission. (2008a). *Comprehensive accreditation manual for hospitals: Management of information standard 6.50.* Oakbrook Terrace, IL: Author.

The Joint Commission. (2008b). *National patient safety goal 2A.* Retrieved September 27, 2008, from http://www.jointcommission.org/PatientSafety/NationalPatientSafetyGoals/08_hap_npsgs.htm

Wachter, G. W. (2002, May). *Telemedicine and telehealth articles: Interstate licensure for telenursing.* Retrieved September 27, 2008, from http://tie.telemed.org/articles/article.asp?path=articles&article=telenursingLicensure_gw_tie02.xml

Whittington v. Episcopal Hosp., 768 A.2d 1144, 1149 (Pa. Super. 2001).

Chapter 29

Event Reporting

Katherine Dempski

Common Barriers to Event Reporting

- Lack of time (I'll do it at the end of my shift)
- Lack of ease in reporting (long forms, difficulty in accessing electronic systems)
- Lack of anonymity (lingering feelings of punitive process)
- Lack of understanding of value of identifying "near miss" events (no serious patient harm resulted, "no harm, no foul")
- Lack of feedback by organization to reporters of systems improved from reporting
- Lack of real or perceived confidentiality of reports (reports can be discoverable)
- Lack of understanding of purpose of reports for systems review rather than individual performance (feelings of "telling on" a coworker)

Event reporting is the vehicle through which quality and risk management departments identify areas for process improvement, identify potential claims, minimize harm, and prevent recurrences through early intervention. Institutions that create a culture of reporting adverse events to analyze systems to improve quality of care and a safe environment of care will have the most effective reporting system. Successful reporting systems are based on a collaboration between providers, environment of care management, and leadership (see **Figure 29-1**). To that end, institutions must have policies in place with definitions of reportable events, including an emphasis on near miss events, and an approach to addressing barriers (ease of reporting, address fear of reprisal) with a clear system for trending and analyzing event data. Staff should be given a clear understanding of the reasons to report

events internally (see **Figure 29-2**). When the internal reporting system identifies that an adverse event caused serious patient harm, regulatory, accrediting, and state statutes may require external reporting to outside agencies.

■ DEFINING ADVERSE EVENTS

An *incident* or *adverse event* is an unexpected occurrence or variation in a system process with unintended results that has the potential to put the institution at legal risk. Adverse events most often involve an injury or a potential injury to a patient, patient's family member, staff member, or visitor or damage to property. Examples of events are burns, medication errors, abuse, equipment failure (with or without an injury), criminal activity, patient or visitor falls, and bloodborne pathogen exposure. Organization policy will dictate which department is responsible for

Trend: Tracking and trending event types and causes gives the organization the ability to implement process improvements. For example, trending patient falls occurrences to time of day and day of week (early mornings on weekends when patients get up to go to the bathroom) could give rise to changing staffing acuity levels and change in time that diuretics are given. Tracking and trending events leads to implementing current changes to prevent harm in the future. It follows the adage "you can't fix what you do not know."

Defend: Early intervention minimizes patient harm and reduces financial loss to the organization. Early investigation lays groundwork for defenses and responsibility to make appropriate response to patient when liable.

Educate: Knowledge of the event cause leads to organization-wide education on new policies or procedures that are instituted to prevent recurrences, as well as "lessons learned."

Figure 29-2   Reasons to report adverse events through internal reporting systems.

different events, for example criminal activity is security, staff injury is human resources (employee health), injury to a visitor is risk management, and injury to a patient or a process variation (with or without patient harm) could be reported to risk and quality/performance improvement departments. Incident reports assist the organization in identifying areas of risk to patients and staff and to prevent incidents from recurring. Additionally, the reports identify system problems and act as an investigative tool for finding solutions. The staff member who is involved in, discovers, or witnesses the event should make the report. Typically, it is the nursing department that makes the most event reports. However, security (patient or visitor violent behavior), clinical engineering (equipment failure or misuse), and patient/guest relations (complaints of care/services) provide event reports.

■ REPORTING PROCEDURES

The institution will provide a form with typical information necessary, including names of any other persons with knowledge of the event or process experts to be consulted. A nonbiased account of the facts leading up to the events and the patient's outcome are the basis of the report. *Sequestering* equipment or medications and IV bags involved in the event are often overlooked by staff but are a vital component of a thorough investigation. Forms may be specific to the event type (usual with electronic systems), such as a medication event or equipment failure event. Specific event reporting forms are part of a robust reporting structure because adverse events tend to happen in high risk areas where processes are complex. To meet the criteria of minimizing recurrence through process improvement by trending and analyzing as well as identifying liability risk, event reporting systems must identify system failures and external reporting requirements. Therefore event-specific forms efficiently gather the pertinent facts and information necessary to investigate these complex system events.

A complete report includes the physician notified, the patient assessment, supervisors and other departments notified depending on the nature of the event, such as blood bank or clinical engineering. Electronic forms offer a quick time-stamped notification to other departments involved as well as departments that need to receive the report, including quality and risk.

Failure to follow organization policy for reporting adverse events will reflect on the nurse's professionalism. A nurse who was fired for a list of failures to follow institutional policies claimed the firing was a pretext to discrimination. The nurse testified she was aware of the event reporting policy and understood the purpose of the policy and the need to provide safe care to the patient, yet she acknowledged that she failed to file a report following an adverse event. She pulled a discontinued tube and noted that the mercury tip was missing and was most likely in the patient. However, she failed to notify the physician or a supervisor or note the missing tip in the medical record so patient harm could be minimized through interventions. The court held she provided no evidence that her firing was a pretext to discrimination. The hospital had this and several other incidents as reason to dismiss her (*Williams v. St. Francis Hosp.*, 1995).

■ DEFINITION OF SENTINEL EVENTS

The most serious of adverse events are sentinel events, identified by the National Quality Forum (NQF) as "Serious Reportable Events." In 2002 the NQF published a list of 27 adverse events they consider to be serious and preventable (National Quality Forum, 2008). A committee was established to keep the list current. Examples are serious injury or death to a patient from a fall, medication error, incompatible blood products, patient serious injury associated with the patient's elopement, stage III or IV pressure ulcers, or the unintended retention of foreign bodies.

The Joint Commission defines a sentinel event as an "unexpected occurrence involving the death or serious physical and psychological injury or the risk thereof that is not related to the natural course of the patient's illness or underlying condition."

- "Serious injury" is the major permanent loss of function of sensory, motor, physiologic, or intellectual impairment not present on admission.
- "Risk thereof" is a near miss. It is a process variation that did not affect the patient's outcome, but should the same or similar facts occur again, patient harm could result.
- "Not related to the natural course of the patient's illness or underlying condition" means the loss of function related to the treatment or lack of treatment of the condition.

These events are called sentinel because they signal the need for an investigation into the occurrence to prevent further harm. Not all sentinel events occur from an error, and not all errors are sentinel events.

■ EXTERNAL REPORTING: MANDATORY REPORTING

Almost half of all states have mandatory reporting of medically related adverse events to state departments of public health, and several others have voluntary reporting. These reporting laws are based on the state's prevailing interest in protecting the public health and welfare. Reportable events are outlined in each state statute and may be similar to the NQF list of "Serious Reportable Events" or the definition of sentinel events determined by The Joint Commission.

To facilitate a full accounting of the investigation, causes of the event, process improvements made, and patient outcome, states protect the report from being discovered, subject to subpoena or being introduced into evidence in any judicial or administrative proceedings.

■ ACCREDITATION REPORTING

The Joint Commission requires that institutions improve safety and quality of care by collecting data on sentinel events and monitoring measures for success in improvements to processes associated with such events. To maintain public confidence in the accreditation process, the commission may perform an unannounced survey on an institution that experienced a sentinel event to review the institution's response from the internal report made, the investigation to factors involved, system improvements put in place to minimize recurrence, and the measures instituted to evaluate success of the improved processes. Appropriate responses to sentinel events include:

* Root cause analysis (RCA): Identifies the factors within systems that caused the event. The focus is on system errors, not individual performance. Those involved in the event or have knowledge of the systems involved are usually part of the RCA team.
* Action plan: Identifies the strategies the RCA team determined should be put into place to reduce the risk of a similar event occurring.

■ PATIENT DISCLOSURE

Disclosure of adverse events is the discussion between providers and the patient of clinically significant facts of the adverse event that could result in harm to the patient immediately and in the foreseeable future, including all reasonable information the patient will need to make future healthcare decisions. Not all states with mandatory reporting laws mandate disclosure to the patient regarding an adverse event. The Joint Commission does mandate disclosure of unexpected outcomes of treatment, including any future concerns. Regardless, the reporting of an adverse event externally and the disclosure to the patient are two separate requirements. Disclosure is usually done by the responsible or primary physician who knows the patient well and the providers who are familiar with the event (see **Figure 29-3**).

■ MEDICAL DEVICE REPORTING

Since 1991, the FDA has required facilities using medical devices to report to the FDA any serious injury or death reasonably related to medical device use. Nurses must be aware of this federal reporting requirement because reports must be made within 10 days of the facility becoming aware of the injury. The nurse should make a report to the responsible department (risk, quality, legal, or clinical

---

• Date and time of disclosure
• Those present
• Discussion points (facts of event and clinical effect on patient)
• Assistance offered to correct injury (intervention such as surgery, procedure, treatment, etc.)
• Patient/family concerns
• Future harm anticipated
• Follow-up discussions planned

Figure 29-3   Disclosure documentation.

engineering) under the organizational policy so the event may properly be investigated and a determination can be made as to external reporting requirements. Serious injury is an injury that is life threatening, results in permanent damage, or requires medical or surgical intervention to prevent permanent injury (irreversible impairment). Use of the device must have caused or contributed to the injury or death. The event could have occurred by device failure, malfunction, improper design, manufacture, labeling, or user error.

■ CONFIDENTIALITY

The event report (may be called an incident report) is intended for use within the facility itself—not for distribution to others—and therefore should remain confidential. Documenting "Confidential" on the report may prove the agency's confidential intent of the report. An event report is not part of the patient's medical record, nor should the nurse document in the patient's medical record "event report completed." Doing so incorporates the report by reference into the medical record and therefore could be discoverable in a legal action. The nurse should not give copies of the event report to the patient or family members. Additionally, nurses should not keep a copy of the report for their personal files. This would constitute a breach of confidentiality, may be a violation of the facility's policies and procedures, and may make the report discoverable in a legal proceeding.

The event report may identify an event for which the organization is liable. In most states, general rules of discovery of evidence for judicial proceedings and peer review statutes offer some protection from the opposing side discovering the report and using it during litigation. The organization's insurance company may require a report on certain incidents where there may be liability. If an event report becomes part of the medical record by a breach of confidentiality, courts may allow the opposing side to obtain a copy and use it against the organization and all professionals involved.

To provide protection to event reports from being discoverable in litigation, the institutions must follow the statute defining the protection and clearly identify the purpose for creating the report. A Veterans Administration medical center withheld a "patient safety report" from a defendant's request to produce documents during the discovery phase of a negligence case. The VA claimed the report was privileged under federal protection as a quality assurance activity. The court agreed and denied the plaintiff's motion to compel discovery of the adverse event report, which was created on the day of the event by the operating room nurse. Mrs. Bethel underwent a procedure, was given Versed, and experienced breathing difficulty. A failed attempt at intubation resulted in anoxic brain injury. During litigation, the plaintiff requested the event report, mortality and morbidity (M&M) reports, and peer review and performance improvement records. The court held M&M documents and peer review documents were discoverable for failure to show that each were created under federal protection (*Bethel v. United States and Veterans Administration Medical Center*, 2007).

Unless the state has a specific protection for adverse event reports under ongoing quality improvement, it may be difficult to claim a blanket protection for event reports under peer review privileges. Event reports not created by the peer review committee for the purpose of the committee proceedings will not fall under most state peer review statutes. In *Hayes v. Premier Living, Inc.* (2007), an event report on a patient fall was not privileged under the peer review statute and was discoverable by the plaintiff.

■ DOCUMENTATION OF INCIDENT

Documentation in the medical record when a patient is involved in an incident is similar but with a different focus. The focus is on the incident as it affects the patient's medical status and the medical care rendered and actions taken to ensure patient safety. For example, the nurse records many of the same facts: date and time of the incident, a concise factual description, assessment of the patient, names of family member and physician notified, and all treatment and follow-up care rendered. However, unlike the event report, the medical record does not focus on quality improvement opportunities for avoiding further incidents. The nurse should not assign blame, state opinions, or make statements of facts the nurse has not witnessed. If information comes from the patient then it is best to use quotation marks for the patient's exact words.

■ REFERENCES

Bethel v. United States and Veterans Administration Medical Center, 242 F.R.D. 580 (2007).

Hayes v. Premier Living, Inc., 641 S.E.2d 316 (Ct. App. N.C. 2007).

Institute for Safe Medication Practices. (2008). *USP-ISMP Medication Errors Reporting Program (MERP)*. Retrieved September 27, 2008, from https://www.ismp.org/orderForms/reporterrortoISMP.asp

Johns Hopkins University, Department of Anesthesiology and Critical Care Medicine, Quality & Safety Research Group. (2005). *Intensive Care Unit Safety Reporting System (ICUSRS)*. Retrieved September 27, 2008, from http://www.safetyresearch.jhu.edu/QSR/Research/Projects/project_ICUSRS.asp

National Quality Forum. (2008). *Serious reportable events in healthcare: 2005–2006 update*. Retrieved September 27, 2008, from http://www.qualityforum.org/projects/completed/sre

The Joint Commission. (2008). *Comprehensive accreditation manual for hospitals: Sentinel events*. [See also ethics, rights and responsibilities, standard RI 2.90.] Oakwood Terrace, IL: Author.

Williams v. St. Francis Hosp., 1995 U.S. Dist. LEXIS 9927 (D.C. Ill.) (1995).

Chapter 30

Forensic Issues

Susan J. Westrick

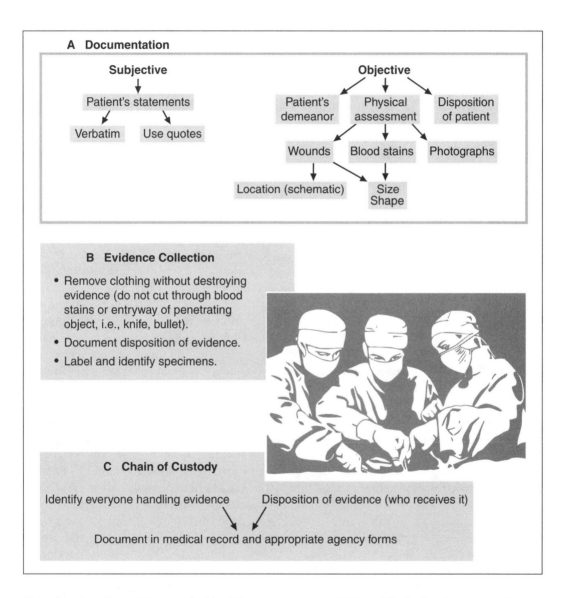

A Documentation

Subjective → Patient's statements → Verbatim, Use quotes

Objective → Patient's demeanor, Physical assessment, Disposition of patient

Physical assessment → Wounds, Blood stains, Photographs

Wounds → Location (schematic), Size Shape

Blood stains → Size Shape

B Evidence Collection

- Remove clothing without destroying evidence (do not cut through blood stains or entryway of penetrating object, i.e., knife, bullet).
- Document disposition of evidence.
- Label and identify specimens.

C Chain of Custody

Identify everyone handling evidence

Disposition of evidence (who receives it)

Document in medical record and appropriate agency forms

Forensic means "pertaining to the law." Forensic issues arise with victims of domestic violence or sexual assault and patients injured by trauma and accident. The victim's initial contact with the healthcare system is usually the nurse, and for this reason nurses share a responsibility with the legal system and must be familiar with basic forensic concepts.

Every hospital accredited by The Joint Commission is required to formulate written policies and procedures related to the collection of evidence. In fact, the commission has recommended that a forensic nurse be available on every shift in the emergency department. Nurses should be familiar with and adhere to an institution's guidelines on forensic evidence collection.

■ DOCUMENTATION

Completeness and accuracy are the hallmarks of a properly documented medical record that subsequently might be used for legal proceedings (see Figure **30-1A**). The nurse's note should be factual and nonjudgmental and include the nurse's observations of the patient's appearance and demeanor. Statements of the victim should be noted in quotation marks and should be verbatim. These statements, if made for purposes of medical treatment, are usually admissible in later legal proceedings. Generally, they are obtained when taking the history from the injured patient or victim.

Documentation of the nurse's findings on the physical assessment should include a detailed description of all body wounds and marks. The use of a "body map" or a schematic of the body is a valuable tool to depict the locations of wounds and marks. The description should include the shape, size, and color of the wounds and marks. General descriptions such as "laceration" can be improved by describing wound edges as "jagged," "smooth," or "deep." Any blood stains or bloody fingerprints should be described. Physicians may report findings of a physical exam to the nurse, who should record them accurately and completely. Proper documentation also includes treatment and the patient's response to the treatment as well as the demeanor of the patient.

Any photographs obtained or physical evidence collected should be carefully documented in the medical record. A photograph taken before surgery or treatment may be important in establishing facts related to the incident as based on the wound or injury.

■ EVIDENCE COLLECTION

The Emergency Nurses Association's 2003 position statement on Forensic Evidence Collection indicates that performance of forensic procedures is a component of emergency nursing practice. Defined in these skills is the emergency nurse's role in helping to preserve the evidence collected, in addition to providing physical and emotional care to clients. This document recognizes that during the course of ED evaluation, evidence can be lost, damaged, or overlooked.

Increasingly, forensic nursing has become a specialty for RNs who provide comprehensive examination, care, and management of patients with forensic implications. Because of their advanced education and training in forensics, these nurses often provide expert testimony and are titled forensic nurse examiners (FNE). A nurse who is specially trained to provide forensic and medical examination and care to victims of sexual assault is a sexual assault nurse examiner, or SANE nurse. These specialty nurses are also trained to minimize the emotional trauma for victims. Emergency rooms and healthcare organizations typically have one of these nurses on call if not onsite.

Treatment of life-threatening injuries takes precedence over evidence collection. At all times, evidence collection should not interfere with treatment. Nurses should always maintain standard precautions in collecting specimens. Each item collected should be handled and packaged separately. Most emergency departments have rape kits available for the collection of evidence in sexual assault cases. Nurses should be familiar with the proper and complete use of these or other kits for evidence collection.

Ordinarily, clothing and shoes are given to the patient's family; however, they may be evidence depending on the situation. Shoes may be very important evidence of where a victim has been and should be treated as such. When removing clothing that has blood stains or other evidence of injury, the nurse should cut away from the site of injury or cut on the seam lines, not through the site. Any foreign bodies, such as bullets or knives, should be handled as little as possible, being careful not to mark these items.

Any evidence collected should be labeled accurately and completely, identifying the specimen as well as who collected it (see Figure 30-1B).

■ EVIDENCE PRESERVATION

After collection and labeling of the evidence, the chain of custody must be documented, identifying anyone who has handled the "evidence" and the responsible agency (e.g., police or medical examiner) or individual who receives the evidence (see Figure 30-1C). This information should be contained in the medical record for use in later legal proceedings. The number of individuals handling specimens should be kept to a minimum to ensure the integrity of the specimen.

Many emergency departments have a chain-of-custody form that is used when evidence is obtained from the patient. It documents the name of anyone who has had access to the evidence and serves as a log of where the evidence has been and who has handled it. This chain of custody becomes important as to the admissibility of the evidence at trial.

■ SUSPECTED DRUG ABUSE OR POSSESSION

When a nurse finds drugs in a patient's possession while searching for something else (such as identification), the nurse should follow hospital policy for this situation. Often the drugs need to be confiscated, and security officers should be involved. If the nurse thinks that a patient is abusing drugs, and this is interfering with treatment, a search may be warranted. Documentation should objectively state behaviors or symptoms that

lead to this suspicion. Again, the nurse should request the assistance of security officers before any search is completed, and all policies should be adhered to strictly. The physician also should be notified of the facts because this information may affect the patient's treatment.

■ ACCIDENT OR TRAUMA INCIDENTS

Forensic nursing concepts are important in cases of accidents, trauma, or even death, not just where crimes are suspected. Thorough histories and assessments are invaluable to others trying to establish facts surrounding the incidents. Identification of bodies involves forensics, and nurses may participate in interviewing families of the deceased. Any suspicions of abuse of children or others calls for careful application of the principles of assessment, identification of any wounds, statements, and evidence collection. It may be the nurse who suspects that some aspects of either the family's or victim's statements do not "match" with other data.

■ TESTIMONY

As a consequence of involvement in care and treatment of an injured victim, the nurse may be called upon to testify in legal proceedings. Competency and credibility as a witness cannot be undermined if the nurse adheres to the basic principles of evidence collection and preservation as well as accurate and complete documentation in the patient's medical record.

In *State of Delaware v. Albert Johnson* (2005) the emergency room triage nurse testified at the criminal trial as to the demeanor of an elderly woman who had been sexually assaulted. The nurse's descriptions of the victim as "shaky," "tearful," and "wringing her hands" and report of the incident as "the worst night of my life" were admissible at trial as statements made for the purposes of medical diagnosis or treatment. Hearsay rules for excluding evidence may apply if the court determines that the statements were made to gather forensic evidence. Therefore, the court excluded statements that the victim later made to the SANE nurse, partly because the investigating detective was present for this interview.

In another similar case, *State of Ohio v. Kevin Young* (2003), the court also found an exception to the hearsay rule in allowing a nurse's testimony to help identify the minor victim's assailant. The court also admitted a sexual assault/abuse form documented by the nurse as a business record that had information entered in the section entitled "Assault/abuse was by:". Both of these crucial pieces of evidence provided by documentation and testimony of the emergency room nurse, as well as results of DNA testing from samples obtained by the nurse using a sexual assault kit, were used to convict the defendant.

Both of these cases underscore the importance of careful, complete, accurate, and descriptive documentation in these circumstances. Thorough assessment and interview of the victim, as well as collection of samples following hospital protocols, provides essential and probative evidence at trial.

■ REFERENCES AND BIBLIOGRAPHY

Emergency Nurses Association. (2003). *Position statement: Forensic evidence collection.* Retrieved September 27, 2008, from http://www.ena.org/about/position/PDFs/ForensicEvidence.PDF

Hammer, R., Moynihan, B., & Pagliaro, E. (2006). *Forensic nursing: A handbook for practice.* Sudbury, MA: Jones and Bartlett.

International Association of Forensic Nurses. (2006). *Homepage.* Retrieved September 27, 2008, from http://www.iafn.org

State of Delaware v. Albert Johnson, 205 Del. Super. LEXIS 253 (2005).

State of Ohio v. Kevin Young, 2003 Ohio 4706; 2003 Ohio App. LEXIS 4258 (2003).

Part III Review Questions

1. The nurse is making rounds when she notices Mr. Jones is not in his room. Mr. Jones is a 77-year-old diabetic patient who recently underwent debridement to improve healing on his left foot. He is being seen by a physical therapist to assist him with use of a walker. The therapist commented on the trouble Mr. Jones is having adjusting to the walker. As the nurse walks farther down the hall, she sees Mr. Jones lying flat on the floor with his walker on top of him. There is a small puddle on the floor next to him. Mr. Jones states, "I slipped on that wet spot and I can't seem to use this walker thing." The best way to document this incident is to write:

   (A) "Mr. Jones is having a difficult time adjusting to his new walker and fell in the hallway and landed flat on his back. Vital signs are stable."
   (B) "Mr. Jones was using his new walker in the hallway when he slipped on a puddle landing on his back. Vital signs are stable."
   (C) "Mr. Jones was found in the hallway flat on his back with his walker on top. A puddle was beside him. Vital signs are stable."
   (D) "Mr. Jones is having a difficult time adjusting to his new walker and slipped on a puddle, landing on his back."

2. At 3:00 p.m., the nurse ends his rounds and notices he forgot to document in his 7:00 a.m. note that a patient's left ankle was swollen at 7:00 a.m. To document, the nurse should:

   (A) Put a line through the 7:00 a.m. note and rewrite the assessment to include the swollen ankle
   (B) Write a 3:00 p.m. addendum to the 7:00 a.m. note
   (C) Write a 3:00 p.m. late entry to the 7:00 a.m. note
   (D) Any of the above

3. The nurse manager arrives on the patient unit at 6:45 a.m. He notes that the computer terminal at the nurses' station is displaying a screen used to enter patient progress notes into the patient record. There is no one at the terminal. He asks all of the staff on duty if they had brought this screen up. All answer in the negative. The only other person on duty, a nurse, had left to go home at 6:30 a.m. The nurse manager should:

   (A) Restart the computer and clear the screen so the computer terminal will be ready for the day staff's work
   (B) Isolate and freeze all activity at that terminal and call the system administrator for instructions and procedures to be followed
   (C) Call the nurse who left to see whether she finished making her entries

before restarting and clearing the computer workstation

(D) Ask the unit secretary to print a copy of the work displayed on the screen and then restart the computer workstation

4. A staff nurse working on a busy acute care medical unit is approached by a professional-looking woman who requests that the nurse bring up the lab result computer screen of a particular patient so she can view and print the patient's laboratory study information. The nurse does not know the woman and asks for identification and the purpose of her request. She said she is a consulting physician who has been asked to review the record of the patient in question. She has a driver's license but no other type of identification. What should the nurse do?

(A) The nurse should comply with the request because the driver's license confirms her identity as she has stated

(B) The nurse should call the patient's attending physician to confirm that the woman has been requested to perform the consultation, and when verified, the nurse then complies with the request

(C) The nurse should tell the woman that because she is unable to produce anything other than a driver's license, and the nurse does not have knowledge of her authorization to view the record, the nurse cannot comply with her request without additional authorization

(D) The nurse should check the patient record to see if such a consultation is ordered, and if it is, the nurse should comply with the request

5. Do-not-resuscitate orders:

(A) Are indefinite

(B) Protect nurses and physicians from any liability

(C) Must be in writing

(D) All of the above

6. A nurse believes the physician incorrectly diagnosed a patient as having a urinary tract infection. The patient is having intractable right-upper-quadrant pain not relieved with narcotics. The nurse documents his assessment in the patient's medical record. His duty to the patient is:

(A) Complete upon documenting his findings in her medical record

(B) Complete when he medicates her for pain and makes her more comfortable

(C) Complete when he notifies the medical director that his assessment differs from that of the physician

(D) None of the above

7. A patient falls in the hallway and fractures his hip. The nurse records the events in the patient's medical record. The nurse completes an incident report. The patient's family requests a copy of the incident report. What should the nurse do?

(A) Give the patient's family a copy because it is part of the patient's medical record

(B) Give the patient's family a copy and chart in the patient's medical record that a copy of the incident report was given to the patient's family

(C) Refuse to give a copy to the family but give a copy to the patient

(D) Refuse to give the family a copy and explain that the form is for the facility's use only

8. The nurse is making rounds when she hears a "thud" followed by a groan. Upon entering the next room, she notices Mrs. Smith lying on the floor next to her bed. Her feet are tangled in the sheets. Both

side rails are raised. When filing the incident report, the nurse documents that:

(A) Mrs. Smith tangled her feet in the sheets and fell out of bed and onto the floor

(B) Mrs. Smith attempted to climb back into bed, tangled her feet on the sheets, and fell to the floor

(C) The nurse found Mrs. Smith on the floor beside the bed with the sheet around her feet, and both side rails were raised

(D) Mrs. Smith attempted to climb over the raised side rails, tangled her feet in the sheets, and fell to the floor

9. A nurse assessing a patient in the emergency department suspects that the patient is a victim of a crime. Which of the following is an essential nursing intervention?

(A) A thorough and descriptive assessment of all injuries including "body mapping"

(B) Telling the victim's family of the nurse's suspicions

(C) Reporting the situation to the police before verifying any more facts with the patient

(D) Notifying the risk manager because there may be litigation involved

10. A nurse suspects that a patient may have drugs in his possession. Which of the following would the nurse *not* be advised to do?

(A) Enlist the help of security officers before any other steps are taken

(B) Take control of the situation quickly and confiscate the drugs when the patient is not looking

(C) Determine whether the patient is placing either himself or others at risk

(D) Notify the physician of the outcome of the situation if drugs are found

Part III Answers

1. *The answer is C.*

   A, B, and D are incorrect because they make an assumption about facts that were not witnessed by the nurse who documented the incident. Even though Mr. Jones explains what happened, it is best to place the patient's own words in quotes and then describe objectively what the nurse witnessed. C is correct because it does not make any assumptions on the facts.

2. *The answer is B.*

   An addendum is the best way to add to or correct a note. Late entry is used when no note was written but one is needed. A line may be placed through an incorrect entry, but this nurse's entry was not incorrect. A note should be corrected, not rewritten.

3. *The answer is B.*

   The workstation is showing a confidential document that was accessed using a password with privileges assigned at least to that level of information. It appears that either the user had not logged out before leaving the computer station or someone gained access with another person's password. Thus, information of a highly confidential nature could have been accessed and even changed. The nurse manager should immediately, following the organization's procedure, notify the system administrator of the situation, take steps to safeguard the privacy of the information, and prevent any use of the station until an investigation is properly under way. The nurse manager and system administrator will need to conduct a detailed investigation that will include at least identification of the user who signed into the computer; ascertainment of exactly when that user last logged in; ascertainment of how and when the station was left in the unsecured manner; interview of all other staff as necessary to determine if any other persons had used the station; and isolation and review of all records to determine via the system's monitoring and tracking mechanism the timing of entries during the time the station was left unsecured. In addition, the nurse manager should review procedures and training of all staff as to proper use and security procedures. Corrective procedures may also include password changes. A situation like this could be very serious because unauthorized access to the system may have occurred.

4. *The answer is C.*

   The nurse is correct in not permitting access to the record as requested based on the information provided by the woman making the request. To make the confidential information available to the requester, the nurse must be assured that this is a proper disclosure. If the nurse fails to do this and the use and disclosure turns out to be improper, the nurse may be liable for the resulting damages. Therefore, the nurse must ask the individual to wait while the nurse takes the necessary steps to ensure the propriety of the request. The nurse should notify the superior and request guidance in managing the request. This would involve at least ensuring that this physician has been duly consulted to review this record; that the identity of the consultant is verified; that the record is not under any particular protections requiring additional consent or approval; that such consultation requests and information disclosure are proper and done according to facility guidelines; and that the necessary procedure for providing a printout is followed. This aspect is more likely to be responded to by the medical record administrator who, in most facilities, oversees any record release. Facilities should have a system in place to manage and respond to requests for information access and disclosure.

5. *The answer is C.*

Although verbal orders are acceptable practice, verbal DNR orders are not. The DNR order requires careful documentation of the patient's wishes, family involvement, and clearly defined orders of which, if any, medical interventions are to be implemented. A is incorrect because DNR orders are renewed every few days according to agency policy. B is incorrect because DNR orders do not necessarily protect healthcare providers from liability (the order may be carried out incorrectly).

6. *The answer is D.*

The nurse should take his concerns up the chain of command starting with the physician, who may be accessible and open to the nurse's assessment and findings. C is incorrect because the duty is not complete until after meeting a satisfactory outcome. A and B are incorrect because a nurse's duty to exercise independent judgment requires the nurse to do more than document and medicate.

7. *The answer is D.*

Incident reports are confidential records, and A, B, and C breach that confidentiality.

8. *The answer is C.*

C documents the facts as the nurse witnessed them. The nurse could add Mrs. Smith's subjective statement, "I tried to get over the side rails, tangled my feet, and fell to the floor," to explain what happened, but to document A, B, or D makes assumptions about facts the nurse did not see. If the nurse documents that Mrs. Smith fell out of bed because she told you, then the nurse should document, "Patient states she fell out of bed" or use the patient's own words in quotes.

9. *The answer is A.*

This is an essential step to confirming the nurse's suspicions and preserving evidence through documentation. The nurse will assist in gathering other information also. Answer B is incorrect because family members may be involved in the incident, and the nurse does not have enough information to inform them yet. The nurse needs to obtain information from them but not suggest causes at this point. Answer C is incorrect because the nurse does not yet have enough information to do this. The nurse needs to talk to the patient or family first, and hospital protocol may prohibit the nurse from notifying the police. Answer D is incorrect because it is premature, even though there could be litigation involved later.

10. *The answer is B.*

The nurse should not place himself or herself in danger and risk an unpredictable situation. Therefore, this would not be an appropriate action. Answer A is a correct action because security should be involved. Answer C is a correct step because the nurse needs to assess any danger in the situation for the patient or others and take any steps to ensure their safety without undue personal risk. Answer D is a correct action because the physician may need to modify the patient's plan of care based on this information.

PART IV

Employment and the Workplace

Chapter 31

Employer and Employee Rights

Susan J. Westrick

A Employee at Will
Cannot terminate for:
- Public policy violation
- Refusal to partake in unlawful/unethical conduct
- Whistle-blowing

C OSHA Mandates for Healthcare Providers
1. Develop an exposure control plan, updated annually.
2. Take precautions to protect employees from exposure to bodily fluids.
3. Provide adequate hand-washing facilities.
4. Provide protective equipment such as disposable gloves, gowns, goggles, etc.
5. Provide appropriate containers for the disposal of needles and sharp instruments.
6. Communicate presence of HIV and hepatitis hazards to employees.
7. Offer hepatitis B virus vaccinations to employees.
8. Offer postexposure evaluation if an employee has been exposed.

B Rights OSHA Grants to Employees
1. To question unsafe conditions and request an investigation.
2. To assist OSHA inspections.
3. To assist a court in determining whether certain imminent, dangerous conditions exist.
4. To bring an action to compel the Secretary of Labor to seek injunctive relief against an employer.
5. To refuse to perform hazardous job activities where there is a reasonable belief there is danger of death or serious injury and no time to seek administrative action to remedy the danger.
6. To access safety records including records disclosing the identity of toxic substances or harmful physical agents.

D Family Medical Leave Act
$\geq$50 employees

12 weeks paid/unpaid leave for:

Birth of child	Adoption or placement of foster care child	Serious medical illness	Care for family with serious illness

---

Generally, nurses are employees at will of the agency they work for unless they have a contract specifically defining the terms of the employment. How an employee and employer terminate the relationship depends on the type of employment involved. Therefore, nurses need to be aware of the differences in the law governing their employment situation. Additionally, nurses should know the state and federal laws that grant employees certain rights within the work environment.

■ EMPLOYMENT AT WILL

Employment is considered to be at will when the employer or employee is free to terminate the employment relationship at any time, with or without reason, and with or without notice. Employment is considered at will unless there is a contractual agreement between the employee and employer or there is a statute dictating the terms of employment. Accordingly, an employer is under no obligation to retain an employee any more than an employee can be compelled against his or her will to work for the employer.

Exceptions to the at will doctrine are when there is (1) an express or implied contract to employ for a particular time period or (2) an express or implied contract to terminate only for certain reasons or through specific procedures. An express contract is typically a written agreement setting forth the terms and conditions of employment, including duration of employment and cause for termination. An implied contract may be found when there are written or oral promises made to the employee to employ for a particular time or to terminate only for certain reasons or through certain procedures. Statements made in employer handbooks and policy manuals have been construed to create a binding commitment on employers to discharge only for cause (i.e., willful violation of policy, inadequate job performance, job-related misconduct, business needs) or through specific disciplinary procedures.

Another exception to the at will doctrine arises when the termination of employment violates public policy, such as when the employee refuses to do something unlawful or reports the employer for unlawful or improper conduct (see **Figure 31-1A**).

■ STATUTORY REGULATION AND PROTECTION

There are several statutes restricting the employment at will doctrine or that give rise to employee rights in the workplace:

1. The *Occupational Safety and Health Act* (OSHA) of 1970 provides that places of employment are to be free from recognized hazards that are causing or likely to cause serious physical harm or death to an employee. Employers must comply with occupational safety and health standards promulgated by the agency. Some of the rights OSHA grants to employees are listed in Figure 31-1B. OSHA prohibits discrimination or retaliation against an employee who has filed a complaint, testified in a proceeding under the act, or exercised any of the previously mentioned rights. It is unlawful for an employer to terminate an employee who exercises his or her rights under OSHA. With respect to healthcare providers, see Figure 31-1C.

2. Employers must provide their employees with employer-paid benefits for on-the-job injury, known as *workers' compensation*. Benefits include payment of a portion of wages while the worker is disabled, medical care and/or payment to healthcare providers, a specific payment for permanent injury, death benefits, and in many states vocational rehabilitation when the employee cannot return to his or her previous job due to permanent restrictions or disability. These remedies are available to the employee without regard to employer or employee fault. In most states, workers' compensation is the sole remedy against an employer for worker-related injuries. In other words, an employee is precluded from bringing a civil action against an employer for work-related injuries and damages. In most states it is unlawful for an employer to retaliate against an employee for filing a workers' compensation claim.

3. The *Fair Labor Standards Act* (FLSA) of 1938 is federal legislation that sets minimum wages and maximum hours of employment, including payment of overtime at 1.5 wages of regular pay for work over 40 hours in a 7 day period. There are some exceptions for healthcare workers and others who may work 80 hours in a 2 week period. Professional employees are exempt from this overtime rule when they are compensated by a salary. Typically, professionals perform work requiring knowledge of an advanced type, and their work requires consistent exercise of discretion and judgment.

   The FLSA and the Ohio Minimum Fair Wage Standard Act were at issue in a case involving nurse Elwell's payment for nursing services by her employer in *Wendy Elwell v. University Hospitals Home Care Services* (2002). Nurse Elwell worked as a home care nurse who was paid through a combination of fee payments and hourly compensation. She often worked in excess of 40 hours per week but did not receive compensation at the 1.5 hourly overtime rate. In 1995 the employer changed its compensation for home care nurses and began to pay them on a per-visit rate. They eliminated additional hourly pay that nurses had received for documentation and eliminated its previous policy of reimbursing home healthcare nurses of "Not Home/Not Found" visits. They also reduced compensation for infusion visits. To be considered full time, nurses had to complete a minimum of 25 visits per week because the actual time spent with patients, completing documentation, travel time, discussions with other health professionals, and meetings would constitute 40 hours per week. According to Elwell, the 25 visits she was required to make per week actually took 39 hours, and she regularly worked an average of 60 hours per week to complete the required documentation and telephone calls to patients and physicians. Additionally, she often accepted and volunteered for additional visits during the week but was paid regular work visit rates. Elwell did not receive compensation for any of the hours she worked in excess of 40 hours per week.

In 1998 she resigned and a year later filed a lawsuit alleging violations of the FLSA and the Ohio statute. The university moved for summary judgment on the ground that she was a professional and exempt from the FLSA. The district court ruled in her favor and the jury awarded her damages, interest, and attorney's fees, but not liquidated damages because it found the university had "acted in good faith and had reasonable grounds to believe it was not violating the FLSA." On appeal to the US Court of Appeals for the sixth district, the court affirmed that Elwell was entitled to liquidated (but not interest because it would be duplicative) and other damages on the basis of this hybrid payment structure, by which she was paid for components of her work that tied compensation to the number of hours worked. The court did not accept the employer's view that Elwell was a professional and therefore exempt from the overtime when she was paid by this structure.

4. In 1993, Congress enacted the *Family Medical Leave Act* (FMLA), which mandates that employers with 50 or more employees grant up to 12 weeks per year of leave during a 12-month period to an employee for any of the reasons shown in Figure 31-1D. Although leave may be unpaid, if the employer provides health benefits to the employee, the employer must continue to provide the same or similar benefits while the employee is on FMLA leave. An employer may require or an employee can elect to substitute all or any part of the statutory 12 weeks of unpaid leave with any accrued paid vacation leave or personal disability leave under the employer's personnel policies. An employee who has been denied leave or has been terminated for exercising leave under FMLA may file a complaint with the Department of Labor or file a civil action. Upon return from family medical leave, most employees must return to their original (or equivalent) position with equal pay, benefits, and other terms of employment in place prior to leave. Many states have similar statutory provisions. Some state provisions are more generous than the federal medical leave and may be applicable to employers with less than 50 employees.

Nurse Woodson, who worked as a charge nurse, filed a lawsuit against her employer alleging that she was terminated from her job and retaliated against in violation of the FMLA (*Wanda Woodson v. Scott and White Memorial Hospital*, 2007).

After receiving a "final warning" alleging wrongdoings in the workplace, Woodson became very emotional and was given the day off. These incidents included her reading coworkers' e-mails and in one case printing an e-mail and making allegations about her supervisor having an affair with another employee. It was also alleged that after she left work, Woodson continued to gossip about this. Thereafter she suffered severe anxiety, a panic attack, and depression. She did not return to work but provided two doctor's notes to excuse her absence. After nurse Woodson left work, her supervisor ran an audit of her access to medical records, which showed she had accessed her own and other employee's medical records, a violation of defendant hospital's policies. Seven days after her "final warning" she was terminated from her position. Woodson claimed that one day prior to her termination she had informed her supervisor that she wanted FMLA paperwork sent to her doctor and that she could not work. The employer stated it did not receive this paperwork until the day after her termination. Woodson made claims against her employer for discrimination under the Americans with Disabilities Act (ADA) and the FMLA for retaliatory discharge. The trial court had dismissed her ADA claim and she appealed her FMLA retaliation claim. However, the appeals court affirmed the trial court and also denied the FMLA claim. They found that the employer had legitimate nonretaliatory reasons for terminating Woodson because her final warning was given before she applied for FMLA leave. The court determined that the close timing of the events did not overcome the employer's right to discharge her under these facts.

In another case, *Throneberry v. McGehee Desha County Hospital* (2005), the plaintiff nurse asserted that her FMLA rights had been interfered with by her employer. According to the FMLA, an employee taking this leave is not entitled to any right, benefit, or position of employment, other than the employee would have been entitled to if the employee had not taken the leave. The FMLA does not require an employer to retain an employee on FMLA leave if that employee has no right to return to work. Therefore, if an employer was authorized to discharge an employee if the employee was not on FMLA leave, the FMLA does not shield an employee on FMLA leave from the same lawful discharge. Nurse Throneberry was a staff home health nurse at defendant hospital. After several years of employment, her deteriorating mental health gradually affected her work relationships and job performance. Throneberry was taking several prescription drugs and began having mood swings and emotional outbursts on the job, causing disruption among coworkers and in the work environment. Administrators gave her a leave of absence, but she continued to come to work while dressed and acting inappropriately. At one point her family was called to pick her up at work after an especially improper incident. Her supervisor was told by other management personnel that "you need to let [Throneberry] go." This would have required reporting her to the Board of Nursing, so she was asked to resign, but Throneberry initially refused to do so. Later she signed an agreement allowing her to resign at a later date but continuing some benefits while she was on leave of absence.

After her resignation, her former coworkers reviewed her unopened mail, some from 5 months before, and found she had billed Medicaid for services without proper documentation. The hospital had to repay over $40,000 due to these errors. Based on these additional performance issues, her supervisor testified that she would have discharged Throneberry before her resignation date took effect. After a jury trial found against her on her claims for retaliatory discharge, she appealed the decision. The jury did find that the employer had interfered with her FMLA leave, and she asserted on appeal that this meant the court must also find in her favor for the discharge claim. The appeals court did not agree and found that although this may have occurred, the employer still had a legitimate reason to terminate her and that the FMLA does not impose strict liability on the employer under these facts. Additionally, the jury's finding was that Throneberry would have been discharged by the hospital even if she had not exercised her FMLA rights.

■ HEALTH BENEFITS

Health insurance is a benefit that an employer is under no obligation to provide. However, if an employer does provide health benefits, the employer must offer an employee who leaves the position or is terminated the opportunity to purchase health insurance at the employer's group rate for an 18-month period.

■ PROTECTION FROM DISCRIMINATION

The federal laws listed in **Figure 31-2** protect employees from discrimination. Mirroring the federal laws, many states have enacted laws to address discrimination based on race, age, disability, and gender, and some states have gone further in adopting laws prohibiting discrimination because of sexual orientation, marital status, and ethnicity.

To prove discrimination, the employee generally must prove (1) that he or she is a member of the protected class; (2) that he or she is qualified for the job or promotion or other beneficial action; and (3) that the job or promotion or other benefit was instead given to a member of a different class. Members of a protected class are individuals who share the characteristics of the class of individuals the antidiscrimination statute seeks to protect. When the employee proves the three elements previously referenced, the employer has the burden of proving a legitimate and nondiscriminatory reason for either not selecting or terminating the employee. If the employer proves a legitimate, nondiscriminatory reason for termination, the employee has the burden of proving that the legitimate, nondiscrimina-

* Equal Pay Act of 1963 — mandates that employers pay equal wages to men and women for equal work
* Civil Rights Act of 1964 — as amended (commonly referred to as Title VII) prohibits employers from discrimination based on race, color, religion, natural origin, and/or sex including sexual harassment
* Age Discrimination in Employment Act of 1967 (ADEA) — forbids discrimination in employment of persons > 40 years old
* Americans with Disabilities Act (ADA) — prohibits discrimination against qualified individuals with disabilities and requires an employer to make reasonable accommodations to disabled individuals
* National Labor Relations Act (NLRA) — prohibits an employer from discriminating against an employee who encourages or discourages membership in a labor union
* Fair Labor Standards Act (FLSA) — bars discrimination against employees who assert rights under the FLSA

Figure 31-2   Federal laws protecting employees from discrimination.

tory reasons offered by the employer are a mere pretext for discrimination.

The general elements of a discrimination claim are slightly modified in cases brought under the Americans with Disabilities Act (ADA). Under the ADA, the employee must prove that he or she (1) is a qualified individual with a disability (i.e., has a physical or mental impairment that substantially limits a major activity); (2) has a record of having such a physical or mental impairment or being regarded or perceived as having an impairment; and (3) can perform the essential job duties with or without reasonable accommodation. When an employee has shown that he or she is a qualified individual with a disability (able to do the essential functions of the job with or without reasonable accommodation), the employer is liable for an adverse employment decision (i.e., termination, refusal to hire) unless the employer can prove that the accommodation would pose an undue hardship on the employer.

In the following two cases, former employee nurses alleged discrimination in violation of the Age Discrimination in Employment Act (ADEA) when they were terminated from their positions. In *Sherryl Perry v. St. Joseph Regional Medical Center* (2004), a 55-year-old nurse had been employed as the Director of the Emergency Department for the past 26 years. Nurse Perry was told by her supervisor, Ms. Watson, that she needed to improve her skills in several areas to meet federal emergency room (ER) standards and that she was dissatisfied with her performance. The employee contended that her age was a determining factor in her dismissal because she was replaced by a younger person, she previously had received favorable evaluations, and that Ms. Watson had made comments about her that were age related. These included that the plaintiff nurse might be "burned out" and "she was not going to be able to change her old ways." Other job-related issues that she was informed of included that nurse Perry lacked enthusiasm for her job, gave priority to her volunteer activities

instead of her job, did not adequately support ER staff, and failed to follow through with critical ER issues or to fix them. Watson was temporarily replaced by her second-in-command coworker, who was 38 years old, but her permanent replacement, hired before her discrimination complaint, was 54 years old. The appellate court affirmed the court below in finding that regardless of her age, she could not show that the employer's reasons for termination were not legitimate. The testimonies that the ER did not meet federal standards and that the employee was unproductive and unable to change were not necessarily related to her age.

Another case involved an age discrimination claim under the ADEA and also ADA discrimination, when the employee was transferred to a temporary position that was eventually eliminated. In *Eileen M. Simonson v. Trinity Regional Health System* (2003), nurse Simonson was employed at defendant's hospital from 1972 to 1999. Since 1994 Simonson had suffered a number of work-related injuries that required accommodation. In 1999 the hospital closed the section where she formerly worked and then assigned her to a temporary position working on a hospital computer system. The hospital eventually informed her that this position had ended and there was no longer a job for her. The appeals court agreed with the district court that her ADA claim failed because her temporary work restrictions had been imposed upon the employee and did not suggest she was "regarded as having a disability" under the ADA. Also Simonson did not make an adequate showing for her ADEA claim because it was not established that she was replaced or that an available job was filled by a younger person. Furthermore, there was no evidence of any inappropriate comments about her age.

These cases underscore the need to be careful not to make age-related comments in the workplace, especially by supervisors. While these comments are not actionable in and of themselves, they can be evidence of discriminatory intent on the part of the employer.

■ COLLECTIVE RIGHTS

Under the National Labor Relations Act and Labor Management Relations Act (NLRA), employees have the right to form a union (self-organize) and to engage in concerted activities without coercion, restraint, or interference from the employer. It is an unfair labor practice for employers to interfere with the right to self-organize. The National Labor Relations Board (NLRB) enforces the act and conducts hearings to settle issues when there are disputes between employers and employees who are protected by the act.

■ ENVIRONMENTAL HEALTH
   AND SAFETY

Hospitals and other healthcare organizations are increasingly responsive to concerns raised about environmental health and safety in an effort to protect workers and patients. Various organizations, including the American Nurses Association (ANA) have joined to form "Hospitals for a Healthy Environment," which is a national movement advocating for environmental sustainability in health care. This has led to efforts to "green" healthcare organizations. Another group working to improve environmental health and safety is the nonprofit group Health Care Without Harm (HCWH). Nurses play a key role in the organization's efforts, and there is a HCWH nurses work group that is dedicated to implementing environmentally responsible practices in their hospitals. Initiatives include elimination of mercury and reduction or elimination in the use of toxic chemicals, such as PVC and DEHP contained in vinyl plastics used in medical devices such as feeding tubes. Consumer protection groups and professional organizations have also advocated for improved labeling of medical devices to warn of these dangers. In 2002 the Food and Drug Administration (FDA) issued an advisory recommending the avoidance of using medical devices containing PVC and now warns healthcare providers to use non-PVC devices on at-risk patients. Medical supply companies have responded by developing environmentally preferable medical products, such as latex and PVC-free products.

Other workplace exposures of concern include lead and thimerosal (used as a preservative in multiple-dose vaccines) exposure for pediatric patients and pregnant healthcare workers and exposure to hazardous chemicals, such as chemotherapeutic agents, while on the job. In one Massachusetts hospital, nurses and other employees experienced headaches and wheezing during floor stripping and waxing procedures. The Massachusetts Nurses Association, as the collective bargaining agent, worked to have HEPA filter fans used to absorb the fumes during this process after there was an unsatisfactory response from managers. Nurses are advised to document and inform managers of any symptoms related to hazardous workplace exposure (Watts, 2008). Such harmful exposures would also likely violate Occupational Health and Safety (OSHA) standards. In any case employees are entitled to information contained in Material Safety Data Sheets (MSDS) about any chemicals they are exposed to. The National Institute for Occupational Safety and Health (NIOSH) has listed occupational asthma as a high priority concern.

In 2001 Brooks, a surgical technician in an operating room (OR) sued the manufacturer of a bone cement for failure to warn of product dangers that she was exposed to for several years (*Carol Jean Brooks v. Howmedica, Inc.*, 2001). Brooks was exposed for about 4 days and 10 surgeries per week from 1982–1992 during the mixing process for Simplex P Radiopaque bone cement (Simplex). During the mixing process a liquid and powder are mixed releasing vapors classified as hazardous by OSHA. Brooks developed a cough in 1990 and in 1991 was told she had asthma. An occupational health physician at the hospital reviewed the Material Safety Data Sheet (MSDS) for the chemicals in the cement and talked with the manufacturer's chemist, but the investigation did not link her cough to Simplex. The employer did restrict her exposure to the chemicals in Simplex thereafter. However, Brooks was later diagnosed with occupational asthma caused by exposure to the chemical in the bone cement and was unable to work after 1995. Her employer, St. Luke's Hospital, intervened in the lawsuit seeking to recover compensation from defendant manufacturer Howmedica for workers' compensation benefits and other costs paid to Brooks.

Defendant Howmedica introduced evidence of stringent premarket approval for a New Drug Application (NDA) by the FDA, which approved its product labeling and package insert before the product was released to the market in 1971. This insert contained warnings of the highly volatile and flammable nature of the liquid requiring adequate air circulation and to prevent excessive exposure to the vapors that may produce irritation to the respiratory tract, eyes, and possibly liver. Subsequently they added more warnings for possible contact dermatitis and damage to soft contact lenses through exposure, as well as recommending eliminating the maximum amount of vapor with adequate ventilation. Brooks testified that she had never read the product warnings in the package. The appeals court affirmed the judgment of the district court and granted summary judgment for the defendant manufacturer. The court found that federal laws regulating safety and labeling of medical devices and drugs (the 1976 Medical Devices Amendments to the Federal Food, Drug, and Cosmetic Act) preempted any state claim that would require different labeling and standards. Because this area is already regulated by the federal government, states cannot impose different regulations that may conflict with federal regulations. These different

and conflicting state requirements could arise during lawsuits.

Even though Brooks was not able to successfully pursue a claim against the manufacturer, individual rights may arise under different theories of liability. Nurses are cautioned to be aware of workplace exposures to chemicals and to read all product labels and warnings. Nurse managers and supervisors should also be advocates of environmental health and safety to avoid any claims of corporate liability as a result of employee injury, and to ensure that OSHA and other standards are met.

■ REFERENCES

Carol Jean Brooks v. Howmedica, Inc., 273 F.3d 785; 2001 U.S. App. LEXIS 26357; CCH Prod. Liab. Rep. P16, 208 (2001).

Eileen M. Simonson v. Trinity Regional Health System, 336 F.3d 706; U.S. App. LEXIS 14201; 92 Fair Empl. Prac. Cas. (BNA) 470; 84 Empl. Prac. Dec. (CCH) P41,444; 14 Am. Disabilities Cas. (BNA) 1118; Accom. Disabilities Dec. (CCH) 11-026 (2003).

Sherryl Perry v. St. Joseph Regional Medical Center, 110 Fed. Appx. 63; 2004 U.S. App. LEXIS 18165 (2004).

Throneberry v. McGehee Desha County Hospital, 403 F.3d 972; 2005 U.S. App. LEXIS 5865; 150 Lab. Cas. (CCH) P34,973; 86 Empl. Prac. Dec. (CCH) P41, 906; 10 Wages & Hour Cas. 2d (BNA) 807 (2005).

Wanda Woodson v. Scott and White Memorial Hospital, 2007 U.S. App. LEXIS 24702 (2007).

Watts, N. (2008, Winter). Massachusetts RNs address hazards of environmental cleaning chemicals. *NENA Today*, 3.

Wendy Elwell v. University Hospitals Home Care Services, (2002). 276 F.3d 832; 202 U.S. App. LEXIS 23; FED App. 0017P (6th Cir.); 145 Lab. Cas. (CCH) P34, 429.

■ ADDITIONAL RESOURCES

Hospitals for a Healthy Environment: www.h2e-online.org

National Institute for Occupational Safety and Health (CDC): www.niosh.org

Health Care Without Harm–The Campaign for Environmentally Responsible Health Care: www.noharm.org

Chapter 32

Contracts

Susan J. Westrick

A Elements of a Contract

1. Offer — must be definite and certain
2. Acceptance of the offer must be clearly communicated
3. Consideration or something of value that is bargained for (quid pro quo)
4. Mutual assent or consent to the terms of the offer
5. Capacity to contract

C Termination of the Contract

- Fulfillment of the terms and conditions
- By mutual consent of the parties
- Release of the contract obligations due to changed circumstances
- Breach of contract by 1 party not fulfilling its terms

B Defenses to Contract Enforcement

- Lack of any essential element of the contract
- Duress or undue influence of a party
- Illegal contract
- Unequal bargaining power between the parties

D Remedies for Breach of Contract

- Monetary damages including compensatory and special damages
- Specific performance for contract involving unique goods, but not for personal services
- Injunction to prevent action by 1 party
- Mediation
- Arbitration

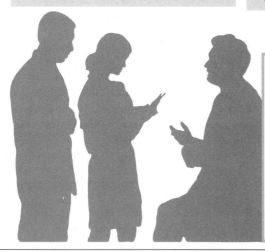

E Practice Pointers

- Do not make specific promises about outcomes of care or guarantee results from treatment.
- Be aware you may be an agent of your employer and may be contracting on his or her behalf.
- Check and follow any agency policies on contracting or witnessing contracts.
- Contract principles will be used in individual or collective bargaining for employment.

Contract law governs agreements between parties to do or refrain from doing something. A contract is defined as a legally binding and enforceable agreement between two or more parties. Contracts between parties are usually made and enforced as part of a business relationship. Nurses most often are involved in contracts that affect their employment. However, it is increasingly common for nurses to be involved in direct contracts with patients or others as part of an agreement to provide services. When operating a business, a nurse may be involved in contracting with others for goods or services.

ELEMENTS OF A CONTRACT

To be legally binding a contract must have certain elements (see **Figure 32-1A**). In addition, there are other rules covering contract formation and enforcement, such as whether modifications can be made orally and whether certain types of contracts must be in writing to be valid. State and federal statutes would need to be considered in particular situations.

TYPES OF CONTRACTS

Express contracts are those in which the terms and conditions have been given orally or in writing by the parties. The terms are expressed in this type of contract. Note that oral contracts are just as valid as written agreements. *Implied contracts* involve terms and conditions that were expected to be a part of an agreement by the parties. A patient going to a physician's office for services constitutes an implied contract, even though no expressed agreement takes place. It is mutually understood by the parties that this is the nature of their implied agreement. *Formal contracts* are those that the law requires to be in writing (e.g., wills, contracts that cannot be performed in less than 1 year, and contracts for the sale of land). The idea is to prevent fraud from occurring with these types of agreements. Most other types of oral contracts are equally as binding and enforceable as written contracts but are often harder to prove. Any agreement that involves substantial consideration (value) by the parties is recommended to be in writing.

DEFENSES TO CONTRACT ENFORCEMENT

Various defenses can be asserted to challenge the validity of a contract (see Figure 32-1B). For example, one could claim that one of the essential elements was not present in the formation of the contract and that the contract

should be null and void. It could be claimed that one party to the contract was under duress or some type of undue influence that should void the agreement. The contract could be illegal and thus unenforceable. In some cases the courts may not enforce an agreement if it finds there was unequal bargaining power between the parties and one party was taken advantage of.

TERMINATION OF THE CONTRACT

A contract may be terminated by various means, one of which is fulfillment of the terms and conditions of the contract (see Figure 32-1C). Another way for the contract to terminate is for one or more of the parties to be released from the contract. A contract may be rescinded by the parties when they both agree they do not want to complete the contract. Another way that a contract can be terminated is by one party breaching the agreement. This occurs when one party fails to perform terms or conditions of the agreement. The nonbreaching party must be able to show that he or she was willing to keep performing the contract and that the breach was unilateral.

In *Thompson v. Friendly Hills Regional Medical Center* (1999), a nurse was discharged for allegedly falsifying her time sheets. She alleged breach of an oral contract not to discharge her without good cause, based in part on statements in an employee handbook. Although the handbook stated that the employer was an "at-will" employer, there were specific grounds and steps outlined for dismissal. The jury agreed that there was an oral contract and that the nurse was wrongfully discharged. Damages awarded to the nurse were upheld after two appeals.

Courts do not always support an employee manual as creating an express contract. In *Pavilascak v. Bridgeport Hospital* (1998) a licensed practical nurse had received an employee handbook upon being hired by the defendant hospital. The nurse asserted that because this manual contained the employer's benefit plan, wage increases, and periodic performance review material that the manual, in effect, created an implied contract. However the court did not accept this argument and furthermore pointed out that the employee manual permitted the hospital to discharge employees "with or without cause, at any time." Thus, the court reasoned that it would be illogical to infer that the hospital had made a promise to keep employees as long as they performed satisfactorily.

■ REMEDIES FOR BREACH OF CONTRACT

The nonbreaching party to a contract may have certain remedies available in a claim for breach of contract against the breaching party (see Figure 32-1D).

1. Monetary damages, the most common type of remedy, may include not only compensatory damages for the loss of the value of the contract but also special damages, such as punitive damages meant to punish a party for wrongdoing or bad faith in the agreement. The type of damages that each party is entitled to may be spelled out in the agreement and is referred to as liquidated damages.
2. Specific performance of the contract may be ordered by the court when no other remedy is appropriate. This may be the remedy when the contract called for a special order or unique goods. Contracts for personnel services are not usually enforceable by specific performance.
3. Injunction or an order to prevent a party from doing something might be ordered.
4. Mediation is a process that allows the parties to settle a dispute, which may be based on a contract, without going to court. A mediator is a neutral third party who works with the parties to reach a mutually satisfactory settlement.

5. Arbitration is another process used to avoid litigation. A neutral third party (an arbitrator) is appointed to consider both parties' interests. The arbitrator is empowered to settle the dispute in the fairest way for both parties.

■ NURSES AND CONTRACT LAW

Nurses may be involved in negotiating a contract for employment either individually or as part of a union, which involves a collective bargaining process. During these proceedings the nurse is aided by a basic knowledge of the principles of contract law. By making the terms of the contract explicit, there will be less chance of misinterpretation in the employment situation. The rights and duties of each of the parties to the agreement will be clearer and easier to enforce.

The terms of any contract must be complied with by employees. In *Villarin v. Onobanjo* (2000), a home health aide allegedly left the home of a severely disabled man before the shift was over. The aide worked for an agency that had contracted to be with the patient when family members were not present. After the aide had left and before a family member arrived home, a fire broke out in the house. When the family member rushed in to save the man, they both died in the fire. The court found that if the facts as alleged were true, both the aide and the agency could be liable for the patient and family member's deaths. The agency had a duty to ensure that the actual services were provided as specified in the contract. The appeals court reversed the dismissal of the lawsuit and allowed the case to go to a jury.

Some types of promises that a nurse makes to a patient could be viewed by the court as creating a contract (see Figure 32-1E). For example, a nurse should not promise any particular cure or outcome when agreeing to provide services. Nurses who contract individually with patients may be more subject to this risk than those who are employees. However, a nurse may be considered an agent of the employer and able to contract on behalf of the employer. One needs to exercise caution in entering into contracts with patients for direct services; seeking legal advice is recommended. Agency policies also may give guidelines concerning responsibilities in contracting with patients, such as in the home care situation.

It is especially important in home care to make sure that patients are terminated properly from service because this may become a contract issue. In *Winkler v. Interim Services, Inc.* (1999), several elderly and disabled patients were notified that services were being terminated by the agency. The patients alleged that this constituted abandonment and breach of contract by the agency. Because they heavily used services, these patients claimed that they were terminated because they were economically undesirable to the agency and were being discriminated against. The court found that the patients were terminated when new Medicare reimbursement rules went into effect and that they were protected by the federal Rehabilitation Act of 1973. In finding for the plaintiffs, the court stated that the home health agency had no right to unilaterally and arbitrarily suspend its obligation under the contract just because it was not profitable to service these clients.

■ REFERENCES

Pavilascak v. Bridgeport Hospital, 48 Conn. App. 580 (1998).

Thompson v. Friendly Hills Regional Medical Center, 71 Cal. App. 4th 544, 84 Cal. Rptr. 2d 51 (1999).

Villarin v. Onobanjo, 276 A.D.2d 479; 714 N.Y. S.2d 90; 2000 N.Y. App. Div. LEXIS 9892 (2000).

Winkler v. Interim Services, Inc., 36 F.Supp. 2d 1026 (M.D. Tenn. 1999).

Chapter 33

Corporate Liability

Susan J. Westrick

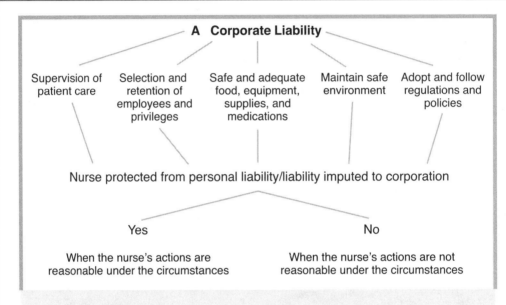

A Corporate Liability

- Supervision of patient care
- Selection and retention of employees and privileges
- Safe and adequate food, equipment, supplies, and medications
- Maintain safe environment
- Adopt and follow regulations and policies

Nurse protected from personal liability/liability imputed to corporation

- **Yes** — When the nurse's actions are reasonable under the circumstances
- **No** — When the nurse's actions are not reasonable under the circumstances

B Suggestions to Protect Nurses Employed by Corporate Employers

1. Be familiar with the corporate employer's rules, regulations, and policies and follow them as closely as possible.

2. Notify the corporate employer verbally and in writing of the lack of adequate and safe equipment, medications, food, and supplies.

3. Keep a lookout for an unsafe environment, taking the patient's needs into consideration. Take appropriate steps to notify the corporate employer and ensure correction of unsafe condition.

4. Notify the corporate employer of known incompetence in accordance with policies.

Corporate liability is the corporate employer's legal accountability for matters beyond the employee's control and in certain circumstances for wrongful conduct of employees. Corporate liability also encompasses the con- cept of a collective failure of the corporate employer to adopt and implement reasonable policies. In the healthcare arena, corporate employers include but are not limited to hos- pitals, healthcare agencies, HMOs, and professional corporations. Five basic duties relative to the delivery of health care apply to all such corporate employers (see **Figure 33-1A**). The legal standard for determining whether the corporate employer is satisfying these duties involves a reasonableness test: whether the corporate employer knew or had reason to know that a question exists. Nurse managers and administrators play a key role in the institution to ensure that proper policies are in place and that staff members follow them.

■ RESPONSIBILITY FOR SUPERVISION OF QUALITY OF PATIENT CARE

The concepts of corporate liability and negligence regarding a hospital's duty to supervise its staff were articulated by the Illinois Supreme Court in the landmark case of *Darling v. Charleston Hospital* in 1965. In this case a patient with a broken leg had increasing signs and symptoms of circulatory impairment, indicating that his cast was too tight. Although the nurses documented their findings including color changes and other significant patient complaints for several days, the physician did nothing to relieve these increasingly dangerous symptoms. Subsequently, the patient's circulation was so compromised from the cast that his leg had to be amputated. The nurses asserted that they had documented their findings and informed the physician, thus ending their duties. The court found, however, that the hospital, through its employee nurses and staff, has a corporate duty to ensure safe care for patients. As part of the evidence it was revealed that there was a hospital policy that staff were to go to their supervisors or beyond if they knew or should have known there was a threat to patient safety. Therefore, the nurses had a duty to go beyond the physician if there was not an adequate response to protect the patient. Part of the corporate responsibility is to provide compe-

tent qualified healthcare providers and to monitor and enforce its patient care policies.

Supervision of patient care includes the obvious professional and nonprofessional employees as well as independent contractors to whom the corporate employer has granted privileges (e.g., nurse midwives, nurse anesthetists, and nurse practitioners who are self-employed by some other professional corporation or medical/surgical group). The corporate employer has a duty to exercise reasonable care to find out if a question exists as to the competence of these individuals. The corporation may be put on notice by a particular reported event, such as a nurse anesthetist being impaired. However, even if there is not an actual notice, the corporation has a duty to affirmatively discover any such problems. Hence, the nurse may be either required or asked to participate in quality assurance practices so that problematic trends can be detected.

■ CORPORATE LIABILITY FOR ACTS OF EMPLOYEES

Courts may take different views as to what extent and under what conditions the corporation will be liable for the acts of employees. In *Whittington v. Episcopal Hospital* (2000) the appeals court affirmed the judgment of the trial court in finding corporate negligence and direct liability for failure to formulate, adopt, and enforce adequate rules and policies to ensure quality care for patients. Plaintiffs filed a wrongful death and survival action following decedent's death at the hospital. The patient had presented at the hospital at term with classic signs and symptoms of preeclampsia pregnancy-induced hypertension (PIH), including headaches, edema and 2+ proteinuria. Plaintiff's physician expert witness testified that instead of admitting her and delivering the baby as required by the standard of care, she was discharged and came back 8 days later to have labor induced. He further opined that additional breaches of the standard occurred when after the patient returned she was left in the waiting room for 13 hours instead of being admitted immediately to labor and delivery. Patients with PIH were to be admitted and monitored immediately, according to defendant hospital's own protocol. There were delays in starting her on antihypertensives in spite of consistently elevated blood pressures. After undergoing an emergency C-section she developed pulmonary edema and acute adult respiratory syndrome resulting in her death. The hospital was held liable for a portion of the damages under a corporate negligence theory, in part because the plaintiff's expert testified that the nurses should have prevented the patient from being discharged the first time as a high risk patient who had been incompletely evaluated. The expert opined that

> the nurse has an obligation to go to her supervisor and inform the supervisor of this problem that has developed. And the supervisor takes it from there to resolve this conflict of discharging the patient. It's called the chain of command. And it has to be used. It should be used. And the chain of command can go all the way to the chairman of the department or the director of nursing. (Whittington v. Episcopal Hospital at p. 460; emphasis added in case report)

In contrast, in McDonald v. Chestnut Hill Hospital (2005) an expert witness testified that the hospital nursery staff nurses negligently failed to follow hospital protocol as to when a glucose "heel stick" should be performed. The parents alleged that the hospital and personnel had failed to timely diagnose signs of hyperinsulinism in their newborn, which resulted in permanent brain damage. However, the court pointed out that there was no criticism of the protocol itself or that the staff was unaware of it. Without more evidence of the hospital's direct part in this, the court said it would not extend corporate liability for

alleging that particular nurses had not followed the protocol. This testimony failed the test of the hospital having "had actual or constructive notice of the defects or procedures which created the harm" in addition to a deviation from the standard of care.

■ DUTY REGARDING SELECTION AND RETENTION OF EMPLOYEES

The corporate employer must exercise due diligence in investigating the background of those working in the facility, including professional and nonprofessional staff and independent contractors (e.g., physicians, nurse practitioners, and midwives with privileges who are not employees). Investigating the background involves ordinary care in checking references, past employment history, skill and educational levels, criminal background checks, and licensure. This duty includes checking the National Practitioner Data Bank (NPDB) that became effective in 1990. The NPDB includes all actions taken by a state against a practitioner's license. Other information available through this resource includes medical malpractice payment awards and Medicaid or Medicare exclusion lists. Any facility or hospital responsible for credentialing employees is allowed access. Another data bank, the Health Care Integrity and Protection Data Bank (HIPDB), was created as part of HIPAA legislation in 1996 to protect against fraud and abuse in the delivery of health care. It reports similar information, including criminal-related healthcare convictions, state disciplinary actions, or licensure actions. Insurance companies or self-insured agencies must also report payments made for judgments or settlements.

If such investigation reveals or even suggests a question concerning the individual's qualifications, the corporate employer has a duty to limit or deny that individual's application. Liability can also attach to nonemployees who actively participate in any such decisions. For example, a nurse serving on a review committee, board of directors, or search committee may be held personally liable for decisions made as a member of the same.

■ DUTY TO PROVIDE ADEQUATE AND SAFE EQUIPMENT

In addition to adequate and safe equipment, the corporate employer has a duty to the patient to provide, maintain, and select adequate and safe medications, food, and supplies that are reasonably suited for the purpose for which they are intended. The nurse regularly deals with issues concerning equipment, medications, food, and supplies. For example, under a reasonableness test a cardiac monitor used by the nurse need not be state of the art as long as the patient's needs are met. In considering whether food is reasonably suited for its purpose, preparation of the food and suitability of the diet are paramount issues, as is whether the food is served to the patient at a proper or improper time.

Part of the employer's responsibility includes training staff to properly use the equipment. In *Chin v. St. Barnabas Medical Center* (1998), a patient undergoing a hysteroscopy in the OR died as a result of improper connection of a hose to an exhaust line instead of the suction line. Although the OR nurse was not responsible for the improper connection, she testified that she was not familiar with the equipment and had not been trained how to use it. The hospital, through its employees, was held liable for the improper use of the equipment in the OR on a corporate liability theory.

If the employer does provide adequate and safe equipment and the nurse elects to utilize some other equipment or improperly uses the equipment provided, it is unlikely that liability will be attached to the corporate employer. Instead the nurse will likely be held liable for his or her own actions.

■ DUTY TO MAINTAIN SAFE PREMISES

The corporate employer has a duty to maintain a safe environment. The legal standard relative to maintaining a safe environment is the reasonableness test. The corporate employer must take reasonable care to maintain the premises safely. This duty incorporates a duty to protect patients, employees, and others lawfully entering the premises. It includes protection from known dangers as well as inspection of the premises for the purpose of discovering and correcting dangers. Particular emphasis must be placed on maintaining an environment appropriate for the unique infirmities of the patients (e.g., railings in hallways, wheelchair ramps). Oftentimes the employer requires that the nursing staff keep a log of defects in the patient care unit (e.g., broken side rails or wheelchairs, malfunctioning monitors or oxygen outlets) and then notify the appropriate department for rectification. If the nurse discovers an unsafe condition, steps must be taken to correct the unsafe condition and include but are not limited to such actions as removing malfunctioning equipment, blocking off spills on the floor, and notifying the supervisor or other departments.

■ DUTY TO ADOPT AND FOLLOW PROPER REGULATIONS AND SAFETY PROCEDURES

The corporate employer has a duty to adopt and follow safety procedures that are reasonably calculated to protect patients and others, including the protocol for inspecting, discovering, and correcting dangers to maintain a safe environment. In addition, this pertains to the duty to reasonably anticipate safety procedures necessary to prevent attacks and injuries caused by another person, to prevent escape, and to prevent self-injury. The nurse should expect the corporate employer to have security measures in place to protect the nurse from attack in all areas on the premises, elevators, and parking areas. Furthermore, there must be protocols and policies in place for the nurse to follow when caring for a combative or self-abusive patient. Policies and procedures concerning restraints are also crucial. A claim may be brought against a corporate employer for failure to adopt and enforce proper regulations.

■ NURSES' RISKS AND REMEDIES

As discussed, notwithstanding corporate liability issues, a nurse's negligent actions will prevent liability from being imputed to the corporate employer. Whether the nurse is an employee of a corporation or is granted privileges by the corporation, corporate liability will not protect the nurse from personal liability arising out of the nurse's own negligent

actions. However, if liability arises out of matters beyond the nurse's control, the nurse will be protected under the corporate liability theory of law. The suggestions in Figure 33-1B will help protect the nurse when employed by any type of corporate employer.

■ REFERENCES

Chin v. St. Barnabas Medical Center, 711 A.2d 352 (N.J. Super. A.D. 1998).

Darling v. Charleston Memorial Hospital, 33 Ill.2d 326; 211 N.E. 2d 253; 14 Atl.3d 860 (1965).

McDonald v. Chestnut Hill Hospital, 2005 Phila. Ct. Com. Pl. LEXIS 273 (2005).

National Practitioner Data Bank (NPDB). (n.d.). *Homepage.* Retrieved October 7, 2008, from http://www.npdb-hipdb.com

Whittington v. Episcopal Hospital, 2000 Pa. Dist. & Cnty. Dec. LEXIS 361;44 Pa.D.&c.4th 449 (2000).

Chapter 34

Employment Contracts and Unionization

Susan J. Westrick

Rights of Employees

Employee at Will	Contract, Union, or Collective Bargaining Agreement
1. Employment may be terminated at will of employee or employer without cause.	1. Terms of agreement specify rights and responsibilities.
2. Employee manuals usually outline rights and responsibilities.	2. Union represents employees in contract negotiations.
3. There is a public policy exception to firing an employee without cause.	3. Private sector employees are governed by NLRA and NLRB.
4. Firing related to complaints about the employer and violations of health and safety statutes may be protected by whistle-blowing statutes.	4. Staff nurses acting as supervisors of assistive personnel may be excluded from unions.
	5. Grievances are filed when employee asserts a contract violation.
	6. All steps in grievance procedure must be strictly followed.

Nurses comprise a substantial part of the employee workforce in health care and need to know basic rights and responsibilities related to their employment status. These are influenced by the type of employment agreement, whether there is a formal contract governing the relationship, and whether or not the nurse belongs to a union. In addition, various state and federal laws and regulations impact particular situations.

■ CONTRACTUAL EMPLOYEE

Most nurses are employed under the terms and conditions specified by a written contract. A *contract* is a legally binding, enforceable agreement between two parties. It should specify basic features of the employment relationship, such as specific duties and obligations of the employer. It should include benefits, salary, terms of employment, evaluation methods, and terms and conditions of discharge or termination. Each party must adhere to the terms of the contract. Breach of contract by one party would give rise to rights by the other party, perhaps to terminate the agreement. For example, if an employee agrees to float to various work sites but then refuses to do so when properly trained, a breach of contract by the employee has occurred. As long as a contract is in place, both parties are bound to its terms and conditions. If any changes in the contract are desired, they must be negotiated, agreed to, and become part of the contract.

■ EMPLOYMENT AT WILL DOCTRINE

If a nurse does not have a contract of employment, the employee at will doctrine governs (see **Figure 34-1A**). Under this doctrine employees are free to take a job or not, and the employer is free to terminate the employee at will. This concept gives employers freedom to hire, retain, or terminate employees with or without just cause (even if they have excellent performance evaluations). Conversely, the nurse can quit the job for any reason at any time. However, it is customary to give either party a reasonable notice to this effect, normally a period of 2 weeks.

■ EXCEPTIONS TO THE EMPLOYMENT AT WILL DOCTRINE

Over the years courts and laws have carved out exceptions to this doctrine that have eroded its sometimes harsh effect (see Figure 34-1A). One of the major exceptions to termination at will is the *public policy* exception. Under this exception the court has found the discharge to be wrongful if the employee was fired while promoting a desirable public policy or performing a public duty. An example is when an employee reports violation of a statute by the employer or has been terminated for serving on a jury. Usually the court requires the public policy to be grounded firmly in constitutional or statutory rights, and some courts have cautioned against further erosion of the doctrine. Specific *whistle-blowing statutes* protect employees who report health and safety violations of employers. Currently there is variation among states and courts as to when this exception is allowed, and decisions based on similar fact patterns have differed in various jurisdictions.

Another exception is when the employer has an employee manual that specifies conditions before termination. The court will require the employer to follow the manual even if it is not a formal written contract. Some courts have supported an exception based on the doctrine of "good faith and fair dealing" that protects against grossly unfair terminations.

■ UNIONS AND COLLECTIVE BARGAINING AGREEMENTS

Recently, more nurses have become employed in organizations where employees are unionized (see Figure 34-1B). Federal or state laws govern federal government and public employees. Other employees in the private sector are governed by the National Labor Relations Act (NLRA) and the board that implements this federal legislation, the National Labor Relations Board (NLRB). Unions bargain collectively for the nurses represented by them. In most cases nurses are in their own bargaining unit, which facilitates negotiations related to their unique concerns (mandatory overtime, patient–staff ratios, salary, benefits). The collective bargaining process joins together employees and generally results in greater benefits for all than could be achieved by an individual.

As part of the collective bargaining process, both management and the union must bargain in good faith until settlement on the issues takes place. Often there is mediation or arbitration in the process by a neutral party appointed by both sides to represent them. Binding arbitration is when an arbitrator chosen by both sides makes a final decision, which is then binding on both parties. The final contract is enforceable and gives rise to significant rights by both parties to the agreement. Nurses must be familiar with the terms and conditions of any collective bargaining agreement in place where they are employed.

■ REPRESENTATION OF NURSES

Nurses may be represented by an independent union, a state-affiliated nurses' association, or the United American Nurses (UAN) of the ANA as the bargaining agent. The UAN was formed in 1999 as an association of state nurses' associations that represent nurses. It also serves as a representative for nurses in states where the state nurses' association does not engage in collective bargaining.

When forming unions or engaging in collective action, employee nurses follow rules established by the NLRB or federal or state law that govern the election process. Generally a majority of employees in an institution must support unionization and selection of the bargaining agent. Formal steps must be taken by employees to ensure compliance with the process. It is an unfair labor practice for an employer to prevent or retaliate against employees who are attempting to organize a union when this is permitted by law. However, rules and procedures need to be followed as set forth by the official governmental agency, usually the NLRB.

Many nurses who favor collective bargaining prefer to be represented by the state-affiliated nurses' association because these organizations promote high-quality patient care as well as nurses' professional interests.

■ STAFF NURSES AS SUPERVISORS

A recent concern of staff nurses involving their right to be represented by unions is the question of their supervisory status. Under the NLRA, supervisors are excluded from protection because they are considered to be management. The definition of *supervisor* under the act typically has included those who have the right to hire, fire, evaluate, assign, or direct other employees. The courts in some recent cases have supported excluding from the NLRA the LPNs working in nursing homes while supervising aides. This is of concern to nurses who also delegate and perform some of the tasks defined as *supervision*.

In 2001 the US Supreme Court examined the issue of supervisory status of staff nurses

in *National Labor Relations Board v. Kentucky River Community Care, Inc.* (2001). Kentucky River Community Care (KRCC) refused to bargain with the union, which had won the election at a residential center for services for the mentally ill. Among those certified in the bargaining unit by the NLRB were registered nurses (RNs), licensed practical nurses (LPNs), and rehabilitation counselors and assistants. KRCC asserted that the nurses were supervisors and thus were improperly included in the bargaining unit. The Sixth Circuit Court of Appeals rejected the NLRB's reasoning for inclusion of the nurses in the bargaining unit and determined that RN tasks, such as directing aides in patient care and acting as the highest ranking employee in a building, were not routine but supervisory in nature. Furthermore, they found the RNs could "write up" rehabilitation staff, call employees in to work, and supervise the work of LPNs.

On appeal the Supreme Court supported the position that the party asserting supervisory status (normally the employer) has the burden to prove the supervisory status of the employees in question. Additionally, the Court affirmed the Sixth Circuit's decision to exclude RNs from the bargaining unit but differed in its interpretation of whether the use of "independent judgment" made the RN duties not merely routine or clerical in nature. The Supreme Court found that nurses use independent judgment and act as supervisors, even when they use their professional training, and not hierarchical authority to direct others. The Court also determined that the NLRB used an incorrect test to determine supervisory status and that use of the NLRB test would remove almost everyone from the definition of supervisor.

The result of this case indicates that the issue of RNs as supervisors remains dependent on a fact-specific basis because only general guidance was provided, but many feel that the result represents a threat for unionization of nurses in the future. The Court did not determine that all staff nurses are supervisors but left open other avenues to evaluate their status.

During this case, the American Nurses Association advocated for nonsupervisory status of the RNs and filed an amicus brief with the Supreme Court to support the NLRB position. The ANA and other professional nursing organizations are currently working on clarifying this issue and are advocating to keep staff nurses under the protection of the NLRA.

■ GRIEVANCES

An employee who feels that the terms and conditions of employment have been violated

by the employer can file a grievance. If a union is involved, the grievance is handled through union representatives. If there is no union, the employee manual should specify steps and rights in the grievance process. In all cases the employee must follow the steps carefully and adhere to all deadlines. Courts require employees to exhaust all these available internal remedies before any legal action can be taken. If there is no formal grievance procedure, nurses are advised to provide documentation in writing to their supervisor in a timely manner.

■ REFERENCE

National Labor Relations Board v. Kentucky River Community Care, Inc., U.S.121 S.Ct. 1861, 149 L.Ed.2d 939 (2001).

Chapter 35

Employment Status Liability

Susan J. Westrick

A Vicarious Liability

1. Respondeat superior — employer's liability for negligent acts of employees
2. Ostensible agency — implied by the law when circumstances reasonably lead patient to conclude a non-employee is acting for the employer

B Independent Contractor

1. One who is hired for a specific purpose, usually to provide a service
2. Responsible for own liability in most cases; may share liability under some circumstances

C Employment Relationship/Setting Liability

1. **Supervisors** — liable for own decisions related to hiring and assignment of staff as well as providing supervision; not liable for acts of competent worker under supervision
2. **Student nurses** — individually liable for acts they are competent to perform; instructor or preceptor may share liability; held to standard of reasonable prudent nurse
3. **Private duty nurses** — usually independent contractors with individual liability; work as coworkers with staff nurses but does not have employment status with the institution
4. **Agency nurses** — employed by an agency that contracts with a third party for temporary employment; agency usually carries malpractice insurance; must follow NPA for state practicing in; work as coworkers with staff
5. **School nurses** — usually employed by school board but may work for a public health agency; respondeat superior typically applies with employer; employer usually carries insurance
6. **Government employed nurses** — may have special doctrines or immunities; federal employees protected by Federal Tort Claims Act, which makes the government the defendant

---

The employment status and practice setting of nurses impact on issues related to liability. As an employee, the nurse retains individual responsibility for actions but usually shares this liability with the employer. The patient or plaintiff is not allowed a double recovery for damages but can sue more than one person or party in alleging that an injury occurred through negligence of an employee.

■ VICARIOUS LIABILITY THEORIES

In addition to the principle of personal liability, there are several theories involving vicarious or substituted liability (see **Figure 35-1A**). Because of a special relationship between the parties, the law makes an additional party responsible for the acts of another. The idea of vicarious liability is to allow the injured party greater access to recovery for damages, usually from the employer for the negligent acts of an employee. This extends liability to the person or agency who hired the individual who caused the harm. Doing so encourages employers to use care in hiring qualified individuals while providing adequate supervision and evaluation of their employees. Employers are usually in a better position to insure against these claims and to share the burdens and risks associated with employment. The employee is usually under the direct control and supervision of the employer, which makes the imposition of vicarious liability equitable. Thus important public policies are encouraged by this practice.

The doctrine of *respondeat superior,* or "let the master answer," is used when it is determined that the servant (or nurse) is under control of the master (or employer) and that the negligent act was within the scope of employment of the employee. Duties for which the nurse is employed would be included in this principle. In contrast, when a nurse acts outside the scope of employment (e.g., removing surgical stitches in an institution where only physicians are allowed to do this procedure), the principle of respondeat superior would not apply.

Another theory of vicarious liability that could be applied is ostensible agency (i.e., an institution can be liable for the acts of a nonemployee under certain circumstances). Ostensible agency is implied by the law when the circumstances indicate to the patient that the individual is representing the institution (e.g., student nurses or other practitioners who are nonemployees but appear to be acting as employees). The implied ostensible agency relationship would make the institution liable for the acts of the nonemployee.

■ INDEPENDENT CONTRACTORS

There is no vicarious liability relationship with the institution when the negligent actor is an independent contractor, a person who contracts with another to provide a service (see Figure 35-1B). A nurse hired to be a private duty nurse by the patient or the institution may be an independent contractor. The key to determining whether one is an independent contractor is whether the person is subject to the control of the other party with respect to completing the task. As nurses move into roles that are more independent and consultative, they will more often become individually liable for any negligence and be removed from shared liability with employers.

■ EMPLOYMENT RELATIONSHIP/ SETTING LIABILITY

The specific employment status of nurses influences their liability to patients. The setting in which nurses work also influences the situation (see Figure 35-1C).

Supervisors

The nurse is often in a situation where he or she is supervising others (e.g., nurse manager or supervisor, staff nurse supervising other nurses, patient care assistants, home health aides, or student, private duty, or agency nurses). In this role the supervising nurse is independently responsible and accountable for supervisory decisions. For example, the nurse would be responsible for decisions related to assigning these individuals to patients and for providing proper guidance and supervision for them. The supervisor is not automatically responsible for any mistakes of these individuals if they become liable for negligent acts. The supervisor has the right to expect others to competently perform tasks while acting within the scope of their employment. The principle of personal liability remains in effect.

Students

A student nurse caring for patients is also individually liable to patients for his or her actions. The student nurse is held to a standard of care that is equal to that of an RN performing the task; patients are entitled to this standard in all their care involving professional nursing interventions, regardless of whether a student provides that care. Instructors, other supervisors, or preceptors who make assignments to the student nurse based on skills and capabilities also may be held liable if they have improperly assigned or supervised the student nurse. Other entities that may be held vicariously liable include the educational institution where the student is enrolled and institutions where student nurses' acts may fall under the theory of ostensible agency. Usually schools of nursing or agencies require student nurses to carry individual liability insurance for their role as a student nurse. Sometimes schools purchase a liability policy that covers all nursing students during their clinical experiences.

In the case of *Austin v. Children's Hospital Medical Center, Susan Hall, and Xavier University* (1996) a student nurse was assigned to care for a 2-year-old postoperatively who had undergone a bone marrow transplant and was in an isolation room. The patient subsequently developed a viral infection that caused his death, and his parents brought a wrongful death action against the hospital, the student nurse Susan Hall (as a named defendant), and the university where the student was enrolled. The university settled with the plaintiff before the case went to trial.

Although the plaintiff lost the case against both defendants on the issue of causation, the facts related to the student nurse's conduct contained substantial issues of negligence and failure to follow the standard of care. Among these were that the student told the patient's mother that she had a "scratchy throat" while caring for the child. The student nurse had also entered the room at least once without a mask on, and then later left early that day because she had a fever. Facts presented in the case raise concerns of individual judgment in caring for a patient when one is showing signs of an illness that most likely would put a patient at risk, especially one who is immunocompromised. It is unclear who assigned the student to this patient, but the faculty supervisor or staff preceptor could be liable for negligent supervision if either had knowledge of the student's illness but allowed her to care for the patient anyhow. However, the student remains individually accountable for following protocols and care standards related to bone marrow transplant patients, which would indicate that potentially infective caregivers should not be assigned to these patients.

Private Duty Nurses

Patients may employ a private duty nurse as an independent contractor who would be solely responsible for his or her own liability. It is prudent for a private duty nurse to have a written contract with the employer. Sometimes a hospital may hire a private duty nurse for a patient, and under certain circumstances the hospital also could be liable for the nurse's negligent acts under the theory of ostensible agency. Staff or supervisory nurses employed by the hospital are still responsible for providing appropriate supervision for the private duty nurse and are still responsible for the patient. However, they all share responsibility for care of the patient. Private duty nurses are advised to carry their own liability insurance policy.

Agency Nurses

Nurses are increasingly employed by proprietary agencies that contract with third parties to provide temporary services. Agency nurses are employees of the agency, which typically provides liability insurance for the nurses. The agency is responsible to hire qualified and competent nurses for particular assignments. Staff and supervisory nurses in an institution remain responsible for the patients cared for by agency nurses and often share liability, even though there is no employer–employee relationship between agency nurses and the institution. Agency nurses must follow the policies and procedures of the institution. All nurses caring for patients on a particular unit need to function in a cooperative atmosphere to ensure the best care for patients. The relationship between agency and staff nurses is one of coworkers, and liability issues remain the same in most instances. Some agencies employ traveling nurses who go to other states for more extended lengths of time but are still in temporary positions. These nurses must be licensed in the state where they will be working. One must also be familiar with the specific NPA in that state and follow its rules and regulations.

In some circumstances, an agency nurse may be considered a "borrowed servant" and thus the "borrower" or employer may become vicariously liable for the negligent acts of the "borrowed" employee. A case in point is *Brown v. Dekalb Medical Center* (1997) where the defendant nurse was an employee of Star Med Staffing, Inc. (StarMed), a medical personnel staffing service that contracted with the hospital for nurse Simmons to work in the hospital's emergency room (ER). The plaintiff's estate alleged that nurse Simmons

negligently administered a dose of Zestril, knowing that the patient, Mr. Brown, was allergic to this medicine. In fact, Mr. Brown (the patient decedent) had come to the ER at 8:30 p.m. the evening before for treatment of an allergic reaction to this same medication and was still a patient in the ER when an additional dose was given. Nurse Simmons apparently administered a dose of Zestril the next morning at 4:00 a.m. after the patient's wife brought the medication to the hospital from home on instructions of the physician. The nurse stated he gave this dose on verbal instructions of the physician, even though the patient's chart indicated the patient was allowed nothing by mouth (NPO). The patient's wife informed the doctor of this administration and expressed concern as to its potential harm, but Mr. Brown was discharged from the ER and told to see the doctor at his office the next morning. The patient experienced another allergic reaction at 5:00 the next morning and died due to airway obstruction from a severely swollen tongue.

In determining who should be liable for this series of allegedly negligent acts, the agency nurse's employer, StarMed, was named as a defendant. The appeals court confirmed the trial court's finding that in these circumstances nurse Simmons was a "borrowed servant" of the hospital and relied mainly on the issue of "control" that the hospital had over nurse Simmons's actions, including the exclusive right to fire him if his performance did not meet the hospital's employment standards. Therefore, the motion for summary judgment that was granted to StarMed was upheld, and the agency had no liability for nurse Simmons's actions.

School Nurses

The nurse who works in a school system is often employed by the school, which shares liability with the nurse. The doctrine of respondeat superior usually applies. Other school nurses are provided by public health agencies to the schools.

Government Employees

If a nurse is an employee of a governmental agency, special doctrines or rules may apply. Some governmental agencies have immunity from liability for their employees. Federal government employees have the protection of the Federal Tort Claims Act, which substitutes the federal government as the defendant in most cases.

In all situations the principle of individual accountability is still present. While liability may typically shift to employers or others, the judgment against a nurse can remain as an individual responsibility. This underscores the need for nurses to be protected adequately with individual or employer liability insurance, or both.

■ REFERENCES

Austin v. Children's Hospital Medical Center, Susan Hall and Xavier University (1996), 92 F.3d 1185, 1996 U.S. App. LEXIS 22329.

Brown v. Dekalb Medical Center (1997), 277 Ga. App. 749; 490 S.E.2d 503; 1997 Ga. App. LEXIS 951.

Chapter 36

Staffing Issues and Floating

Susan J. Westrick

How to Float Safely — Essential Steps

1. Find out as much as possible about the assignment.
2. Assess skill, experience, and training.
3. Limit your assignment to less routine and less specialized tasks. For example, administer only medications that are familiar to you, such as pain medications, but not unit-specific intravenous medications.
4. Utilize all resources. Request to partner with a regular staff member who will mentor and monitor your assignment, or who is coassigned to your patients.
5. Refuse assignment if unqualified and seek alternative sources of care.
6. Express specific concerns to supervisor.
7. Follow up in writing as soon as possible if assignment is refused.
8. Consider whether refusing the assignment leaves the patient without any nurse. Doing so may be considered patient abandonment.
9. Never "walk off" the job.
10. Familiarize yourself with your employer's policies and regulations.
11. Request inservices/training for new information and refreshing skills.
12. Volunteer to cross-train in areas you are most familiar with. For example, cross-train among different pediatric units, or more than one intensive care unit.
13. Indicate you are willing to work on another unit as long as support and guidance are available to ensure patient safety.
14. Follow all institutional guidelines for floating and cross-training, even if accepting an assignment with reservation. Otherwise, you may face employer discipline or discharge.

Always put patient safety first!

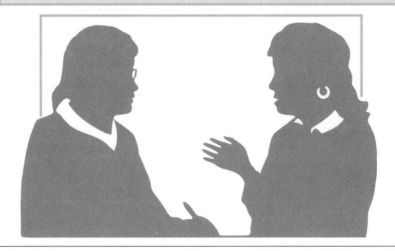

EMPLOYER'S RIGHT TO ASSIGN NURSES ACCORDING TO STAFFING NEEDS

With few exceptions (see the last section in this chapter) employers have the right to designate the nursing unit to which a nurse is assigned in accordance with the needs of the patient population. The employer has a legal duty to provide professional nursing staff in sufficient numbers to meet the needs of the patients. Any unit that does not meet this standard is considered to be understaffed. Therefore, the employer has an affirmative obligation to "float" nurses to units that are otherwise understaffed if there are no other solutions to the problem. Because of the nursing shortage and chronic staff shortages in many patient care areas, the Joint Commission now requires facilities to have a system of cross-training to ensure competency when staff are asked to work on other units. Float staff that have less familiarity and comfort with new areas increase liability for the institution. There are recurring problems with administering medications that are unfamiliar to the nurse and this increases the chance for errors. Therefore, in addition to ensuring competence of any reassigned or floated staff, proper administrative support must also be given to the nurse.

THE NURSE SHOULD BE QUALIFIED FOR THE ASSIGNMENT

Because the employer must provide nursing staff to meet the needs of patients, the nurse must be qualified to meet those needs. First and foremost, the nurse is personally liable for his or her own conduct. This is further articulated in the American Nurses Association's *Code of Ethics for Nurses with Interpretive Statements* (2001) which states that nurses bear primary responsibility for the nursing care that patients receive and are individually accountable for their own practice. If the nurse knowingly undertakes actions for

which the nurse is not qualified, the care provided is likely to deviate from the standard of care. In such an event the nurse is at risk for a nursing malpractice claim. The fact that the employer assigned the nurse to the nursing unit is not a defense. Therefore, the nurse must first ascertain the unit to which he or she is being "floated" and the nature of the responsibilities on that unit. It's imperative that the nurse ask the supervisor as much as possible about the type of unit, diagnoses/needs of the patients, and whether the assignment entails "charge" responsibilities. Nurses accept or reject specific role demands based on their education, knowledge, competence, and extent of experience.

If the nurse is told to provide care for which he or she is unqualified, it's very important for the nurse to ask whether an experienced staff member or in-service instructor is available to instruct or supervise. If so, then the nurse is competent to provide the specialized care under the instruction and supervision of the experienced staff member unless it is established that certification in a procedure or classroom/in-service instruction is mandatory. If an experienced staff member or in-service instructor is available to teach the procedure and answer questions during the nurse's shift, the nurse should consider these factors.

When such information is obtained, the nurse should then assess his or her own skills and experience to determine whether he or she is qualified. If the answer is yes, the nurse must do so. If the answer is no, the nurse must put the employer on notice. In making these decisions, consultation and collaboration with other nurses and health professionals is the key to effective workplace harmony while effectively meeting patient needs.

THE EMPLOYER MUST BE PUT ON NOTICE IF THE NURSE IS NOT QUALIFIED

When the nurse has determined that his or her level of skill and experience is unsuitable for the assignment, the nurse must advise the person making the assignment. This applies regardless of whether the person making the assignment is the charge nurse, nurse manager, supervisor, etc. The nurse should be as specific as possible about the reasons for refusing the assignment rather than simply refusing to take care of the patient. If the person making the assignment will not or cannot change it, and appropriate supervision is not available to the nurse, the nurse should voice the specific concerns to that person's supervisor. Soon after the nurse should document this verbal exchange in the nurse's personal notes. Doing this most often shifts the burden of liability to the employer, who has the control over staff assignments. It's also a good idea for the nurse to keep a personal written account of the events for the nurse's own records, and to establish a pattern or trend through this documentation.

From a practical standpoint, the nurse has only two choices: either the assignment can be accepted or refused. If the nurse accepts the assignment, all efforts should be undertaken to prepare as much as possible. The nurse should utilize all resources available, such as consult with coworkers, review equipment manuals, and review hospital policy and procedure manuals. (See **Figure 36-1** for steps to take when floating.)

If the nurse elects to refuse the assignment, it's imperative to keep in mind that doing so may subject the nurse to disciplinary action or even termination. In most instances, the nurse is an "at will" employee of the employer. This means that the employee can self-terminate at any time for any reason, and the employer can terminate at any time for any reason. However, if the employer has terminated the nurse for refusing an assignment that would place patients at risk, the nurse may have recourse against the employer for wrongful discharge. A wrongful discharge

claim will be successful if the employee can prove an improper reason for the dismissal. An "improper reason" in this context is generally defined as a violation of public policy. In one case, a nurse anesthetist claimed that she was constructively discharged (compelled to resign due to intolerable conditions) from the employer hospital for refusing to work with an impaired anesthesiologist. The nurse asserted that the alleged constructive discharge was in violation of public policy or, in other words, injurious to the public. The court held that there was no violation of public policy because the nurse did not prove that the physician was impaired. Hence the wrongful discharge claim did not prevail because the nurse could not prove the public was at risk because of an impaired anesthesiologist.

■ CASE LAW INVOLVING FLOATING AND REASSIGNMENT

Two cases with different outcomes illustrate concepts involved in floating nurses to units where they did not regularly work. In *Winkelman v. Beloit Memorial Hospital* (1992), a nurse who had worked exclusively in the newborn nursery was asked to float to a postoperative and geriatrics unit. Nurse Winkelman told the supervisor that she did not float and that when she was hired in 1971 she was told she would work only on the newborn nursery. The floating assignment to the other unit was limited, did not include team leading, and followed guidelines established by defendant hospital in 1987 regarding floating from the maternity ward. This guideline required all nurses to float on a rotation basis. Winkelman claimed she told her supervisor that she was unqualified to float to this unit, and that floating would put the patients and her license at risk, and the hospital in jeopardy. According to nurse Winkelman she was given three options: float, find another nurse to float for her, or take an unexcused absence day. Her supervisor,

Linebarger, said she gave her only two options; to float or find a replacement. Winkelman went home and later received a letter stating that her actions constituted a voluntary resignation. She denied that she had resigned and sought reinstatement which the hospital refused.

Winkelman later filed a complaint against Linebarger with the state board of nursing, alleging that she violated board rules by assigning her to float the another unit which was not commensurate with her abilities and could present harm to a patient. The board made an investigation and later dismissed this claim, although board members did not interview nurse Winkelman or her coworkers. Winkelman, as an employee-at-will then sued the defendant hospital for wrongful discharge alleging her employer's actions violated an important public policy. The basis of this public policy is the board of nursing rules and regulations that state that a nurse could be disciplined for performing services for which the licensee is not qualified. The jury found that this was a public policy exception and that Winkelman was wrongfully discharged and awarded damages. The Supreme Court of Wisconsin upheld the judgment and found that a public policy exception could be found in well-established administrative rules, and is not limited to statutes or constitutions. The court further commented that the nursing rules allowed a nurse to refuse an assignment in a questionable area, and that the employer should provide for the nurse's further education and training to work in that area.

In another similar case, nurse Francis was asked to float to an orthopedics unit from his regular assignment to the intensive care unit (*Francis v. Memorial General Hospital*, 1986). Nurse Francis refused to float because he did not feel competent to act as charge nurse on that unit, and was suspended for two days. Upon his return he gave notice that he would

not float if he felt incompetent to take an assignment. The hospital offered to orient him to all other units to facilitate his ability to float. He declined this offer and was suspended indefinitely. In his claim for wrongful discharge, the court found that the employer was permitted to discharge Francis since he was offered a solution to become competent for floating assignments, but refused. Unlike in *Winkelman*, discussed above, the hospital in *Francis* fulfilled its duty to assist an employee for cross-training and helping employees to gain competence to work on other patient care units.

■ PATIENT SAFETY COMES FIRST

The paramount priority for both the nurse and the employer is the safety of the patient. The hospital/employer has a duty to provide *adequate* staff. The nurse has a duty to exercise a *reasonable* degree of care and skill. Less than optimal staffing requires a balancing of safety issues. Remember the standard for care is not perfection but rather is a standard requiring reasonable care. If no other option for the patient exists, the nurse should accept the assignment and proceed in a manner as safe as possible.

■ EXCEPTIONS TO THE EMPLOYER'S RIGHT TO FLOAT NURSES

There are limited exceptions to the employer's right to float nurses. If the nurse is a member of a collective bargaining unit (union), the collective bargaining unit's contract with the employer may specify if and when a nurse may be floated. The nurse should be familiar with the terms of the contract. In the event that an employer attempts to float a nurse in contravention of the terms of any such contract, the nurse should still express concerns to the person making the assignment as previously described. In addition, the collective bargaining unit will very likely have an established procedure for the nurse to follow under these circumstances.

The other exception is if the nurse has an employment contract directly with the employer. If so, the terms of the contract control. If the contract is silent relative to the floating issue, the best course of conduct is for the nurse to proceed in the manner previously described.

It's important to be aware that an employee handbook can be the basis for an implied contract between the employee and the employer, especially if the employee relies on the information and policies therein. Therefore, it's always prudent to refer to the handbook and, if not already available, this document should be requested.

■ REFERENCES

American Nurses Association. (2001). *Code of ethics for nurses with interpretive statements.* Silver Spring, MD: Author.

Francis v. Memorial General Hospital, 104 N.M. 698; 726 P.2d 852 (1986).

Winkelman v. Beloit Memorial Hospital, 168 Wis. 2d 12; 483 N.W. 2d 211; 1992 Wisc. LEXIS 197; 7 L.E.R. Cas. (BNA) 686 (1992).

Chapter 37

Americans with Disabilities Act

Katherine Dempski

A Americans with Disabilities Act

- Title I prohibits employers from discrimination against disabled but otherwise qualified job applicants. All aspects of employment are covered including the application process, hiring, training, promotion, compensation, and any other terms, conditions, or privileges of employment. It applies to private employers with ≥15 employees, state and local governments, and labor unions.
- Title II prohibits state and local government programs and activities from discrimination against disabled individuals including structural accessibility requirements.
- Title III prohibits private entities that provide public accommodations and services (such as health-care institutions and physician's offices) from denying their goods and services to disabled individuals based on the disability. Structures must be accessible.
- Title IV requires that telecommunication devices and services such as interpreters be available for the hearing and speech impaired.
- Title V includes the miscellaneous provisions necessary for the construction and application of the act.

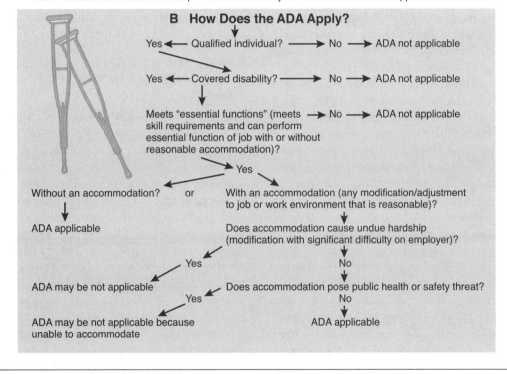

B How Does the ADA Apply?

Qualified individual? — Yes / No → ADA not applicable

Covered disability? — Yes / No → ADA not applicable

Meets "essential functions" (meets skill requirements and can perform essential function of job with or without reasonable accommodation)? — No → ADA not applicable / Yes

Without an accommodation? → ADA applicable

or

With an accommodation (any modification/adjustment to job or work environment that is reasonable)?

Does accommodation cause undue hardship (modification with significant difficulty on employer)?

Yes → ADA may be not applicable

No → Does accommodation pose public health or safety threat?

Yes → ADA may be not applicable because unable to accommodate

No → ADA applicable

Congress passed the Americans with Disabilities Act (ADA) in 1990 with the goal of encouraging disabled individuals to participate in work and social environments by discouraging discrimination. The law is intended to balance the needs of disabled citizens with the ability of public and certain private entities to reasonably accommodate those needs without causing an undue hardship. The act does not give an individual any unfair advantage. It seeks to end discrimination of qualified disabled individuals by removing barriers that would prevent them from the same opportunities as others. The ADA has five titles (see **Figure 37-1A**).

■ COVERED DISABILITIES AND REASONABLE ACCOMMODATIONS

The ADA applies to those with an impairment that substantially limits major life functions. A disability is defined as a mental or physical condition that substantially limits a major life activity, such as seeing, hearing, speaking, walking, breathing, performing manual tasks, learning, caring for oneself, and working. The act is more clear on what it does not cover, such as nonchronic illnesses and impairment from current illegal drug use. Covered impairments are constantly evolving, but generally the act applies to alcoholism, epilepsy, paralysis, HIV infection, AIDS, mental retardation, and specific learning disabilities.

A qualified individual with a disability is one who meets the skill, experience, education, or other requirements of employment and can perform the "essential functions" of the position with or without a "reasonable accommodation." The term *essential functions* refers to the ability to perform the job requirements with the exception of marginal or incidental job functions. *Reasonable accommodation* is any modification or adjustment to the job or work environment that will assist the qualified individual to perform essential job functions. This includes adjustments that give the qualified individual the same rights and privileges enjoyed by the employees. When a qualified individual can perform essential job functions except for marginal functions, the employer must consider whether the individual could perform those functions with a reasonable accommodation. The employer is only required to accommodate a known disability. Employers are not required to lower the quality of standards and are not obligated to create a position that does not exist. *Undue hardship* is an "action

requiring significant difficulty or expense." An accommodation for the qualified individual must not pose an undue hardship on the employer. Undue hardship is not the only limitation on an employer's requirement to reasonably accommodate a qualified individual. Public safety and health must always be considered (see Figure 37-1B).

Hospitals are not required to eliminate essential job functions, such as lifting, moving, or positioning patients or equipment. Therefore, a reasonable accommodation did not exist when the nurse had an injury that limited her ability to perform these functions (*Gunertne v. St. Mary's Hospital*, 1996; *Stafford v. The Radford Community Hospital Inc.*, 1995). An offer of inferior position with less benefits is not a reasonable accommodation (*Norville v. Staten Island University Hospital*, 1999).

■ HOW THE ADA AFFECTS NURSES AS EMPLOYEES IN THE PREEMPLOYMENT PHASE

The employer may not ask an applicant to take a medical examination before a job offer is made. Employers may not make a preemployment inquiry into a disability but may ask about a disability as it applies to the performance of specific job functions. Employers may condition job offers on a post-job offer physical examination that is required of all employees at the same level. The reason for not hiring an applicant after a post-offer physical examination must be related to business necessity. Testing for illegal drug use is not considered a medical examination; therefore, an employer may test and make employment decisions based on the results. However, this information must be treated the same as a confidential medical record.

An employer may establish qualifications standards that exclude qualified disabled individuals, such as HIV positive people, who pose significant risk of substantial harm known as a "direct threat" to the health and safety of others but only if the direct threat is not eliminated or minimized by a reasonable accommodation. The employer must use objective medically sound reasoning to establish the risk.

How the ADA Affects Nurses as Employees

Employers are only required to accommodate a known disability; therefore, the employee is responsible to tell the employer of a need for an accommodation. The employee may disclose only as "a disability under ADA" with the need for accommodation, but the employer may ask for medical documentation. The employer is then required to take steps to ensure confidentiality by separating medical records from the employee personnel file.

Uniformly applied leave policies do not violate the ADA when there is no apparent discrimination to the disabled worker. However, the employer may be required to modify a leave policy upon a qualified individual's request unless it would cause an undue hardship.

The ADA differs from workers' compensation programs in that workers' compensation applies when an employee is injured on the job. A work injury would have to fit into the act's criteria for "qualified disabled individual" to fall under the protection of the ADA.

■ PUBLIC ACCOMMODATIONS IN THE HEALTHCARE SETTING

Physicians' offices, pharmacies, inpatient and outpatient healthcare institutions, and long-term care facilities fit into the act's definition of *public accommodations*. The act also considers establishments that provide a "significant" amount of social services to be places of public accommodations. Therefore, certain group homes, independent living centers, and retirement communities will come under the act if they provide enough social services.

As public accommodations, healthcare providers must provide access to these services by accommodating "service animals"

that are trained to perform tasks for the handler. Service animals differ from therapy animals that provide comfort. Therapy animals are recognized as clinically beneficial but do not provide a task under the ADA.

■ HOW THE ACT AFFECTS NURSES AS HEALTHCARE PROVIDERS

Public accommodations, such as healthcare institutions and physicians' offices, must provide auxiliary aides and services. Individuals with hearing impairments should be provided with qualified interpreters, assistive listening devices, note takers, or written material. Vision-impaired persons must be provided with qualified readers, taped texts, or large print or braille materials.

There are limits to the length a public accommodation must go to reasonably accommodate disabled individuals, such as a direct threat to public health and safety or a fundamental disruption to services provided. Service animals are a medical necessity for the handler; therefore, local health codes that prohibit animal entry for infection control and food service safety do not apply. Accommodation of the service animal in the healthcare setting includes ensuring there is no direct threat to public safety and health by consulting infection disease, providing a private room, and reassigning staff members who have allergies. Staff members are not required to care for the animal because the handler is responsible to provide care or make care arrangements if he or she is unable to do so personally. The accommodation need only be reasonable and not cause a fundamental disruption to providing healthcare services (see **Figure 37-2**).

As patients' advocates, nurses must always be aware of their institution's policy on providing auxiliary aides to a disabled patient or the patient's disabled family member. Having such a policy in place did not shield a hospital from liability when the nurses did not know how to implement the policy.

May do:

- Ask "is this a service animal?"
- Ask what tasks the animal is trained to perform.
- Ask the handler to remove a service animal that is out of control of the handler or that poses a direct threat to the health and safety of others.
- Require the handler to provide water, food, and exercise to the animal.
- Require the handler to ensure that the animal is taken to a proper location to relieve itself.

May not do:

- Ask the handler about his or her disability.
- Ask for "certification" or other proof of service dog status (there is no requirement that the animal must wear a vest or tags that identifies it as a service animal).
- Deny accommodations based on another's allergies or discomfort (allergies that fit under "disability" must be accommodated as well as the handler's disabilities).

Figure 37-2   Service animals.

■ REMEDIES FOR NONCOMPLIANCE

The ADA provides plaintiffs in private causes of action with an injunction against the defendant. Upon finding a violation of the act, the court may order an injunction, which prohibits the defendant from continuing the unlawful behavior or commands the defendant to correct any wrong done to the plaintiff. Monetary remedies are not generally available under the act except in specific circumstances. The attorney general must be involved in the case and make a request in federal court for the plaintiff to be awarded monetary damages. The attorney general usually makes the request in cases where the defendant has established a pattern of discriminatory behavior or exhibits discriminatory conduct that rises to the level of public concern. In those cases the court may grant an injunction, award monetary damages to the aggrieved party, and assess a civil penalty. The court will take into consideration any good faith effort by the defendant to comply with the act.

■ REFERENCES

Aikens v. St. Helena Hospital, 843 F.Supp. 1329 (N.D. Cal. 1994).

Gunertne v. St. Mary's Hospital, 943 F.Supp. 771 (S.D. Tex. 1996).

Norville v. Staten Island University Hospital, 196 F.3d 89 (2d Cir. 1999).

Schmidt v. Methodist Hospital, 5 AD Cases 1340 (7th Cir. 1996).

Stafford v. The Radford Community Hospital Inc., 908 F.Supp. 1369 (W.D. Va. 1995).

Chapter 38

Employees with AIDS/HIV Infection and Exposure to Bloodborne Pathogens

Katherine Dempski

Source Testing

- Employee is responsible to wash skin, flush mucous membrane, notify supervisor, initiate medical evaluation, and complete a worker's injury report
- Medical management includes evaluation and treatment within a few hours of exposure to determine bona fide exposure
- Initiate risk assessment and request that the employer have a physician seek the source's consent to be tested
- Initiate postexposure prophylaxis based on risk no more than 2 hours postexposure per policy

---

Nurses have a duty to not negligently expose patients to infectious diseases, including diseases from other patients as well as from the nurses themselves. Although there are state and federal statutes that protect the confidentiality of HIV-positive employees, HIV-positive nurses must find the balance between maintaining their own confidentiality and not exposing others to the infectious disease while performing professional duties. Likewise, healthcare agencies have a duty to not negligently expose employees in the performance of their duties and must have in place policies and procedures for exposure prevention as well as a robust postexposure procedure.

■ OCCUPATIONAL EXPOSURE

Healthcare facilities may be liable to healthcare providers and others within the facility when exposure to HIV occurs due to negligence. The viability of the case depends on the individual facts, the legal theory the case is brought under, and the state's laws. A plaintiff will have to prove either that actual exposure (such as a needlestick with HIV positive blood) to the infectious disease occurred or that the fear of becoming HIV positive due to the exposure is "reasonable." Usually under tort law a plaintiff cannot sue for mental anguish unless it is associated with a physical injury, but some courts have ruled that the reasonable fear of being HIV positive is a compensable injury.

A nurse who sued for negligent infliction of emotional distress after being exposed to a needlestick from an AIDS patient had her case dismissed for failure to show that her emotional distress was based on an actual exposure and was based on a reasonable response to the actual medically demonstrated risk of contracting the disease. The nurse was tested periodically and after 6 months had not contracted the virus. Medical testimony was admitted that if she were to test positive, there was a 95% chance of it happening in the first 6 months. Beyond that 6 months, any emotional distress was, as a matter of law, unreasonable (*Ornstein v. NYC Health and Hospitals Corp.*, 2006).

To qualify for workers' compensation, individual state laws require employees to provide documentation on the circumstances of the work-related exposure. To rule out preexisting HIV infection, the employee will be required to have a confidential HIV test within a few days (usually less than 10) of the exposure.

A nurse who claimed emotional distress causing a mental impairment was entitled to a percentage of workers' compensation after a needlestick injury. The court heard testimony on both sides as to the feasibility of the nurse converting to HIV positive but held there was no evidence that she suffered a mental impairment (*Stout v. Johnson City Medical Ctr.*, 1995).

The Needlestick Safety and Prevention Act (2001) requires employers to document and review annually their exposure control plan that shows the evaluation and implementation of safer needle devices, and they are required to involve nonmanagerial employees in identifying and choosing safer devices. The employer must maintain a confidential log of injuries from contaminated sharps that includes:

1. Type and brand of devices
2. Department in which the injury occurred
3. Explanation of how the injury occurred

The act applies to any facility under OSHA where employees may be exposed to blood or other infectious materials.

■ NURSES' RIGHTS WITH A BLOODBORNE PATHOGEN EXPOSURE

Healthcare providers must follow strict statutory guidelines when obtaining a patient's informed consent for HIV testing. Even nurses who are exposed to a patient's blood products must receive the patient's informed consent before testing the patient. When the patient refuses to have an HIV test, the exposed healthcare provider may seek a court order but must show that he or she has a bona fide exposure and his or her rights to the informa-

tion of HIV status from the known source outweighs the source's right to refuse.

The statutes vary in each state, but the following is a general example of the process (see **Figure 38-1**). The healthcare worker must have a "bona fide exposure" during his or her occupational duty. A bona fide exposure is generally defined as exposure to blood, visibly bloody fluid, or other potentially infectious material to a puncture wound that breaks skin, mucous membrane exposure (such as splash to the eye), or prolonged exposure to skin (which may be cut or abraded). An incident report describing the incident and identifying witnesses must be completed. OSHA requires that the employer attempt to obtain voluntary consent to the HIV test, and a physician must seek to obtain the consent. Upon refusal, the exposed healthcare provider will need to submit to a baseline HIV test. An evaluation committee made up of impartial healthcare providers will review the incident. This group determines whether the statute's criteria have been met. The healthcare provider may need to seek a court order. The employer of the exposed nurse bears the cost of this process. When the test is done, the confidentiality statute must be followed. The test results may not go into the patient's healthcare record unless the results relate directly to the current medical care. If the patient wishes to receive the test results, then HIV counseling must be offered including the source's right to confidentiality and mandatory disclosure of the results to meet state infectious disease reporting requirements.

■ NURSES' RIGHTS AS EMPLOYEES TO CONFIDENTIALITY

The HIV confidentiality statutes that protect patients give healthcare providers the same rights (see **Figure 38-2**). A hospital has a duty to keep the results confidential under the HIV confidentiality statutes. The ANA supports confidentiality regarding the HIV-positive nurse.

- Right to confidentiality as an employee and a patient
- Right to maintain employment status while competently performing professional duties (HIV is protected disability under the ADA)
- Right to anonymity following an exposure to a patient
- Right to be free from mandatory HIV testing

Figure 38-2   Rights of HIV-infected nurses.

AMERICANS WITH DISABILITIES ACT

HIV-seropositive employees are protected from job discrimination under the ADA. An employer may not fire an employee solely because he or she is HIV seropositive. An employee may be excluded from his or her job position if the infection becomes so disabling as to prevent the employee from competently performing the job functions.

An employer may establish qualifications standards that exclude otherwise qualified disabled individuals, such as people who are HIV positive, when there is a significant risk of substantial harm to the health and safety of others. To exclude the qualified individual, the employer must show that the significant risk poses a "direct threat" to safety and that this direct threat is not eliminated or minimized by a reasonable accommodation. The employer must use objective and medically sound reasoning to establish the risk to others. For example, because HIV is transmitted by exposure to affected blood and not by casual contact, the employer would need to show a work environment where a potential to blood exposure is legitimate.

THE HIV-INFECTED NURSE

Healthcare providers are not required by law to reveal personal information on their health status, including their HIV status. In the absence of a legal duty, however, professional organizations, such as ANA and the American Dental Association, have issued position statements on the ethical obligation of disclosure. The ANA believes that HIV-positive nurses may deliver safe and effective care without compromising the patient and should not be removed from patient care based on HIV status alone.

All nurses have a duty to protect their patients from harm. Therefore, the HIV-infected nurse should avoid exposure-prone invasive procedures. If an exposure to a patient does occur, the HIV-infected nurse has a duty to inform the patient of the exposure and potential risk for HIV infection. This can be done while protecting the anonymity of the nurse. The HIV-infected nurse must understand the duty to not compromise patient care by remaining in a high-risk area of practice for blood exposure (see **Figure 38-3**). Universal precautions as recommended by the CDC must always be followed to minimize risk. Nurses with personal risk factors for HIV have an ethical obligation to know their own HIV status so steps can be taken to minimize risk to their patients.

AGENCY HIV POLICIES

The primary goal of HIV policies is to ensure the health and safety of all employees, patients, and visitors. Policies should reflect the most up-to-date medical and scientific information on the prevention of HIV transmission, postexposure

- Health and safety of patients is primary duty.
- Safeguard patients and the public from spread of HIV.
- Use universal precautions and follow agency policy on proper disposal of infectious waste.
- Avoid high-risk areas of practice for blood exposure and invasive procedures.

Figure 38-3   Duty of HIV-infected nurses.

management, and the implementation of infection control. Staff education and training should focus on infection control and the HIV-positive individual's right to privacy, whether as a patient or employee. Staff members must have useful guidelines on postexposure protocols, such as HIV testing for those who are involved in hazardous waste cleanup. Agency policy must be written to comply with the federal laws involving HIV, such as the ADA and the Rehabilitation Act as well as state laws on workers' compensation and HIV informed consent/confidentiality.

■ **REFERENCES**

American Nurses Association. (1992). *ANA position statement: HIV infected nurse, ethical obligations and disclosures.* Washington, DC: Author.

Cushing, M. (1992). The courts confront occupational HIV. *American Journal of Nursing, 92*(10), 26–27.

Ornstein v. NYC Health and Hospitals Corp., 806 N.Y.S. 566; 2006 N.Y. App. Div. LEXIS 34 (N.Y. 2006).

Stout v. Johnson City Medical Ctr., 1995 Tenn. LEXIS 601 (Tenn. 1995).

The Needlestick Safety and Prevention Act, H.R. 5178, 106th Cong. (2001).

Chapter 39

Impaired Nurses

Susan J. Westrick

A   Indications of an Impaired Nurse

1. Physical and mental
   - Slurred speech
   - Unsteady gait
   - Flushed face
   - Reddened eyes
   - Rapid mood swings
   - Poor personal hygiene
   - Smell of alcohol on breath

2. Work performance
   - Difficulty concentrating or remembering
   - Tardiness or frequent absences
   - Inability to complete work in a timely fashion
   - Prolonged use of private areas and bathrooms
   - Illegible documentation
   - Failure to follow through on tasks and assignments

3. Evidence of diversion
   - Patients complaining of ineffective pain relief
   - Frequent trips to the medication room or cart
   - Discrepancies in narcotic count
   - Reports of excessive waste, breakage, use of prn medications, and illegible or altered medical records
   - Volunteer to administer medications

B Do's	Don'ts
• Carefully consider/monitor and document suspicions by way of *factual*, nonjudgmental information (i.e., discrepancies), patient complaints, and observations and then report information to nursing management for further review and follow-up. • Participate in education and peer assistance programs to increase personal awareness and to assist in the impaired nurse's reentry into the workplace. • Strive to prevent legal implications involving yourself and your employer by responding to the impaired nurse in a timely and professional manner.	• Enable by excusing, ignoring, defending, or justifying. • Confront nurse on your own. • Allow personal beliefs, judgments, or feelings of betrayal interfere with your professional responsibility to assist the impaired nurse. • Look the other way and fail to address the issue of an impaired colleague in the hope you can avoid professional or legal involvement.

One indirect but not insignificant issue that must be considered in patient care is the impaired nurse. As a pattern of impairment unfolds and evolves, the impaired nurse becomes increasingly unable to function cognitively, physically, and emotionally, resulting in unsafe practice. This places patients and the public at significant risk, and the results can be personally and professionally devastating for all involved. The state board of nursing becomes involved, and the licensee can be subject to sanctions including license suspension or revocation.

■ DEFINITION OF IMPAIRMENT/ABUSE

The definition of *impairment* typically includes a dependency on alcohol, drugs, and/or other chemical substances. Impairment also has been associated with psychiatric illness, psychological conditions, and excessive fatigue. *Substance abuse* generally refers to overindulgence or dependence on addictive substances, especially alcohol and drugs. *Dependency* is defined as a state of psychological or physical addiction to a chemical substance. Using prescribed medications such as sedatives, amphetamines, or tranquilizers without a prescription or in greater quantities than prescribed is a form of *drug misuse* that often leads to more serious abuse. Impairment results from the use of these mood-altering substances and leads to an inability to perform professional duties with reasonable skill or safety.

■ INCIDENCE AND ETIOLOGY

According to the American Nurses Association (ANA) up to 10% of nurses have alcohol and/or drug abuse problems and 6% of nurses have problems that are serious enough to interfere with their practice. Because it is well known that these problems are underreported, the actual numbers are likely higher. In most states the majority of nursing disciplinary hearings involve allegations of substance abuse. Some commonly abused drugs are meperidine hydrochloride (Demerol), Vicodin, Percocet, and morphine with workplace theft or diversion noted as the most frequent means of obtaining drugs.

Although no definitive conclusion has been reached as to why nurses become impaired, the frequently cited reasons include chronic pain, low self-esteem, depression, job stress (especially related to critical care nurses), sense of powerlessness, increased workload, extended shifts, and loneliness. Likewise, researchers have struggled to find an explana-

tion as to the process by which impairment occurs. While some believe that chemical dependency is a disease process grounded in physiological and psychological factors, others believe that social factors (e.g., peer influence, exposure to high-risk behavior, ready access to chemical substances, awareness that drugs are effective in solving patient problems, such as pain and anxiety, shift in work setting to less supervised areas, such as outpatient and community health) also play a role.

■ CURRENT ATTITUDES AND FOCUS

In 1984, the ANA took steps to publicly recognize substance abuse as a problem among nurses. Since then, the direction has been to treat and rehabilitate the impaired nurse and to allow the individual to safely return to practice. These goals have found support in a variety of other professional models including state Nurse Practice Acts (NPAs) and the National Council of State Boards of Nursing (NCSBN). Both the ANA and the NCSBN have established formal resolutions seeking the implementation of assistance programs, as well as an increase in education and research. Additionally, many hospitals have enacted policies and procedures governing and addressing issues related to the impaired nurse.

The ANA has supported creating nondisciplinary, peer-assisted programs for nurses across the country. This less punitive approach has been accepted by many state boards of nursing that now allow nurses to enter voluntary assistance programs as an alternative to having their licenses acted upon. Typically the nurse is monitored closely for 2 or more years and must meet all conditions of the program, such as random urine drug screen tests. While in the alternative program and fully complying with its requirements, the nurse will likely be allowed to continue working, possibly with certain restrictions. Employers are informed of the nurse's participation in the program so that reasonable accommodations can be made in the workplace, if possible.

For example, Connecticut has recently passed a law that provides for an alternative to licensure discipline for healthcare professionals, including nurses, who participate in an assistance program, with certain exceptions (Public Act No. 07-103, 2007). The program offers confidential treatment for chemical dependency related to drugs or alcohol. An oversight committee monitors quality assurance of the assistance program and may take corrective action if required. Such laws that incorporate various healthcare professionals and disciplines typically take many years to pass but help to ensure consistency and fairness in the process, as well as more efficient use of resources.

■ IDENTIFICATION OF AN IMPAIRED NURSE

Typically there are signs and symptoms that signal impairment or substance abuse. These most often include changes in physical appearance, work performance, or personal relationships. Additional indicators of drug diversion in the workplace include patients' frequent complaints of inadequate pain relief, or missing doses of narcotics. **Figure 39-1A** lists signs indicating impairment and diversion.

■ ETHICAL AND LEGAL OBLIGATIONS

Coworkers of an impaired nurse often struggle with the ethical issue of whether or not to report their suspicions. Reasons cited for not reporting include loyalty, uncertainty, fear of jeopardizing another's job or license, fear of being labeled a "whistle-blower," and feelings of inadequacy regarding what to do and say. By failing to report, nurses engage in enabling behavior (e.g., ignoring or excusing the activity, taking blame for the situation, defending or justifying the impaired nurse's actions), which serves as an inadequate and improper response.

The ethical dilemma has been resolved, however, by the legal obligation to report, as mandated by many state reporting laws. Such laws generally require that drug and alcohol abuse be reported to the state licensing board. Likewise, the ANA Code of Ethics for Nurses mandates intervention when patient safety is at issue. Provision Three provides that "The nurse promotes, advocates for and strives to protect the health, safety, and rights of patients" (ANA, 2001). Within this provision, how to address impaired practice is presented and suggestions are offered to deal with such a situation. In all instances, patient safety is the overriding concern, but there is also a strong recognition that the impaired nurse or other healthcare practitioner should be advocated for as a colleague who needs appropriate assistance and treatment. The code mandates that in any case where the impaired practice poses a threat or danger to self or others, the nurse must take action to report the individual to persons who are authorized to address the problem.

The guidelines for handling the situation and for reporting are presented in Figure 39-1B.

■ CASE LAW AND LEGAL CLAIMS

1. Retaliatory discharge/reporting impaired nurse: In *Serena Rucker v. St. Thomas Hospital* (2007), a nurse who worked as a patient relations coordinator (PRC) claimed that she was terminated from this position in retaliation for reporting a nurse who was impaired while working at defendant hospital. The Tennessee court of appeals did not agree and affirmed the lower court that nurse Rucker was an employee at will who was offered another nursing job by the hospital but turned it down, and she left the hospital. Furthermore, the hospital offered ample proof of work performance issues including "overstepping her bounds" on several occasions, including

the incident regarding the impaired nurse. A patient in the ICU had reported to nurse Rucker that a nurse caring for her husband had returned from lunch acting strangely and in a manner that led the patient's wife to think the nurse was impaired. Apparently nurse Rucker handled the situation inappropriately by not getting risk management involved and by interfering with the unit manager's ability to handle the situation. Nurse Rucker claimed that this was yet another incident in which she was harassed in her role as the PRC.

2. Americans with Disabilities Act (ADA): The following two cases involve issues related to the ADA, which protects persons from discrimination who have past substance abuse problems or who are currently undergoing treatment. The act does not cover those who currently abuse drugs or alcohol and would present a direct threat to patient health and safety in the workplace.

In *Mary Ann Jones v. HCA Health Services of Kansas, Inc, and Suzan McNett* (1998), nurse Jones claimed she was discharged and discriminated against by not recognizing her drug dependence on Demerol as a disability protected by the ADA. She also claimed that her supervisor, defendant McNett, invaded her privacy in a number of respects. Plaintiff Jones was working at defendant hospital under a Kansas State Nurses Association (KSNA) written agreement as part of a peer assistance program. This program had certain participation conditions and requirements to avoid being reported to the nursing board for disciplinary action. Jones had read and signed the "Peer Assistance" contract, and the employer agreed to conditions specified in the contract. Jones was a clinical manager who worked nights, and as part of her duties she was monitoring a new

graduate nurse whose patient-controlled analgesia (PCA) machine continued to alarm. Nurse Jones borrowed the keys to unlock the PCA machine and to troubleshoot the cause of the problem. Taking control of the keys to any narcotics and signing for "wasting" of medications violated conditions of the peer assistance program. This same day nurse Jones also signed the narcotic log representing that one-half of the drug had been wasted, but in fact she told the new graduate to "save" it in case the patient later requested the other half. This action resulted in the narcotic count being incorrect after the shift. After supervisor McNett suspected that the plaintiff may be impaired because she appeared to be sleepy and glassy eyed (although Jones said she was "wiped out"), she required Jones to provide a urine sample for a drug screen, which later turned out to be negative. The hospital nursing administrator, after reviewing all the facts, decided to terminate Jones. One reason for termination was Jones's violation of the peer assistance contract prohibiting her from handling the narcotic keys or signing for these medications. The district court granted the hospital's summary judgment motion for dismissal, and the plaintiff lost the case on all of her claims, including those related to invading her privacy.

The case of *Jeanne Dovenmuehler v. St. Cloud Hospital* (2006) was also based on ADA claims. Nurse Dovenmuehler applied for a position as an RN in the defendant's Children's Center, one unit of which was a neonatal intensive care unit (NICU). The NICU had private rooms and curtains so that there was no direct visibility into most rooms. After she was hired and 6 weeks into her employment, she revealed that she was under a Minnesota Health Professionals

Services Program (HPSP) plan but did not reveal that she was chemically dependent. She did disclose that she had been terminated from her previous employment for diverting narcotics. The hospital terminated the plaintiff because it determined that it could not assist her in complying with the terms of the HPSP plan. Specifically the defendant employer could not provide for the restriction related to supervised narcotic access in the NICU. Although the plaintiff claimed that the hospital did not reasonably accommodate her disabilities, the court determined that she did not even inform the employer of her impairment and alleged disability, thus they could not reasonably accommodate it. In fact the court also determined that she was not qualified to perform this particular job because the HPSP could not be complied with to provide for patient safety.

3. Evidence of "on the job" impairment/ diversion of drugs in workplace: A nurse was terminated by her employer based on several warnings and incidents related to deficits in patient care activities, including medication administration (*Deborah Alford v. Genesis Healthcare*, 2007). Nurse Alford contended that she was fired for filing a workers' compensation claim after a back injury and sued defendant Genesis Healthcare for wrongful discharge, defamation, and other torts. A few months after this back injury, she told an evening administrator that the medication she was taking for anxiety was making her "woozy." The unit manager then informed her she would have to go home as long as she was impaired. Additional incidents were related to patients' complaints that they did not receive their medications when Alford was on duty and responsible for their care. Other nurses corroborated

that there were medication discrepancies when Alford was working those days, and she did not "count" medications when leaving her shift as required by Genesis. The medication errors were reported to the Maryland State Board of Nursing as required by law. The board gave Alford a choice of facing possible disciplinary action or voluntarily enrolling in a rehabilitation program for nurses facing substance abuse and other illnesses. Alford chose to enter the program and eventually got another nursing position. The district court upheld the defendant employer's motion for summary judgment and found that Alford was discharged for violating defendant's procedures and placing patients' safety at risk. The court also found that the employer had a "qualified privilege" to report to the nursing board and that the reporting statute grants immunity to those who do report in good faith.

4. Off duty conduct considered/refusal of chemical screen test: The North Dakota State Board of Nursing suspended Bonnie Kraft's nursing license for 1 year, and she appealed this decision to the Supreme Court of North Dakota (*Bonnie Kraft v. North Dakota State Board of Nursing*, 2001). The board found that there was ample evidence that nurse Kraft was likely impaired while at work and considered her refusal to submit to chemical testing as an admission of a positive result. On a particular day, she was observed by two doctors and three nurses to have slurred her speech, mispronounced two easy first names of patients, shown problems with equilibrium, laughed frequently, and her breath smelled like alcohol or acetone. After being sent to the ER to be checked, she refused a blood test and was observed by nurses to be red faced with dilated and red-rimmed eyes and to have difficulty

speaking. The defendant medical center's published policy was that refusal to submit to a drug or alcohol test shall be considered a positive test and insubordination, which may result in termination. Kraft contended that she has asthma and sinusitis and had been using inhalers, antibiotics, and cough syrup on the day in question. Additionally, the board of nursing considered her simple assault conviction (that occurred at her home) to be a violation of nursing standards and was related to the practice of nursing. The North Dakota statute permitted the board to take disciplinary action against a registered nurse to suspend, revoke, place on probation, refuse to issue or renew a license, or to reprimand a license if the nurse "has been arrested, charged, or convicted by a court, or has entered a plea of nolo contendere to a crime in any jurisdiction that relates adversely to the practice of nursing and the licensee or registrant has not demonstrated sufficient rehabilitation" (*Kraft*, p. 6).

The court affirmed the board's suspension of her nursing license for 1 year, ordering her to obtain chemical dependency and psychiatric evaluations and assessing a $1000 penalty.

5. Defamation/false accusations of impairment: In a case involving erroneous accusations of diverting and abusing drugs, a nurse unsuccessfully sued her former employer for defamation and intentional or negligent infliction of emotional distress (*Suzanne Govito v. West Jersey Health System, Inc.*, 2000). The court found that the defendant employer's statements were privileged, and the allegedly defamatory statements were made to appropriate recipients in the workplace. The plaintiff nurse could not prove that the speaker knew the information was false or spoke in reckless dis-

regard of its falsity in order to meet the required standard of proof. Plaintiff nurse Govito was an RN in the intensive care unit (ICU) and was working the day an empty morphine tubex syringe was found in the ICU nurses' lounge. After investigating, the head nurse found that the plaintiff had signed out 37% of morphine over the past several months when working. Several days after finding the empty syringe, nurse Govito was led to a meeting with state investigators from the New Jersey State Department of Law and Public Safety, who questioned her about procedures related to morphine administration. Plaintiff told them she had been awake for 24 hours and was too tired to talk to them. On her way out of the meeting she was met by a group of people, including a nurse supervisor and another nurse she knew to be a recovering alcoholic and drug addict. They were there to take part in an "intervention" and proceeded to tell her they knew she had a problem and had a room ready for her at a recovery center. When plaintiff refused this, they attempted to prevent her from leaving, stating that persons in these circumstances often commit suicide. Plaintiff then announced that she quit her job and drove home. Hospital personnel had notified Govito's husband of the situation.

Later blood tests and exams were all negative for any evidence of substance abuse. The state investigator's report included many errors by Govito in signing out and documenting narcotics over a lengthy period of time, and although this behavior is typical of a drug diverter or user, she continued to deny that she was either. She did consent to a 2 year suspension of her nurse's license for documentation infractions but did not reactivate her license because she felt her reputation was irreparably tarnished.

Interestingly, the court also found that a nurse, although not a "public figure," does fall within the scope of "public interest" because the public has an interest in effective delivery of health services. Part of this interest extends to having nurses in the workplace who are not impaired and thus not jeopardizing patient safety. Finding that nurse Govito could not support any of her claims against her former employer, the lawsuit was dismissed.

6. Violation of employee handbook/unemployment benefits: In *Janovsky v. Ohio Bureau of Employment* (1996), a nurse was fired after she was found to have an open bottle of wine in her car in violation of the employee manual's prohibition of having alcohol on the premises. Her employer, Walnut Creek, called the police after a coworker's tip that Janovsky possessed an open bottle of wine in her car. A coworker also alleged that the nurse often went to a grocery store nearby and then was seen drinking from a container in a brown paper bag in the back of her car. After Janovsky turned over the open bottle to the police, she was fired by an administrator for violating the policy, and this constituted just cause for her dismissal. Janovsky subsequently applied for unemployment benefits, which were initially granted by the Ohio Bureau of Employment Services (OBES), finding no just cause for her dismissal. However, the appeals court reversed the trial court and the OBES order and found that the plaintiff Janorsky was at fault. No individual discharged for just cause could receive unemployment benefits, so this was denied for nurse Janovsky.

■ EFFECTIVE PROGRAMS

The key to helping an impaired nurse succeed in recovery and return to practice is an effective diversion program. More than 25 states have implemented such programs, which have been defined by the NCSBN as voluntary, confidential alternatives to licensure disciplinary action. The goal is to enable the nurse to regain productivity, health, and self-esteem.

Additionally, many facilities offer employee assistance programs, which generally provide the employees and family members with access to free, confidential counseling, evaluation, and referral. Sometimes the state board of nursing implements similar programs. The programs usually consist of networks of supervisors who refer the nurse for rehabilitation and document the course of treatment and compliance. In addition, they provide the employer with assurance that the employee is receiving effective treatment and will be able to return to the clinical setting as a solo practitioner.

In addition to a monitored employee assistance program, other tools have been effective in aiding the recovery of an impaired nurse: (1) random urine testing for drugs and alcohol; (2) mandatory attendance to Alcoholics Anonymous/Narcotics Anonymous meetings; (3) back-to-work agreements outlining conditions of continued employment; and (4) restricted practice areas to preclude high stress, high medication usage, and unsupervised shifts and settings. Failure to participate in these programs may prompt the employer to report the RN to the state board of nursing for possible disciplinary action.

■ COSTS AND CONSEQUENCES

A coworker and the healthcare facility may invite litigation if they fail to reasonably recognize an impaired nurse and follow through in an appropriate manner. The implementation of organizational policies and procedures, as well as the promotion of staff education, will aid in effective rehabilitation of the impaired nurse and the avoidance of liability.

Given that impaired nurses commonly divert medication from the workplace as a means of supporting their habit, healthcare facilities should use this cost as a further incentive to timely identify and treat these individuals. Likewise, the financial losses associated with the amount of management time devoted to the issue, as well as the rate of employee turnover or retention, should hasten the decision to implement an effective assistance program.

Certain intangible costs associated with impaired nurses, such as staff morale, quality of care, and erosion of public confidence, are crucial and must be prevented.

■ REFERENCES

American Nurses Association. (2001). *Code of ethics for nurses with interpretive statements*. Washington, DC: Author.

Bonnie Kraft v. North Dakota State Board of Nursing, 2001 ND 131; 631 N.W.2d 572; 2001 N.D. LEXIS 152 (2001).

Connecticut Public Act No. 07-103. An Act Concerning a Professional Assistance Program for Health Care Professionals. (2007).

Deborah Alford v. Genesis Healthcare, 2007 U.S. Dist. LEXIS 26196 (2007).

Janovsky v.Ohio Bureau of Employment, 108 Ohio App. 3d 690; 671 N.E.2d 611; 1996 Ohio App. LEXIS 184 (1996).

Jeanne Dovenmuehler v. St. Cloud Hospital, 2006 U.S. Dist. LEXIS 86914; Am. Disabilities Cas. (BNA) 1561 (2006).

Mary Ann Jones v. HCA Health Services of Kansas, Inc., and Suzan McNett, 1998 U.S. Dist. LEXIS 4419 (1998).

Serena Rucker v. St. Thomas Hospital, 2007 Tenn. App. LEXIS 722 (2007).

Suzanne Govito v. West Jersey Health System, Inc., 332 N.J. Super. 293; 753 A.2d 716; 2000 N.J. Super. LEXIS 249; 16 I.E.R. Cas. (BNA) (2000).

Chapter 40

Sexual Harassment in the Workplace

Susan J. Westrick

A Rights and Responsibilities of Employees and Employers

Employee

- Right to a workplace free of sexual harassment including a nonhostile environment
- Right to have a clearly defined policy by management against sexual harassment in the workplace
- Responsibility to confront harasser, document incident, and report to supervisor
- Right to confidential and timely investigation of a claim by employer
- Right to potential remedies under the law including damages, injunctive relief, and disciplinary action against the harassing employee

Employer

- Responsibility to communicate a clearly defined policy against sexual harassment to employees
- Responsibility to consistently enforce the policy
- Responsibility to conduct fair, confidential, and timely investigation of complaints
- Right to expect employees to report incidents of sexual harassment and to cooperate fully with all investigations
- Responsibility to take steps to prevent incidents of sexual harassment in the workplace

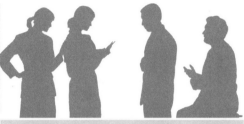

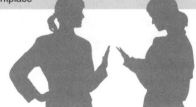

B Steps to Take When Sexual Harassment Occurs

1. Confront the harasser and make it clear that the specific behavior is unwelcome and is interfering with your work performance. Do not send out ambiguous messages through your behavior that could be misinterpreted. Some authorities recommend that you send a return-receipt letter to the harasser so that there is no question that the person has received a clear message.

2. Document the incident in your own notes so that you have a record of the incident or incidents. Record any witnesses to the circumstances and include who you notified of the incident. If the harasser is a patient, you should document the facts objectively in the patient's record and the outcome. In any event, you should keep your own notes of the incident. Employers may have other policies that you need to follow in these situations.

3. Report the incident to your supervisor, who will then be on notice of the situation. If you have a union contract, you may need to report the incident to a union representative who will help you resolve the issue, perhaps through a grievance process.

4. Keep other evaluations of your job performance to show that you have evidence of performing well on the job, if a claim is made by the harasser about your poor job performance in retaliation for your claim of sexual harassment.

Sexual harassment in the workplace has become a growing concern for employees and employers in healthcare settings. Both the intimate nature of contact with patients and a work environment in which there is often power disparity among workers contribute to this problem. Almost all claims of sexual harassment involve complaints by females against male harassers, but females also may be the subject of a complaint. Same-sex harassment can also occur and may be the basis of a valid claim. Sex role stereotypes, socialization of males and females, and traditional power disparities between men and women have contributed to making sexual harassment a sometimes pervasive and underreported situation.

■ SOURCES OF PROTECTION

The primary source of protection against sexual harassment in the workplace is Title VII of the Federal Civil Rights Act of 1964, which bans job discrimination on the basis of sex, race, color, national origin, and religion. Prior to 1980, Title VII did not clearly include sexual harassment as a form of sexual discrimination. Throughout the years courts have extended protection under this law so that various forms of sexual harassment are included. The Civil Rights Act of 1991 contains definitions of sexual harassment that are operative at this time. The Equal Employment Opportunity Commission (EEOC), a federal agency that enforces Title VII and with which a complaint would be filed, has further clarified definitions of conduct and circumstances that constitute sexual harassment. These definitions have been upheld in the federal courts. Additional information and guidelines on sexual harassment are found at the EEOC Web site www.eeoc.gov.

Many states have laws that provide an additional source of protection for workers. Union contracts for employees may explicitly deal with this issue, and most employers provide employment manuals with explicit policies on sexual harassment.

■ DEFINITIONS AND TYPES

Sexual harassment is defined as unwelcome sexual advances or requests for sexual favors or other verbal or physical conduct that unreasonably interferes with job performance.

There are two major categories of sexual harassment as defined by the Civil Rights Act of 1991:

1. *Quid quo pro* or "this for that" sexual harassment involves conditioning job privileges or advancement on granting of sexual favors by the other party. It occurs most often when there is a supervisor relationship with the victim of harassment, and the supervisor has control over the victim. The alleged harassment must have resulted in a loss of job benefits or in a detriment to one's job. Employers have been held strictly liable for the acts of their supervisors in such circumstances. The EEOC guidelines specify that the unwelcome sexual advances may have been made explicitly or implicitly a condition of the job.

2. Sexual harassment in a *hostile work environment* involves sexual conduct such as dirty jokes or lewd remarks, sexual remarks or gestures, pinup calendars or posters, or even sexually suggestive looks or job assignments. The EEOC has included conduct that has the purpose or effect of unreasonably interfering with an individual's work performance or creating an intimidating, hostile, or offensive work environment. Victims of this type of harassment do not need to prove that they suffered an economic loss. It is enough to show that the conduct affected the psychological well-being of the victim. The victim does not have to be the person harassed but could be anyone affected by the offensive conduct. The EEOC has supported claims where pervasive sexual conduct creates a hostile work environment for those who find it offensive, even if the targets of the conduct welcome it and even if no sexual conduct is directed at the persons bringing the claim (*Spencer v. General Electric*, 1988).

The conduct or behavior complained of is viewed from the perspective of the victim, and courts have used the "reasonable woman standard" if the victim is a female. Although there is no universal standard to determine what specific conduct or behavior falls within these definitions, the courts have interpreted the language broadly.

■ EMPLOYER'S LIABILITY

Sexual harassment can occur from supervisors, fellow employees, or patients. Employers have a duty to investigate complaints by employees in a timely manner, maintain confidentiality of complaints, and document claims and their outcomes (see **Figure 40-1A**). It is also unlawful to retaliate against an individual for opposing employment practices that discriminate based on sex or for filing a discrimination charge, testifying, or participating in an investigation, proceeding, or litigation under Title VII. Along with strict liability for supervisors, employers have been found liable for acts of their employees if they knew about the conduct or behavior but did not respond appropriately. Successful claims can result in large legal expenses for employers and have been cited as a cause of impaired productivity, emotional distress, absenteeism, and high turnover of employees.

Employers can be found liable for the acts of nonemployees (or independent contractors) if the conduct creates a hostile work environment for employees and the employer does not address the situation adequately. In *Lisa Dunn v. Washington County Hospital and Thomas J. Coy* (2005), the plaintiff Dunn, a former employee at defendant hospital, alleged that defendant Coy, a physician who had staff privileges, made life miserable for her and other women (but not men) on the staff. Dunn worked as a nurse at defendant hospital, a small hospital of 59 beds, and contended that Dr. Coy, the head of obstetrics and emergency services, repeatedly engaged in conduct of a sexually harassing nature. Dunn filed a claim against him with her employer. The trial court had granted summary judgment for the hospital ruling that the hospital could not control his conduct as an independent contractor and thus was not liable for it. The appeals court, however, ruled that the employer has direct liability to provide a

nondiscriminatory work environment and that they must conduct an appropriate investigation and have a response to the situation. They reversed the lower court's decision on the sex discrimination under Title VII and remanded the case for further proceedings. Part of the evidence of harassing conduct included Coy's statement to Dunn that "paybacks are hell" in implying he would do what he could to impede her career for her filing the claim against him. It was alleged that the hospital did nothing despite similar complaints by other nurses because they didn't want to alienate a "prized rainmaker." At one point in the decision, the court noted that "Dunn did not offer evidence that Coy had damaged other nurses' careers; instead the record shows that she stood up to a windbag." The dissent supported allowing an additional claim for retaliatory discharge because throughout her nearly 2 year period between her complaints to the employer and her resignation, she stated that Coy was pressuring her to withdraw her statement against him. She had informed her supervisors of this and they did nothing. In her deposition Dunn quoted statements from the CEO of also being frightened by Coy's actions and threats.

This case demonstrates that although employers can be held liable for the discriminatory environment created by an independent contractor, the plaintiff nurse will have to bring forward concrete proof of harm. Even though the claim for sexual harassment may be sustained, further proof is needed to hold an employer liable for retaliatory discharge because of it.

At issue in the case of *Gary Hamner v. St. Vincent's Hospital and Health Care Center* (2000) was whether his termination was in retaliation for filing a sexual harassment claim against a physician. Hamner, a charge nurse at defendant hospital, alleged he was harassed by Dr. Edwards, the medical director on his unit. The harassment conduct by Edwards included lisping at Hamner, flipping his wrists, and making jokes about homosexuals.

Hamner filed a grievance with the hospital, which was investigated. After the investigation, Hamner was sent a letter stating that Edwards had been spoken to about the complaints and that Edwards acknowledged his "irreverent" humor and that he would be more mindful of Hamner's concerns in the future. Three days after receiving this letter, Hamner was fired for falsification of a hospital document, the Physician's Order Sheet, where he recorded a patient's code status notation as: "Code C: To be approved by Dr." Hamner alleged in his lawsuit that he had been fired in retaliation for submitting a sexual harassment grievance in violation of Title VII. However, the US court of appeals for the seventh district found that the evidence indicated that the harassment was directed toward the plaintiff's sexual orientation, and not his gender as a male, and therefore was not prohibited conduct under Title VII. The court affirmed the defendant employer's motion for judgment as a matter of law.

Facts involved in another case filed by a plaintiff nurse and former employee were not as clear in terms of proving sexual harassment after she resigned (*Nurse "BE" v. Columbia Palms West Hospital Limited Partnership d.b.a. Palms West Hospital*, 2007). There was evidence that other employees had observed the plaintiff nurse O'Brien having sometimes flirtatious behavior with Dr. Chaparro, the person who had allegedly sexually harassed her. Four nurses and a physician and unit secretary testified about O'Brien's sometimes inappropriate wardrobe and her openly flirtatious behavior with physicians and other staff members. O'Brien testified that she had rebuffed his advances and invitations and had complained to her supervisor about his "harassing" phone calls asking her for dates. She later resigned in light of an investigative report about her complaints that she felt downplayed Chaparro's conduct, and conflicts over her scheduled shifts. O'Brien then filed a lawsuit against Dr. Chaparro alleging

assault and battery and intentional infliction of emotional distress. Ultimately, these claims were settled, but the hostile environment and retaliation claims against Palms West went to a jury trial. The jury awarded the plaintiff $10,000 damages on the hostile environment charge and found no liability on the retaliation claim. The appeals court reversed the award for damages and found that the employer was not put on notice of sexual harassment when O'Brien had reported Chaparro's phone calls as only "harassing," and at that time she did not identify who he was. In looking at all the circumstances, the court found that the employer dealt with the incident appropriately by investigating the claims, meeting with Chaparro to let him know his conduct was out of line, granting her a short leave of absence, and moving O'Brien to another unit to avoid contact with him. Accordingly, the district court's decision was reversed as to the court's denial of judgment as a matter of law in favor of West Palms, and the jury award was vacated.

This case illustrates that evidence of inappropriate behavior on the part of the complainant will undoubtedly weaken any later claim of sexual harassment because the totality of the circumstances will be evaluated.

Employers have a legal and ethical duty to provide employees with a safe work environment, which includes an environment free of sexual harassment. In addition, clear policies against this conduct should be communicated to employees and followed by employers.

■ STEPS TO TAKE WHEN SEXUAL HARASSMENT OCCURS

A series of actions should be taken when a harassment situation occurs (see Figure 40-1B). In all instances the nurse should follow policies set out by the employer for such situations and follow procedures for internal solutions to the problem. If the nurse is not satisfied with this process, he or she can file a complaint with the EEOC and the state human rights commission. If still not satisfied, the nurse may retain an attorney to pursue a civil lawsuit.

■ REMEDIES FOR SUCCESSFUL CLAIMS

When investigating allegations of sexual harassment, the EEOC evaluates the totality of the circumstances including the context of the behavior and the nature of the advances. A determination of the allegations is made on a case-by-case basis.

Injunctive relief in the form of a court order that would require the employer to discontinue the activity or to take steps to prevent the harassment may be available to an employee. If an employee is terminated due to harassment, the court can order reinstatement along with an award of back wages. Courts may grant punitive damages to the employee if the claim involves an especially egregious case against an employer.

Termination of employment of the harasser or transfer to another job is another possible remedy. Disciplinary action of some type is expected against employees who are guilty of sexually harassing other employees. Other types of relief may be granted through state statutes or union contracts.

■ PREVENTION

Both employees and employers can take steps in the workplace to help prevent sexual harassment. One way is for both groups to recognize the seriousness of this issue and its detrimental effects on the work environment. All employees need to know that they have a right to work in an environment free of these concerns (see Figure 40-1A). Employers need to identify high-risk areas for sexual harassment and implement preventative strategies. Staff education regarding specific aspects of the law, as well as prevention strategies, can be an effective way to decrease exposure of employees to situations involving sexual harassment.

There must be top-level commitment to issuing clear and strong policies against tolerating any form of sexual harassment. Employers must strictly enforce these policies and give careful attention and response to alleged claims of sexual harassment. It is unwise to endorse in any way a culture or work environment that condones this type of harassment.

As a victim of sexual harassment, an employee needs to deal with the issue. Not doing so jeopardizes not only the victim's work environment but also that of others. By dealing with the situation, the victim may find that others have been victimized, which makes it easier to establish a pattern of unacceptable behavior or conduct. This prevents the harasser from controlling the situation and will help prevent the physical and emotional cost to the victim and other potential victims.

■ REFERENCES

Davidhizer, R., Erdel, S., & Dowd, S. (1998). Sexual harassment: Where to draw the line. *Nursing Management, 29*(2), 40–44.

Fiesta, J. (1999). When sexual harassment hits home. *Nursing Management, 30*(5), 16–18.

Gary Hamner v. St. Vincent's Hospital and Health Care Center, 224 F.3d 701; 2000 U.S. App. LEXIS 21421; 83 Fair Empl. Prac. Cas. (BNA) 1265; 78 Empl. Prac. Dec. (CCH) P40, 170 (2000).

Lisa Dunn v. Washington County Hospital and Thomas J. Coy, 429 F.3d 689; 2005 U.S. App. LEXIS 24660; 96 Fair Empl. Prac. Cas. (BNA) 1647; 87 Empl. Prac. Dec. (CCH) P42, 181 (2005).

Nurse "BE" v. Columbia Palms West Hospital Limited Partnership d.b.a. Palms West Hospital, 490 F.3d 1302; 2007 U.S. App. LEXIS 16028; 100 Fair Empl. Prac. Dec. (CCH) P42, 882; 20 Fla. Weekly Fed. C 830 (2007).

Spencer v. General Electric, 697 F.Supp. 204 (E.D. Va. 1988).

US Equal Employment Opportunity Commission. (2008). *Sex-based discrimination.* Retrieved October 13, 2008, from http://www.eeoc.gov/types/sex.html

Chapter 41

Violence in the Workplace

Susan J. Westrick

A Suspected Violence against a Patient

- Must protect the patient.
- Legal duty is often based on statutes (e.g., child abuse laws requiring mandatory reporting)
- Ethical duty is based on ANA *Code for Nurses.*
- Maintain confidentiality of patient and integrity of evidence.

B Violence by Healthcare Workers

- Includes verbal, physical, or sexual abuse.
- Includes claims for forcing medications, food, or misuse of restraints or medication for control.
- Must be reported to nurse manager or administration.

C Violence against Healthcare Workers

- Exposed to verbal and physical abuse or injury by patients or families in high-risk settings or by colleagues.
- Can recover workers' compensation claim for injury.

D Documentation and Reporting

- Maintain objective record of all events.
- File any required incident, police, or other reports.

E Prevention and Strategies to Minimize Violence

- Detect early and intervene.
- Teach strategies to deal with stress.
- Make referrals to social or mental health agencies.
- Implement emergency protocols such as for restraints.
- Institute workplace safety programs and security devices.

Violence has become an increasing risk for those in the workplace, with healthcare workers among those most at risk for injury. Nurses are especially vulnerable to violence in high-risk areas of practice such as the emergency department and psychiatric settings, but the problem is greater than before in other patient settings, reflecting the increase in violence in society in general. Among the many factors identified as contributing to this problem are short staffing, exposure to increasing numbers of patients with substance abuse issues, and inability to meet patient and family expectations. Patients who are elderly or very young may be exposed to violence by healthcare workers. It is imperative that nurses be able to safely intervene with effective strategies to protect themselves or others. These strategies must incorporate an awareness of legal rights and responsibilities for all involved.

■ SUSPECTED VIOLENCE AGAINST A PATIENT

A nurse who suspects that violence or abuse has occurred against a patient must document the findings, gather more information from the victim or others, and protect the patient (see **Figure 41-1A**). In many instances (e.g., child or elderly abuse) the nurse has a legal duty to report the abuse, based on mandatory reporting statutes. However, in the case of domestic violence or abuse concerning adults, states vary as to whether reporting by healthcare workers is permitted. Many states require permission of the victim before police or state agencies are notified. This is based on the theory that adults can "speak for themselves" whereas those who are vulnerable because of their age cannot do so.

Whether reporting is mandatory or not, the nurse has an ethical duty to protect the patient, as clearly articulated in the ANA Code of Ethics for Nurses (2001). In addition, a malpractice or other claim could be successful against a nurse for not reporting a suspected incident. This can happen if it can be proved that harm came to the victim because of the failure to report.

In all cases, confidentiality regarding the situation and the victim must be maintained. Permission must be obtained if photographs are to be taken of evidence, unless it involves a mandatory reporting situation. Any evidence must be accurately marked, labeled, and stored in containers that will preserve it and not disturb the "chain of custody." The storage of evidence and the names of who has had access to it are extremely relevant to whether it can be used in any subsequent legal proceeding.

■ VIOLENCE BY HEALTHCARE PRACTITIONERS AGAINST A PATIENT

Violence by healthcare workers against a patient can take many forms: physical abuse, verbal abuse, rough handling, and sexual abuse (see Figure 41-1B). Nurses have been charged with calling patients names, using medications or restraints inappropriately to control patients, and forcing patients to take medicines. If a nurse has knowledge of this behavior

against patients it is suggested that the nurse confront the other healthcare worker about the behavior and report it to the nurse manager or appropriate administrator. Each agency should have a protocol as to how to deal with such situations that must be followed.

■ VIOLENCE AGAINST HEALTHCARE WORKERS

Staff may be vulnerable to violent situations because of their practice settings (e.g., community health center in high-crime area, emergency department, psychiatric setting). Nurses can be exposed to physical violence as well as verbal abuse and harassment by patients and their families (see Figure 41-1C). Although nurses should be eligible for workers' compensation from physical injuries incurred as a part of their job, the effects of these injuries can be far-reaching (e.g., change of jobs or practice settings, permanent disability, HIV-positive status). Nurses have suffered posttraumatic stress disorder (PTSD) as a result of these incidents.

Another type of abuse that nurses can be exposed to is physical or verbal abuse by colleagues. Nurse–physician interaction may be a source of interpersonal conflict that occasionally results in violence or abuse. Bullying, intimidation, and threatening behaviors fall within the area of workplace violence. Because of implications that reporting this type of behavior may have on one's own performance evaluation, this type of workplace violence is often underreported. In fact some administrators or institutions may actively try to suppress this type of unfavorable information. The correct course of action is for institutions to actively develop and enforce violence management policies while promoting a culture of respect for colleagues and workplace safety.

The case of *Turner v. Jordan* (1997) illustrates the duty to warn staff of a patient's known violent nature. A patient suffering from a bipolar disorder, who was well known to the psychiatrist, was assessed and admitted by an emergency room resident. The psychiatrist wrote a note less than an hour after admission stating the patient's propensity for aggression, combativeness, and dangerousness. Later that evening, the patient violently assaulted a nurse. The Supreme Court of Tennessee found that the psychiatrist had a duty to assess the patient in terms of his danger to the staff and to warn and protect them from harm by the patient. It was noted that measures should have been taken to control the patient with medication, seclusion, restraints, or transfer to a more secure environment. The court stated that doing so would not only protect the staff but would also better meet the patient's treatment needs.

■ PROTECTING WORKERS— ORGANIZATIONAL/LEGISLATIVE RESPONSES

The National Institute for Occupational Safety and Health (NIOSH) has found that an average of 20 workers per week are murdered and another 18,000 are victims of nonfatal assaults. According to the Bureau of Labor Statistics (2004), healthcare and social service employees have the highest rate of nonfatal assault injuries in the workplace, with nurses having three times as many as others. In response to increasing violence against nurses, the American Association of Critical-Care Nurses (AACN) published a position paper in 2004 on "Workplace Violence Prevention." This paper states that all too often nurses consider assaults as part of their jobs and that this results in underreporting and multiple negative consequences in the workplace.

Some states have enacted legislation to increase penalties for persons convicted of assaulting healthcare workers. The Occupational Safety and Health Act of 1970 (OSHA) was enacted to assure a healthful and safe work environment, and this includes a violence-free workplace. In 1996 OSHA developed voluntary guidelines to protect healthcare workers. Employers may be penalized by OSHA if they fail to assess potential

risks, provide education and support for staff to prevent and deal with potential violence, and have a system to monitor incidents. Some effective strategies include assigning experienced staff to potentially violent clients, having a buddy system for workers, and educating staff about how to deal with escalating violence. It is best to have written policies for these situations and to provide ongoing in-service education for staff members.

■ VIOLENCE IN THE COMMUNITY

When traveling to agencies or patients' homes in high-crime areas, nurses must be especially vigilant of personal safety. If a nurse is uncomfortable visiting a patient alone, the nurse's employer should request a security escort. The employer has a legal duty to provide reasonable measures to ensure the safety of employees. Some agencies will not permit home visits in especially high-crime areas because of these concerns. The nurse must be aware of and follow all agency policies regarding employee safety.

■ SUSPECTED DRUG POSSESSION

If a nurse has suspicions of drug possession or weapons, the nurse should call security and notify the nurse manager. A nurse should not conduct a search of a patient's or visitor's belongings because doing so would violate the person's right of privacy. However, a nurse may act on knowledge of what is in "plain view" because this does not require a search. The nurse should note in the chart if the patient has symptoms or behaviors that could indicate use of drugs (other than those prescribed) but should not draw a conclusion about the source. As in all documentation, statements must be objective.

If the nurse suspects that a coworker possesses or uses drugs, the same procedures should be followed and the nurse manager notified. The nurse should document the situation in personal notes or wherever required to do so by agency policies. If the situation involves personal risk to the nurse, security should be notified. In no case can the situation be ignored.

■ DOCUMENTATION AND REPORTING

A thorough and objective record of events or evidence involving violent situations needs to be compiled (see Figure 41-1D). Notes should be made in patient records, and incident reports or police reports may need to be completed. In all cases agency or institution policies must be followed. These notes may be used as evidence in subsequent legal proceedings and may be invaluable to successful claims. Reports may need to be filed with state agencies. Employees need to follow through with necessary documentation of work-related injury for workers' compensation claims.

■ RISK MANAGEMENT AND STRATEGIES TO MINIMIZE VIOLENCE

The best way to deal with violence is to prevent it by early detection and intervention (see Figure 41-1E). Nurses should be aware of situations that could become violent and actively work to deter this from happening. Some institutions have multidisciplinary crisis management teams who assist staff with patients identified as potentially violent. Screening tools are used to identify these individuals, and the team then makes periodic rounds on these patients and helps the staff plan appropriate care. Teaching strategies, such as how to effectively handle stress, can help to prevent child or domestic violence. Appropriate referrals to social service or mental health agencies can be made as an early intervention strategy. A nurse who suspects that an employee is abusing patients must deal with the situation promptly.

If a patient or coworker becomes violent, the nurse needs to assertively state that the behavior should stop. Nurse managers and security may need to be called if the individ-ual is not calmed. It is strongly recommended that hospitals and other healthcare institutions have a crisis management team in place, similar to a response team for a cardiac arrest, that can be called when a patient/staff or visitor's behavior escalates. In most instances this will involve a team comprised of behavioral care personnel and security who are specially trained in deescalation techniques. It is often a nurse who takes the lead in these situations and directs when security needs to intervene. Algorithms provide an excellent way to provide consistent and effective intervention. In all cases, personal safety and the safety of others (including the perpetrator) must be considered. If a patient leaves the facility while threatening harm to someone, the police may need to be notified. In some extreme cases, healthcare workers may have a legal duty to warn identifiable third persons.

Workplace safety can be enhanced by in-service education programs that teach employees principles of personal safety and by the presence of physical barriers and security devices designed to prevent unauthorized access to high-risk areas. Protocols and procedures that deal with these situations proactively can minimize problems when they occur.

■ REFERENCES

American Nurses Association. (2001). *Code of ethics for nurses with interpretive statements*. Washington, DC: Author.

Gilmore, J. (2006). President's message—Violence in the workplace. *Nephrology Nursing Journal, 33*(3), 254–255.

Jacobson, J. (2007). AJN reports—Violence and nurses. *AJN, 107*(2), 25–26.

Trossman, S. (2006). Taking action to ensure better care, better workplaces. *The American Nurse, May/June,* 1, 6–8, 13, 15.

Turner v. Jordan, 957 S.W.2d 815 (Tennessee 1997).

U.S. Department of Labor (USDL), Occupational Safety & Health Administration (OSHA). (2003). Guidelines for preventing workplace violence for healthcare and social service workers. Washington, DC: Author.

Chapter 42

Intentional Torts

Susan J. Westrick

A Elements of Intentional Torts

Battery
- Unconsented touching
- Contact with person or objects on or close to them
- May result from lack of permission for a procedure (no informed consent)

Assault
- Fear or apprehension of a battery
- Present, not future harm intended
- Must be a reasonable fear of harm
- Mere words are not enough, need to include an overt act

False imprisonment
- Physical restraint or intimidating words
- Victim aware of restriction of movement
- May include withholding means to leave (car keys, wheelchair)

Intentional infliction of emotional distress
- Conduct that is outrageously distressing
- Victim experiences severe emotional distress

Defenses
- Consent (could be implied)
- Necessity
- Justification
- Self-defense

B Elements of Quasi-intentional Torts

Defamation
- False statements that injure one's reputation
- Libel — by the written word (includes charting)
- Slander — by the spoken word
- Publication to a third party or parties
- May need to show economic harm or business interference
- Claim not usually valid if made in a business relationship to supervisors or others up the chain of command who need to know the information
- Claim not usually valid if statement made by a former employer for a reference — "qualified privilege"

Invasion of privacy
- Interference with right to be left alone
- Revealing private facts publicly
- Using likeness or photos without permission
- Less rights for public figures, based on newsworthiness of private facts

Defenses
- Truth as an absolute defense to libel or slander
- Privilege or qualified privilege in a business relationship
- Public figure or newsworthiness exception

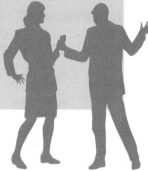

The law of torts protects individuals against private wrongs by another person. A *tort* is defined as a legal or civil wrong committed by one person against the person or property of another, independent of a contract. A tort involves some type of intentional conduct on the part of the actor (who could be a nurse) that invades the interest of another. In situations where the intent is less clear, the tort is termed a *quasi-intentional tort*. The type of intent that is required to prove an intentional tort is that of intent for purposeful conduct on the part of the actor. What is necessary is that the actor intended the act. The actor is then responsible for all the natural consequences that follow from that act, even if the specific harm that resulted was not intended. Intentional and quasi-intentional torts are contrasted with *negligent torts* in which there is no intent on the part of the actor but rather a failure to uphold a standard or duty that was owed to the injured party. No expert witness would be needed in proving intentional tort cases because there is no requirement of a standard to be proved in the situation. Sometimes a particular act (such as a battery) could have criminal as well as civil consequences, although this is not the usual case in healthcare situations.

■ INTENTIONAL TORTS

Figure 42-1A reviews the elements of intentional torts. In healthcare situations, *battery* (unconsented touching) can apply when a patient has not consented to a procedure. This would also then become a claim for lack of informed consent. The unconsented touching does not always have to be direct touching for a claim to prevail. It may include instances of touching the patient's clothing or purse or other objects that are in the person's hands. Nurses are cautioned to ask for the patient's permission in any doubtful situation.

Assault is defined as threat to do harm or the immediate fear of a battery. Usually assault and battery are claimed together even though they involve two separate torts. Mere words are not enough to prove assault. Together with an overt act of threatening, the two factors may be enough. The threat must create a reasonable apprehension, it must be immediate (not in the future), and the victim must be aware of the threat. The actual touching, or battery, does not have to occur for a claim of assault to be successful.

An operating room nurse brought a lawsuit for assault and battery against an orthopedic surgeon who allegedly jabbed her in the back in the OR with the sharp end of a surgical instrument called an osteotome, or bone chisel (*Baca v. Velez*, 1992). Nurse Baca was in charge of the instruments and had a disagreement with Dr. Velez over the osteotome that resulted in the alleged conduct by the doctor. The trial court jury rendered judgment in favor of the doctor on the nurse's assault and battery claim. In upholding the verdict, the Court of Appeals of New Mexico found that one of the essential elements was lacking in her claim because there was no evidence that the plaintiff nurse felt scared *before* (emphasis added) the touching took place. According to the New Mexico statute, for there to be an assault, there must have been an "act, threat, or menacing conduct which causes another person to reasonably believe that he is in danger of receiving an immediate battery" (unconsented touching). The nurse testified that she felt afraid "after the initial jabbing" and wasn't sure if she felt any anticipation that he might injure her further. Thus the court upheld the summary judgment on the assault claim.

False imprisonment is defined as the act of preventing the free movement of a person or detaining a person without legal cause. The patient needs to prove that he or she was restrained physically or by intimidation. Thus, the person must be aware of the actor's intent to restrain movement. It is sufficient to show that there was essential restraint, such as removing the person's outdoor clothing or car keys from the room to prevent him from leaving. Misuse of chemical or physical restraints can result in successful claims of false imprisonment if all other elements are present. However, there are some justifications for physically restraining patients, including preventing harm to themselves or others.

A claim of false imprisonment could probably have been made on the facts of the case of *Remmers v. DeBuono* (1997) where a partially paralyzed patient in a wheelchair was placed in his room by a nurse's aide after several "wandering" episodes. The nurse's aide had "slammed the door" to the patient's room and gone back to her other duties. A nurse who attempted to open the patient's door 1 minute later found it would only open one-third of the way. When the nurse entered his room she found the patient's bed moved across the door on the inside, effectively blocking him in. The case against the nurse's aide by the commissioner of health in New York for patient mistreatment and neglect was sustained by the court. The evidence of the aide slamming the door and the door found barricaded soon after was sufficient evidence to prove the claim. In addition, one could argue that the elements necessary to prove false imprisonment could have been supported as well. It is not clear whether the victim was aware of his restriction of movement, which is an essential element of a successful claim.

Intentional infliction of emotional distress involves outrageous conduct that inflicts severe emotional disturbance on the victim. This situation is rare in the healthcare setting but could occur if a patient was intentionally told some false and extremely upsetting news, such as that he or she had a fatal illness.

Intentional infliction of emotional distress by hospital emergency room nurses was alleged by a patient and her husband in *Roddy v. Tanner Medical Center, Inc.* (2003). The pregnant patient had gone to defendant hospital after having cramps and heavy bleeding, which was evident after she came to the ER. The patient informed the ER nurse that about 5 minutes away from her house she "felt something big pass and the blood kept getting heavier." The nurse subsequently removed several large blood clots from the patient and her clothing. The clothing was placed in a plastic bag by the nurse after the patient said she did not want it thrown away. The patient was transferred to a room and returned home the same day after a D & C procedure. She had suffered a miscarriage at 10.5 weeks into her pregnancy. When she was discharged she took the bloody bag of clothing home, and when doing laundry, she removed her pants from the bag and heard a "thud." She screamed

when she saw the intact fetus in the fetal sac lying on the floor. After this traumatic event she suffered posttraumatic stress syndrome, sleeping trouble, panic attacks, and strain in her marriage. Although the court sympathized with the plaintiffs, it found the evidence fell short of supporting the claim of "intentional infliction of emotional distress" because although the nurse's search of the patient's clothing may have been negligent, there was no showing of intent or reckless disregard.

This case illustrates the need to always be thorough and sensitive to the needs of patients who are in highly distressed situations. Part of the evidence presented at trial was that when the husband called the ER to report what had happened at home regarding the fetus, the ER nurse had treated him "rudely." Fortunately, he then called back and spoke to a labor and delivery nurse who apologized and arranged for proper medical follow-up.

What is more common is when there is *negligent* (but unintentional) *infliction of emotional distress*. Persons with successful claims generally need to show that some damage has occurred, such as inability to work or health problems that resulted from the incident.

A claim of negligent infliction of emotional distress in the employment context was asserted by a nurse whose employment was terminated. Nurse Pavliscak, an employee at will, claimed that her dismissal without advance notice was unreasonable. The appeals court overturned the trial court's finding of negligent infliction of emotional distress as a matter of law and found that judgment should have been directed for the defendant. The appeals court stated that there was no evidence that she was publicly humiliated. She was told in a private meeting that she was being terminated immediately and that she must take her personal items and leave the hospital premises (*Pavliscak v. Bridgeport Hospital*, 1998).

Defenses

One valid defense is that the patient consented. A patient may claim that an assault and battery took place when he or she did not give verbal consent to an injection. However, a valid defense could be that the patient turned over and got in position for the injection, thus inferring consent. Another defense could be necessity or justification when it may have been necessary to touch a patient to prevent the patient from a fall or harm. Self-defense is another defense. Even a claim of intentional infliction of emotional distress could be justified under some circumstances if there was an emergency or disaster that warranted the nurse's action.

■ QUASI-INTENTIONAL TORTS

Figure 42-1B reviews the elements of quasi-intentional torts. *Defamation,* an invasion of the right to one's good name or character, involves the two torts of *libel* (written communication) and *slander* (oral communication). Defamation consists of publication of a false statement to a third party or parties that injures the person's reputation. The defamatory statements must be made as a statement of fact and be of the type that would be seen as derogatory, adverse, or harmful to a person's reputation. The tort is a personal one and only living persons can be defamed. Statements made about a group are not defamatory.

Claims for defamation may arise when false or derogatory statements are made about patients in a public place or written in a chart. Nurses are reminded to chart objectively and to not state opinions that may be considered defamatory.

A claim of defamation also may arise when an employer writes or gives an oral negative reference about a former employee (who may be a nurse). The nurse may claim that a job was not obtained because of this. However, this circumstance involves a qualified privilege by the employer; because of the work situation, the employer is privileged to disclose negative information about former employees and in some instances has a duty to do so. In fact, courts have recognized a qualified privilege for statements made up the chain of command when they are made in good faith. The discussion must be held with supervisors or others who have a legitimate need to know and not just with coworkers or others. One needs to be cautious in making statements about colleagues, physicians, or other workers that could be considered defamatory.

In *Faulkner v. Arkansas Children's Hospital* (2002), the appellant nurse's claim for defamation against her former employer failed, in part, because she did not plead facts showing she suffered any actual damage as required. The appellate courts affirmed the trial court's dismissal of the action. Nurse Faulkner (who was the hospital's ECHMO coordinator) claimed, among other wrongdoings against her, that another nurse slandered her by making unfavorable statements about her performance to another ECHMO coordinator at a different hospital. The statement that Faulkner was no longer the ECHMO coordinator at defendant hospital was found to be true and thus not defamatory. The court also found that the other statements made about Faulkner could be read as a prediction of the future and not capable of being proven true or false. As such, the statements failed another test for defamation that requires the statement to be an objective, verifiable fact.

In *Columbia Valley Regional Medical Center v. Bannert* (2003) a former employee sued a hospital and two managers, including LaMont, for allegedly producing a libelous memo about her that another employee, named Catlett, found on a shared drive of defendant hospital's computer system. The memo was then copied by Catlett to a diskette and given to the plaintiff Bannert. A printed copy from this diskette was then circulated to other hospital employees. The memo, allegedly authored by Bannert's immediate supervisor LaMont, contained statements about her poor performance and the manager's plan to gain her resignation by "creating rumors for un-professionalism, substance abuse, lewdness and . . . enlist Human Resources in documenting the allegations in her Personnel

Record." The trial court jury found for the plaintiff and awarded damages of over $1.5 million in actual and punitive damages for defamation against her by the defendants, who appealed.

The Court of Appeals of Texas reversed this decision finding that the authorship of the memo was not proven. Computer experts found the origin of the memo to be Bannert's computer, written 3 days prior to the date of the memo being placed on the shared drive. LaMont, who denied writing the memo, had started to use a new computer a few weeks prior to when the memo was produced and her old computer had been "reformatted," thus losing prior data. Bannert's expert computer witness had concluded that "To me, the logical conclusion to all this, particularly taking into account . . . the fact that we were given the wrong PC, et cetera, . . . is that Ms. LaMont wrote the letter." But the appeals court found that these witnesses' statements were not supported by his examination of the various computer hard drives and diskette. Therefore, the court held there was no evidence to support the conclusion that LaMont wrote the questionable memorandum. The judgment of the court below was reversed, and the plaintiff Bannert received no award after the appeal.

Invasion of privacy protects the person's interest in being left alone, free from unwarranted intrusions into one's privacy. Claims by patients may include public release of private facts or appropriations of one's likeness without permission. Courts have allowed such claims when pictures of patients have been published in medical texts without their permission. All agencies should have policies for obtaining written permission from patients for photographs, even for publicity purposes.

Defenses

Truth is an absolute defense to a claim of defamation. Another defense could be privilege or qualified privilege. A defendant may also claim that false statements made about another were intended as a joke and that no harm was caused. Sometimes the defense of fair comment in the public interest may overcome a claim of defamation. Consent may be a defense to invasion of privacy. The defendant may also claim that the victim is a "public figure" so that there may be less protection against invasion of privacy. Most courts do embrace this concept because public figures may fall into an exception for "news worthiness" of facts that would otherwise be considered private. Under limited circumstances the public may have a right to know certain information.

■ DAMAGES AND LIABILITY

Damage awards from successful claims of intentional and quasi-intentional torts can be substantial. Some torts require actual damage to be proved, but others do not. In addition to compensatory damages, the court may award punitive damages against an individual for a particularly harmful or malicious act. These intentional acts usually are not covered by malpractice insurance policies, and the nurse would be individually liable if found guilty. In some cases the employer also may be held liable for the intentional conduct of the employee.

■ REFERENCES

Baca v. Velez, 114 N.M. 13; 833 P2d. 1194, 1992 N.M. App. LEXIS 43 (1992).

Columbia Valley Regional Medical Center v. Bannert, 112 S.W.3d 193; 2003 Tex. App. LEXIS 5857 (2003).

Faulkner v. Arkansas Children's Hospital, 347 Ark. 941; 69 S.W.3d 393; 202 Ark. LEXIS 156 (2002).

Pavliscak v. Bridgeport Hospital, 48 Conn. App. 580; 711 A.2d 747, 1998 Conn. App. LEXIS 196 (1998).

Remmers v. DeBuono, 241 A.D.2d 587; 660 N.Y. S.2d 159; 1997 N.Y. App. LEXIS 7240 (1997).

Roddy v. Tanner Medical Center, Inc., 262 Ga. App. 202; 585 S.E.2d 175; 2003 G.A. Appl. LEXIS 868; 2003 Fulton County D. Rep. 233 (2003).

Part IV Review Questions

1. An employee at will reports to a state agency that his employer is violating health and safety codes, and the employer is fined. The employee is subsequently terminated and brings a lawsuit against the employer for wrongful discharge. The likely outcome of the case will be:

   (A) The employer will win because an employee at will can be terminated at any time
   (B) The employee will win because of the public policy exception
   (C) The court will need to look at the employee handbook before any decision can be made
   (D) Because there is not a contract for the employment situation, the NLRB will handle the employee's claim

2. A nursing supervisor who is 62 years old believes she was terminated because of her age. She brings a lawsuit under the Age Discrimination in Employment Act (ADEA). Which of the following is *not* an essential component of the claim?

   (A) She must show she is a member of the protected class
   (B) She must prove she is qualified for her position
   (C) She must show that the position was given to someone else who is not a member of the class that the ADEA seeks to protect
   (D) She must show specific intent on the part of the employer to discriminate

3. A nurse employed by a home care agency is working with a patient in his home. The nurse makes the statement, "I know that if you do these exercises each day your hand will regain all of its former function." This statement could cause a problem for the nurse or the employer because:

   (A) The nurse has created an implied contract for the employer
   (B) The statements of the nurse could be interpreted by the patient as a promise to guarantee results and could create a contract
   (C) There is unequal bargaining power between the parties so a contract has not been created
   (D) Statements such as this can be misinterpreted by the patient and are therefore unethical

4. A patient requests that the nurse take care of him when he leaves the hospital and specifies an hourly rate and other conditions. Which of the elements of creating a contract are *missing* from this scenario?

   (A) There is no offer or acceptance
   (B) There is no consideration (value) that would be exchanged by the parties
   (C) There is an offer but no acceptance or mutual assent
   (D) There is no capacity to enter into the contract

5. A nurse speaks out in the local newspaper about the short staffing at her hospital. She claims that there are violations of

state-mandated nurse–patient ratios on a regular basis by her employer. The nurse does not have an employment contract and is an employee at will. If she is fired because of this:

(A) She will have no recourse against the employer because she is an employee at will

(B) There may be recourse against her employer's action if it is found that she was promoting an important public policy while making these statements

(C) The employer will have to reinstate the employee unless he can show cause as to why the employee was fired

(D) She can win a claim that her employment is secured because she can make any statement she wants as protected speech under the First Amendment

6. Staff nurses who assign other nurses to patients or who evaluate them may be excluded from the protection of unions. This means that:

(A) Some charge nurses could be considered "supervisors"

(B) Nurses should refuse to undertake these duties in the workplace

(C) The employer can keep nurses from joining unions if they perform these tasks

(D) The NLRB cannot rule on a claim that the nurse's rights have been violated if the union refuses to allow nurses to join

7. A nurse is assigned to a patient diagnosed with Alzheimer's disease and requires assistance with all activities of daily living, including eating. The patient is on a "soft" diet and his dinner tray, which is prepared by the hospital, contains tea, pureed vegetables, pureed chicken, and chocolate pudding. The pureed chicken appears somewhat "lumpy" but no more so than usual. The nurse spoon feeds the patient, who thereafter appears to be quite comfortable. Two hours later the patient begins vomiting bright red blood. Radiographs reveal the presence of a very small metal object, probably from the pureed chicken, in the patient's stomach. A claim is brought against the nurse and the hospital and the likely outcome is:

(A) Both the nurse and the hospital are liable

(B) Only the nurse is liable

(C) Only the hospital is liable

(D) No party is found liable

8. The operating room calls for a patient after a 6-hour delay. The nurse helps the patient move onto a stretcher, which doesn't have an IV pole attached to it. The nurse locates one that is too slender to fit into the pole hole in the stretcher. Instead of taking the time to locate the nursing unit's IV pole on wheels, the nurse wraps tape around the base of the slender IV pole until it is thick enough to fit into the hole on the stretcher. During transport to the operating room, the IV pole topples over, lacerating the patient's forehead. A claim is brought against the hospital and the nurse. The likely outcome is:

(A) The nurse is not liable because this is accepted practice on the nursing unit

(B) The hospital is not liable because the stretcher did not have an IV pole

(C) The nurse is liable

(D) Both parties are liable

(E) The hospital is solely liable

9. A nurse midwife is employed by Obstetrics, Inc., a corporation formed by a group of obstetricians. The nurse midwife and all physicians in Obstetrics, Inc. have admitting privileges at Best Hospital. While the nurse midwife is attending

to a laboring mother, she notes that the baby's heart rate has dropped significantly and is concerned that the amniotic fluid will contain meconium. The written policy of Obstetrics, Inc. is that under these circumstances the nurse midwife must call the on-call obstetrician in the group and notify him or her of the situation. Rather than doing so, the nurse midwife follows her typical pattern (as demonstrated at this hospital before) and elects to wait and see what happens. The baby has cerebral palsy. A claim is brought against Obstetrics, Inc. and Best Hospital. Liability is imputed to:

(A) Obstetrics, Inc.
(B) Best Hospital
(C) Both Obstetrics, Inc. and Best Hospital
(D) Neither

10. A student nurse is working at a hospital as a paid nursing assistant. During this time the student performs a negligent act for which liability is found. The student also has clinical experiences at this hospital and sometimes cares for the same patients as a student nurse and as a paid assistant. Which of the following would be true?

(A) The student is personally liable
(B) The hospital would be vicariously liable under a theory of respondeat superior
(C) The hospital is liable under a theory of ostensible agency
(D) The educational institution is liable because it placed the student in this assignment
(E) Both A and B

11. An agency nurse travels across state lines to work. Which of the following factors determines liability for the nurse's actions if negligence is found?

(A) Which agency or individual carries malpractice insurance for the nurse

(B) Whether or not the nurse is licensed by the state where the negligence occurred
(C) Who employs the nurse as well as who controls her practice in this patient situation
(D) Whether or not the nurse has personal assets to satisfy any judgment that the patient may be entitled to

12. A nurse with 10 years of medical nursing experience in the neurology intensive care unit (NICU) arrives at work one night and learns he is being floated to the cardiothoracic intensive care unit (CTICU) for the shift because that unit is short one nurse. When the nurse tells the supervisor that he has never taken care of a CT patient, the supervisor says, "You're an intensive care nurse, you can do it. Besides the whole hospital is understaffed tonight." On arrival in the CTICU, the nurse is assigned to a patient who is due to be admitted directly from the operating room after undergoing a quadruple coronary artery bypass. The nurse's best course of action is:

(A) Explain to the CTICU charge nurse that he or she has never taken care of a CT patient before
(B) Ask if there is a stable patient already in the unit that can be assigned instead
(C) Ask if one of the regular CTICU nurses can be available to assist
(D) Ascertain the procedure for taking care of a fresh, postoperative patient in that unit
(E) All of the above

13. A nurse has an employment contract with the employer hospital. The contract explicitly states that the employer will not require the nurse to float. One day the supervisor approaches the nurse and asks if she will float to another unit that is particularly understaffed. Considering the contract the nurse:

(A) Must refuse to float

(B) May walk out

(C) May agree to float

(D) Must take legal action against the employer

(E) All of the above

14. An employer may be required to perform all of the following as a reasonable accommodation for a qualified disabled nurse *except:*

    (A) Reassign the nurse to another job position

    (B) Create a job position that fits the nurse's skills

    (C) Allow an auxiliary aide animal into the workplace

    (D) Assign someone else the nonessential job functions

15. Which of the following actions by an employer is considered to be unlawful under the Americans with Disabilities Act?

    (A) Preemployment inquiry into a disability

    (B) Job offer conditioned on an examination

    (C) Drug testing of applicants

    (D) Uniformly applied leave policy that causes hardship on a disabled employee

16. After being exposed to a patient's blood products, a nurse may do all of the following *except:*

    (A) Review the chart for the patient's HIV status

    (B) Draw blood on the patient and send it for HIV testing

    (C) Have a physician request the patient's consent to be tested

    (D) Fill out an incident report and submit it to the evaluation group

17. Nurses have a legal duty to:

    (A) Know their own HIV status if they have risk factors

(B) Transfer to a specialty area without invasive procedures if they are HIV positive

(C) Identify safety risks to a patient and take steps to prevent harm if the nurse is HIV positive

(D) Inform their own partners if they are HIV positive

18. An effective substance abuse diversion program includes:

    (A) Automatic termination

    (B) Mandatory treatment including Alcoholics Anonymous/Narcotics Anonymous attendance

    (C) Revocation of license

    (D) Encouragement to seek employment elsewhere

19. In the process of reporting suspicions that a coworker is impaired, the nurse should do everything *except:*

    (A) Document the factual basis for the suspicions

    (B) Confront the nurse with the findings

    (C) Notify the nurse manager

    (D) Participate in substance abuse education programs

20. For a claim of sexual harassment to prevail when a complaint is filed with the EEOC, a victim must:

    (A) Prove there was physical contact between the harasser and oneself

    (B) Have taken steps outlined in any employment policies, unless there are compelling reasons not to do so

    (C) Prove that the alleged conduct resulted in an adverse job-related decision

    (D) Be a federal employee because the EEOC enforces a federal law

21. An acceptable action to take if one is being sexually harassed in the workplace is to:

(A) Ignore the behavior if the harasser is a patient
(B) Calmly state to the harasser that you do not approve of what he or she is doing
(C) Document the incident the next time it happens
(D) Confront the harasser and make it clear that the specific conduct is unwelcome and unacceptable

22. A nurse is assigned to a patient admitted for drug withdrawal on the evening shift. As the nurse enters his room, he quickly shoves his hand under his pillow as if to conceal something. Nursing interventions should include which of the following?
(A) Conduct a search of his room
(B) Tell him he must show what he is hiding
(C) Document the incident and any behavior changes he may have
(D) Notify the supervisor and possibly security if the nurse strongly suspects he is hiding illegal drugs
(E) Both C and D

23. Which of the following is *not* an appropriate action to take if a community healthcare nurse suspects that a patient is being abused by a nursing assistant from her agency?
(A) Document the incidents that led to this conclusion in personal notes
(B) Follow up with any procedures required by the employer
(C) Confront the nursing assistant if it can be done safely
(D) Detain the employee until security or the police can be called

24. The nurse is talking to a coworker in the cafeteria about a physician. The nurse makes statements about the fact that the physician does not know what he is doing and often makes mistakes when treating patients. A visitor in the cafeteria later reveals to the physician that she overheard these statements, and she identifies the nurse who made the statements. Could the physician sustain a successful claim of slander against the nurse?
(A) No because the statement was made in the work environment
(B) No because the statement was just overheard by the visitor and was not published by the nurse
(C) Yes because the statements injured the work reputation of the physician and were spoken so a third party could hear them
(D) Yes because the statements were intended to cause harm to the physician and were only partially true

25. A patient claims that a nurse struck his arm intentionally when she was helping him get back in bed and used threatening language that there was more to come. What claims can be substantiated as based on these facts?
(A) Assault because the nurse made unconsented contact with the patient
(B) Battery because there was threatening language and fear of another harmful touching
(C) Both assault and battery, for reasons included in A and B
(D) No claims because the nurse was only doing what was necessary

Part IV Answers

1. *The answer is B.*

   Reporting bona fide claims to a state agency will most likely meet the standard of the public policy exception to firing at will employees for any reason. An important public policy is served by encouraging these violations to be reported. Answer A is incorrect because of the public policy exception. Answer C is incorrect because the employee manual is irrelevant to the facts given, although some courts may look to it for other exceptions to the employee at will doctrine. Answer D is incorrect because the NLRB only handles claims when there is a collective bargaining agreement governing the employment situation.

2. *The answer is D.*

   It is not necessary to prove a specific intent on the part of the employer to discriminate against the employee. This intent often can be inferred on the basis of proving the other essential elements. Specific intent would place too high a burden of proof on the employee. However, after all the other components of the claim are shown, the employer can present a nondiscriminatory reason for the termination that the court may accept. Answers A, B, and C contain components that must be shown to shift the burden of proof to the employer to present a nondiscriminatory reason for the termination.

3. *The answer is B.*

   The statement could be construed by the patient as creating a promise or a guarantee by the nurse as to specific results if the patient follows the directions. The nurse is also considered an agent of the employer and could bind the agency to the agreement if a contract was found by the court. Answer A is incorrect because this would be an express contract since specific statements were made. Answer C is incorrect because there is no indication of a situation of unequal bargaining power by either party. Answer D is not correct because misinterpretation by a patient is not automatically unethical.

4. *The answer is C.*

   Although there is an offer, it has not been accepted and there is no mutual assent. Answer B is incorrect because there is consideration that would be exchanged—services for money. Answer D is not correct because there is no information in the question to indicate a lack of capacity to contract on the part of either party.

5. *The answer is B.*

   This is the public policy exception to the usual case that the employee at will can be fired for any reason (even for no cause). If these allegations are proved true, the employee has a valid claim against the employer for reinstatement.

Answer A is incorrect for the same reason. Answer C is incorrect because cause does not have to be shown to fire an at will employee. Answer D is incorrect because even though this speech may be found to be protected, it is too broad to state that anything said will be protected.

6. *The answer is A.*

A nurse who is in charge generally performs the tasks described in the question and could be considered a "supervisor" by the courts. Supervisors are considered to be management and would be excluded from participation in a union. Answer B is incorrect because the employer has a legitimate right to expect an employee who is qualified to perform this task, even if union protection may not necessarily be available to the employee. Answer C is not correct because all the circumstances would be looked at, not just these particular tasks. Answer D is incorrect because the NLRB can still rule on the claim even if the nurse eventually would be excluded from participation in the union.

7. *The answer is C.*

The hospital is liable for negligently prepared food because the pureed chicken was not adequate and safe, and it was not reasonably suited for the purpose intended. B is incorrect because there is no indication that the nurse knew or should have known there was a metal object in the pureed chicken. A and D are incorrect for the same reasons.

8. *The answer is C.*

The nurse selected the equipment to be used and did so notwithstanding the fact that an adequate and safe IV pole on wheels was made available for use by the hospital. The nurse knew or should have known that such an injury to the patient

would occur. Therefore, it is not likely that liability will be imputed to the hospital. E is incorrect for the same reasons. B and D are not the best answers because although it could be argued that the hospital failed to provide a stretcher reasonably suited for the purpose intended, a reasonable alternative was provided to the nurse who elected to forego using it. That it was common practice on the nursing unit to tape the IV pole is not sufficient to protect the nurse from liability absent a written hospital policy to do so.

9. *The answer is C.*

Although the nurse midwife has ignored Obstetrics, Inc.'s written policy and Obstetrics, Inc. argues that for that reason it is not liable, the nurse midwife has done this before. Therefore, there is a pattern of conduct on the part of the nurse midwife, and both Obstetrics, Inc. and Best Hospital knew or should have known that there is a question concerning the nurse midwife. A, B, and D are incorrect under the same reasoning.

10. *The answer is E.*

Both A and B are correct statements. A is correct because the principle of personal liability always remains. B is correct because when the negligent act occurred, the student had an employee–employer relationship with the hospital. C is incorrect because the theory of ostensible agency is not applied in the employee-employer relationship. D is incorrect because the student was not participating in clinical experiences when the negligent act occurred, and no one from the school was supervising the student.

11. *The answer is C.*

In addition to his or her personal liability, the employer would be liable under respondeat superior. The institution where the nurse is working could also be liable if it exerts so much control over the nurse's practice that he or she is considered an agent. Also the patient may view the agency nurse as an agent of the institution so that ostensible agency may be implied. A is not relevant to whether liability is found or as to who is liable. The fact of whether one is protected by insurance is not considered in determining liability. B is not correct because liability could still be found even if the nurse was not licensed by the state. D is not a factor to determine liability because the judgment could be satisfied from future wages. The fact that there are no assets or future assets does not determine liability.

12. *The answer is E.*

The actions described in A–D all serve to protect the nurse and protect the patient. As in A, by telling the charge nurse in the CTICU that the nurse doesn't have experience in CTICU nursing, the nurse is giving further notice to the employer that he or she may be unqualified for the assignment. By asking for a more stable patient as in B, the nurse is seeking to take care of a patient for which the nurse is more qualified. In C and D, the nurse is taking efforts to be as prepared as possible to provide adequate, safe nursing care.

13. *The answer is C.*

If the nurse is willing to float and, after obtaining as much information as possible about the assignment believes he or she is qualified, the nurse may float. Absent contractual language to the contrary, that the hospital agreed not to float the nurse does not preclude the request that the nurse do so. If the nurse accepts the assignment, the contract will not protect the nurse from personal liability. All steps must still be taken to provide safe, reasonably proficient nursing care. The

nurse is not obligated to refuse to float as in A. The agreement not to require the nurse to float does not allow the nurse to walk out simply because the employer asks as in B nor does it mandate taking legal action as in D.

14. *The answer is B.*

The employer is not required to create a job under reasonable accommodation. An employer is required to reassign a qualified individual (A) or reassign nonessential job functions (D). The employer must accommodate an auxiliary aide animal (C) unless there is documentation that it poses a health or safety risk.

15. *The answer is A.*

A is unlawful because employers may not make preemployment inquiries into disability but may inquire about ability to perform specific job functions. B is lawful, while an employer may not require an applicant to take a medical exam prior to a job offer, the job may be conditional on a postoffer examination. C is lawful because employers may base job offers on results of drug testing, and D is legal under the act as long as the leave policy is uniformly applied to all employees and does not specifically target disabled employees. If the employee asks for a modification, the employer may accommodate.

16. *The answer is B.*

A nurse may not draw blood for an HIV test without verifying that a physician has properly documented informed consent in the medical record.

17. *The answer is C.*

C is the only *legal* duty (this is the standard of care in nursing). All the other answers are *ethical* duties that should be performed within the bounds of ethics. Ethical duties are often guidelines for nurses to follow and occasionally become the standard of care in certain circumstances. Therefore, under some circumstances A, B, and D could turn from an ethical duty to a legal duty.

18. *The answer is B.*

A, C, and D represent past remedies. Currently, the goal is to encourage recovery through formal rehabilitation including inpatient and outpatient programs (B), random drug testing, education, and back-to-work agreements that define the terms of continued employment.

19. *The answer is B.*

The nurse should not confront the impaired nurse. It is important to make certain that the suspicions are reviewed and confirmed by the nurse manager and that when confronted, a plan is outlined and treatment resources are immediately available.

20. *The answer is B.*

Courts and agencies that deal with claims generally require that an employee exhaust all internal remedies before a claim will be processed. An exception to this would be if an employee could not follow the policy because the immediate supervisor was the harasser. This would constitute a compelling reason for not following the policy. A victim does not have to prove that actual physical contact occurred with the harasser (A) or that there was a negative effect on one's job (C), especially in cases involving a hostile work environment. These elements may be a part of the victim's case, especially in quid pro quo harassment. Title VII of the Civil Rights Act applies equally to private and public employees and employers (D).

21. *The answer is D.*

One needs to be firm and clear about what conduct is unacceptable, and the

first step in doing this is to confront the harasser. A is incorrect because sexual harassment by patients needs to be dealt with in a constructive way. B is incorrect because the message to the harasser is somewhat ambiguous. C is incorrect because each incident of harassment should be documented.

22. *The answer is E.*

The nurse should provide objective documentation of the incident and any assessment of the patient in the patient's record. It is also appropriate to tell him that for his medical care to be effective, the healthcare team needs to know about anything he is taking that is not a part of his care plan. The supervisor should be notified, and if the nurse thinks there is an issue of safety, security should be notified. Answer A is incorrect because a nurse cannot conduct a search without the patient's permission. Answer B is incorrect because a nurse cannot demand that a patient do this because it is the patient's decision. The nurse can ask to see what is under the pillow in a nonthreatening manner.

23. *The answer is D.*

The nurse should not attempt to detain anyone suspected of abuse because doing so could jeopardize personal safety. However, the supervisor or security needs to be notified. Answers A and B state correct actions to be taken to document the incident and follow agency protocols. Answer C is a correct action if it can be done safely. The nurse is putting the employee on notice of the incident and making it clear that the behavior is not acceptable.

24. *The answer is C.*

The statements were made as facts, not just opinion, and were of the type that would harm the business relationships of the physician (although economic harm may need to be shown). Publication has occurred even if the nurse did not intend this because he or she is responsible for the natural consequences that flow from acts. Answer A is incorrect; just because a statement is made in a work environment would not exempt it. Answer B is not correct because publication has taken place. Answer D is incorrect because it does not matter what the specific intent was, and being partially true means that some of the statements were false and thus were actionable.

25. *The answer is C.*

The facts indicate that the elements for both claims of assault and battery are present. There are no facts to support that the actions constituted a necessity or were justified by the nurse, so answer D is incorrect. Answer A or B alone would be incorrect because each only contains one part of the claims that could be sustained.

PART V

Ethics

Chapter 43

Ethical Decision Making

Susan J. Westrick

Moral Principles of Ethical Decision Making

Autonomy — the ability to allow the patient to independently make decisions regarding care and treatment, based on information provided so that the patient can effectively reason in his or her own way.

Freedom — the patient's ability to freely determine what method of treatment is most consistent with protecting his or her autonomy and independence. The nurse has an obligation to ensure that the patient receives the relevant information needed to make these decisions.

Beneficence — the expectation of the patient that the nurse will *do good* and prevent harm to the patient. The patient has a right to expect beneficence.

Nonmalfeasance — to protect the patient from harmful circumstances or decisions and to promote, not ignore, treatments that will not harm and forbid those that will cause harm.

Veracity — information given to the patient must be truthful so that informed decisions can be made by the patient. This protects the patient's autonomy.

Confidentiality/privacy — endorses the theory of self-ownership, the right to privacy and freedom from harm due to a breach of that privacy. The patient expects that this right will not be violated by the nurse.

Fidelity — the patient has the expectation and right to expect that the nurse will remain faithful and trustworthy to each understanding and agreement.

Justice — the nurse's moral obligation to treat all people fairly, without prejudice or regard for their socioeconomic status, personal characteristics, or disease process.

■ NURSE'S ROLE

According to the ANA's *Code of Ethics for Nurses with Interpretative Statements* (2001), the nurse is committed to respect the dignity of each patient and to foster each patient's freedom to make choices to receive that to which he or she is entitled. *Respect for the patient and the primacy of the patient's interests* is the basis for this commitment. As such, the nurse has a duty to respect the patient regardless of socioeconomic status, personal character, or nature of the illness. Every patient should be treated with dignity and worth, taking into account the differences and special needs of each patient.

To further ensure this respect, the nurse must make decisions through a reasoning process that incorporates professional judgments, clinical observations, and the practical matters of technical feasibility. This process is a vital component of nursing. In doing so, the nurse needs to be certain that any approach that is taken does not violate the moral principles that need to be considered when assessing an ethical dilemma.

As part of the process, the nurse needs to consider the consequences of the actions taken and to determine in what manner any objections to the decisions that have been made will be handled. This justifies the decision from a moral standpoint while satisfying all of the principles of decision making. Inherent in the duty to enhance the patient's responsibility to maintain an autonomous existence is the duty to assess and evaluate, in an ongoing manner, the nurse's clinical competence, decision-making capabilities, and clinical judgments.

■ ETHICAL PRINCIPLES

The following ethical and moral principles provide guidelines for the nurse when patient interactions involve ethical decisions or dilemmas (see **Figure 43-1**).

- Autonomy: The nurse allows a patient to maintain character, values, and uniqueness, regardless of the nurse's own values. The nurse helps the patient to understand the nature, extent, and possible outcome of treatment so the patient can make healthcare decisions based on information provided in an easily understood manner. The nurse has the responsibility to continue to provide information to the patient and to evaluate the patient's understanding of that information to satisfy the moral obligation of maintaining

the patient's autonomy. The *informed consent* doctrine is based on the principle of the patient's autonomy.

- Freedom: This enables the patient to function independently and be allowed to freely make informed decisions in an autonomous manner. The nurse cannot interfere with the patient's desires or actions. This means that although the nurse can provide information on alternatives and different approaches to patient care, it is the patient who is allowed to decide the appropriate course of action. The nurse may not agree with the patient's choices but respects the patient's right to make those choices.

- Beneficence: The nurse has a moral obligation to do good, and the patient has a right to expect that he or she will derive some benefit from that good. This obligation also includes preventing harm and reducing the risk of harm. This is not done merely by instructing the patient as to what is good or not good for him or her, but rather providing the information that will enable the patient to reduce the risk of harm or prevent harm from occurring by making informed choices about the best approach, i.e., the one that will "do good." This principle may come into play when the nurse protects a vulnerable client, such as a minor, from risk of harm, possibly from a parent. Thus the nurse must report suspected child abuse to the proper authorities and take protective measures for the child in the healthcare setting. This would benefit the child and remove him from potential harm.

- Nonmalfeasance: The nurse has a moral obligation to avoid harm to the patient. The nurse's primary obligation is always to the patient. Ignoring the treatment and efforts required to protect the patient's well-being or allowing actions that will cause harm to the patient is unacceptable. For example, the nurse in the psychiatric setting seeks help and implements protective measures for patients who display self-destructive behavior as a form of self-harm.

• Veracity: To function in an autonomous manner and make healthcare decisions, the patient expects the nurse to provide truthful information. Without the truth, the patient cannot make informed decisions based on reason, and his or her rights to do so have been violated. Using the principle of veracity, the nurse does not participate in giving placebos unless the patient agrees to their use. It also is enacted by appropriate disclosure of errors by nurses to patients. Nurses are expected to follow institutional guidelines for error disclosure, most often with the involvement of risk management. Referring appropriate error disclosure to risk managers ensures the use of consistent approaches, provides support for the nurse, and leads to more effective correction of conditions that led to the error.

• Confidentiality/privacy: This moral obligation endorses the theory of self-ownership and privacy; that is, the patient has the right to expect that the nurse will guard against the unwarranted or unethical release of information about the patient. This principle protects the patient from harm that may be caused by breach of confidentiality or privacy. Examples of nursing situations requiring protection of confidentiality include healthcare information, records, and personal information of patients or clients.

• Fidelity: The nurse is obliged to stay faithful to the agreement or the understanding reached with the patient regarding the care to be given. This allows the patient to be able to predict his or her environment, based on the expectations of the established trustworthy relationship. This principle includes the obligation of the nurse not to abandon the patient and to ensure continuity of care in patient care activities.

• Justice: The nurse is required to treat all people fairly without regard to socioeconomic status, personal attributes, or nature of the patient's health problems. Personal feelings about certain illnesses or diagnoses cannot interfere with the nurse's duty to care for others. If for some legitimate reason a nurse cannot provide care, as based only on a permitted exception, the nurse assures that the patient does receive care by another healthcare practitioner.

■ ETHICAL FRAMEWORK FOR PRACTICE

Several frames of reference and resources are available to guide nursing conduct and ensure compliance with professional ethical standards.

Patients' Rights

Over the years, several medical and hospital organizations have set forth agendas that enumerate the rights of patients who are under their care. Many of these patients' rights have mirrored the principles involved in ethical decision making: the rights to confidentiality, to truthful information, and to be treated equally regardless of personal circumstances. Although each bill of rights is worded differently, the message is the same: the patient has the right to be treated with respect and dignity and to determine what is to be done with his or her body.

As with most ethical decisions, however, these rights can conflict with the nurse's responsibility to the patient and present a difficult challenge for the nurse. For example, a patient receives truthful information about an anticipated procedure during the informed consent process, but the patient refuses the procedure. Certainly, the nurse's ethical obligation to "do good and avoid harm" would be defeated if the patient does not undergo the procedure. On the other hand, the patient's right to refuse the surgery would be violated if the refusal were ignored. This sort of dilemma requires a reasoning process based on the nurse's observations and clinical judgments. In doing so, the nurse must find a balance between any preconceived notions and acting blindly, without regard for the individual characteristics and needs of each patient, with the solitary goal of influencing the patient. The goal is to reach a decision based on a mindfulness of the patient's rights and freedoms while adhering to the principles of decision making, with a full understanding of the consequences of that decision.

The ANA Code of Ethics for Nurses

The ANA *Code of Ethics for Nurses* (2001) requires that nurses justify their ethical decisions and the consequences of those decisions on universal moral principles, the most basic of which is respect for all humans. The clear mandate of the code is that the nurse's primary commitment is to the recipient of health care, and this includes an individual, group, or community. The code of ethics establishes the ethical standard for the profession and is viewed as a nonnegotiable contract of the profession with the recipients of nursing care. The code has been used in malpractice cases and other litigation to help establish the required standard of care and conduct in particular situations.

Ethics Committee

Healthcare organizations have established ethics committees to serve as a resource in establishing policies, procedures, and guidelines to deal with recurring ethical dilemmas in practice. Some of these areas include end-of-life situations and conflicts between patient, family, or staff views related to appropriate treatment options. These multidisciplinary committees typically serve as a resource for staff and families experiencing serious ethical dilemmas. Nurses should serve on these committees and utilize this resource to help them resolve ethical conflicts in their practice.

■ PROFESSIONAL BOUNDARIES AND RELATIONSHIPS WITH PATIENTS

Nurses' relationships with patients should always remain on a professional level. The nurse must maintain appropriate boundaries with the patient to fulfill professional ethical standards. The nurse's practice should reflect prudent decisions that take into account the vulnerable position of the patient and the power position of the nurse in the nurse-patient relationship. The intimate nature of the nurse–patient relationship where the nurse often learns highly personal information about patients, and the closeness of patient interactions may lead to abuses of this guiding principle to maintain professional boundaries. Areas where this may become a problem include when a nurse reveals personal information about him- or herself or maintains social interaction with a patient, even when not under the nurse's direct care at that time. If these involve significant disclosures and relationships, they may interfere with a present or future caregiver relationship by the nurse. For example, nurses should not accept gifts from patients or involve themselves in situations beyond therapeutic relationships. Doing so makes them at risk for making objective decisions related to patients and could jeopardize a patient's autonomy and self-determination. It also creates a risk for professional discipline of the nurse by the state licensing board. The National Council of State Boards of Nursing (NCSBN) issued a statement in 1996 to clarify and provide guidance for boundary crossings and violations. Similarly, the ANA Code of Ethics for Nurses (2001) mandates that nurses maintain boundaries that establish appropriate limits to patient relationships. The code recognizes that sometimes these boundaries can be blurred but that nurses should always err on the side of caution when doubts or questions arise. Nurses are advised to seek assistance from peers, supervisors, and others to remove him- or herself from situations that potentially threaten this professional value. This may include reassignment to remove the nurse from a situation that could result in boundary violations.

■ CASE LAW INVOLVING ETHICAL ISSUES

The following cases all contain issues related to ethical concerns. In some instances nurses have faced discharge from employment for what they consider to be properly advancing their own ethical beliefs or those related to patient care and safety. When faced with situations such as these, the nurse must make a personal choice of how to proceed, being mindful of the risks and possible adverse employment decisions that may result. Situations involving ethical considerations are not always well defined and are subject to interpretation as based on the specific facts and circumstances.

1. *Patient advocacy/chain of command:* Whether nurses in the emergency room (ER) advocated properly on behalf of a patient was at issue in the case of *Rowe v. Sisters of the Pallottine Missionary Society* (2001). The patient, 17-year-old Brian Rowe, came to defendant St. Mary's Hospital's ER after a motorcycle accident caused extensive injury to his leg. He was examined by an ER physician, who said he found a pulse in the foot of the injured leg, but the nurses documented and stated that they did not find a pulse, even with use of a Doppler machine. Also the patient had no sensation in his foot and could not move it. Nevertheless, the MD sent the patient home with instructions to elevate and

ice the extremity as a "severe sprain [left] knee" with follow-up with an orthopedist several days later. However, during the night the patient's swelling and pain greatly increased, and he visited another hospital's ER the next morning. There he was diagnosed with a dislocated knee, a lacerated popliteal artery, and extensive tissue damage to the leg to the extent that amputation was contemplated. At trial it was asserted that the nurses breached the standard of care in not adequately advocating for the patient when he was discharged with unexplained and unaddressed symptoms. Evidence was presented that St. Mary's had a policy requiring a nurse who "believed that appropriate care [was] not being administered to a patient by a physician" to report the situation to the supervisor, who would discuss it with the doctor. If that did not relieve the problem, the matter was referred "up the chain of command" so that another doctor could evaluate the problem. Instead of following the hospital's policy, the ER nurses simply made notes of their findings in the medical file. When asked about the documentation, one nurse said she documented, "I guess basically to cover myself." The appeals court upheld the judgment and award of damages against the hospital largely because of the conduct of the nurses in not following this internal policy that required patient advocacy. Nurses are cautioned that documentation alone will not protect them when it is determined that further action is required to ensure patient safety.

2. *Personal beliefs versus ethical code requirements:* In a New Jersey case, the court was faced with a question of refusal to provide treatment to a patient as based on a nurse's belief that it violated, in part, the ANA Code of Ethics for Nurses, the ethi-

cal code promulgated by the American Nurses Association (*Corrine Warthen v. Toms River Community Memorial Hospital*, 1985). Nurse Warthen worked in the kidney dialysis unit but refused to provide dialysis for a terminally ill patient. At the time of her refusal, nurse Warthen informed the head nurse that her objection was based on "moral, medical, and philosophical objections." She believed that the procedure was not in the patient's best interest because he had experienced significant complications, such as cardiac arrest and severe internal hemorrhaging, during previous dialysis procedures. The nurse did discuss the situation with the patient's treating physician, who informed the plaintiff nurse that the patient's family wished him kept alive through dialysis and that he would not survive without it. However, nurse Warthen continued to refuse to dialyze the patient.

After seeking a reassignment that was initially granted by the head nurse, a subsequent request at a later date resulted in being informed that her continued refusal would result in termination from her position. As an employee at will, nurse Warthen argued that her adherence to the Code of Ethics for Nurses constituted advancing a "public policy" and thereby created an exception to the employer's right to fire her. The court, however, found that her stated adherence to the code was based on her personal beliefs, and not those advanced as a public policy exception identifying the "clear mandate of public policy" as required by law. The court further stated that the code serves the interests of protecting the nurse and the profession of nursing but not the public at large. In fact, the court found that the code language severely constrains the ethical right of nurses to refuse participation in medical procedures. Particularly pertinent was the portion of the code requiring nurses to care of all persons, irrespective of the nature of their health problem. The case ends its discussion by stating that by refusing to perform the procedure, the nurse may have eased her own conscience but she neither benefited society at large, the patient, nor the patient's family.

This case illustrates that nurses are cautioned to not confuse personal beliefs with ethical code requirements, especially in light of family or patient wishes that contradict these personal beliefs. Ethical principle violations for this conduct may include those for patient autonomy, freedom, and beneficence.

3. *Whistle-blower statute protection:* The following two cases involve the New Jersey Conscientious Employee Protection Act (CEPA) that prevents employee discharge or other disciplinary action in retaliation for making a valid complaint or claim about conduct protected by the statute. In *Higgins v. Pascack Valley Hospital* (1999) plaintiff employee nurse Higgins alleged she was a victim of adverse employment decisions following her complaint of defendant coemployees not complying with paperwork required by state regulations. Nurse Higgins was a per diem employee and member of defendant hospital's Mobil Intensive Care Unit (MICU). In 1991 and 1992 Higgins complained to her supervisor of two incidents. The first was an instance of two coworkers filing incorrect forms after treating a patient, and the second was an allegation that one of these employees had stolen medication from a patient's home during an ambulance call with the plaintiff. The supervisors made investigations of these incidents and found no wrongdoing on the part of these employees. However, nurse Higgins

testified that one of these employees stated he had fabricated the proper paperwork after her complaint. Later seven coworkers sent letters to her supervisor stating they did not want to work with her, citing a lack of trust and fear that she would falsely accuse them. The letters also expressed anger that, contrary to the nursing code of ethics, Higgins did not speak directly with the employee before accusing him of taking the patient's medication. After this, Higgins was transferred to the ER, her working hours were reduced, and she was not hired for either of two full-time positions she was qualified for.

As part of the basis for a claim of defamation, Higgins asserted that a letter from her supervisor of the hospital's conclusions after its investigation of her accusations against the coworker was posted at the hospital by an unidentified person. The court did not accept this as evidence for a defamation claim against either the employer or her coworkers, in part because the supervisor's letter contained true statements and opinions, and truth is an absolute defense to defamation. But the Supreme Court of New Jersey did allow Higgins's claim for protection under the whistle-blower statute for objecting to her coemployee's activity. The employer unsuccessfully argued that it should not be liable when the complaints were about employees and not the employer itself. The trial court's jury award of over $315,000 in compensatory damages and $320,000 in punitive damages to nurse Higgins was sustained by the court on the CEPA claim, but it dismissed claims related to individual named defendants and the hospital for defamation.

In another case based on the New Jersey CEPA, a nurse employee working in a women's prison observed that medical services and medications were being provided to patients without complying with state law (*Fleming v. Correctional Healthcare Services*, 2000). Specifically, inmates were required to pay a nominal fee as a copayment for these services, and the forms were often not being completed. Nurse Fleming verbally reported this to her immediate supervisor and the next in command, who acknowledged that this was true. Nurse Fleming also complained to them that medications were being given to inmates with expired doctor's orders, which she believed violated state and federal law. Eventually the nurse, after having no satisfactory response, wrote a letter to the medical director about these same complaints. The immediate supervisor returned this letter to nurse Fleming stating it would have to go through the two levels of nursing supervisors who would then take it to the medical director. One week later Fleming was fired after receiving a negative work evaluation, telling her that the letter to the medical director was the most important factor in her dismissal. Also cited was the fact that she did not correctly follow the internal "chain of command" in making her complaints. The supervisor considered this to be "insubordination," but Fleming contended that this was retaliation for taking her complaints to a higher-up when her oral complaints to her supervisor had not produced results.

The appeals court looked to the intent of the statute and held that an employer cannot fire an employee for "insubordination" because an employee failed to follow the chain of command established by the employer when the employee is making complaints of illegal or unethical workplace conduct. Allowing this would undermine the intent of the statute in protecting employees, especially when an employer could fire an employee when directing that these complaints must be filed with a lower-level supervisor who had previously ignored the same complaints.

Nurses are cautioned that the chain of command should typically be followed when making complaints, as was not required in the Fleming case because of special circumstances. However, it is important to follow-up verbal statements to supervisors with written documentation before proceeding further. Even so, there may be exceptions, as considered by the New Jersey court, where one may have to go above immediate supervisors and internal chain of command structure when responses at the designated level have been inadequate or the risk to report at that level may be too great for the employee.

Another case arising on the basis of an employer's alleged violation of Ohio's whistle-blower statute and public policy exception to firing an employee at will resulted in summary judgment for the employer. In *McGuire v. Elyria* (2003) nurse McGuire complained about inadequate staffing levels to her supervisors and was eventually dismissed. The Ohio statute required the employee to have a reasonable belief that the violation that

was occurring was a criminal offense or a felony, not merely a hazard to public health or safety. Without more evidence to support strict compliance with the statute, the court denied the nurse's claim as a matter of law, and this was affirmed by the appeals court.

■ REFERENCES AND BIBLIOGRAPHY

American Nurses Association. (2001). *Code of ethics for nurses with interpretive statements*. Washington, DC: Author.

Bensing, K. (2007, July 2). Within boundaries. *New England Advance for Nurses*, 21–25. Retrieved October 14, 2008, from https://nursing.advanceweb.com/ce/testcenter/content.aspx?courseid=609&creditid=1&cc=91497&sid=2186

Corrine Warthen v. Toms River Community Memorial Hospital, 199 N.J. Super. 18; 1985 N.J. Super. LEXIS 1177; 118 L.R.R.M. 3179 (1985).

Fleming v. Correctional Healthcare Services, 164 N.J. 90; 751 A.2d 1035; 2000 N.J. LEXIS 654; 16 I.E.R. Cas. (BNA) 687; 141 Lab. Cas. (CCH) P59,028 (2000).

Higgins v. Pascack Valley Hospital, 158 N.J. 404; 730 A.2d 327; 1999 N.J. LEXIS 744; 15 I.E.R. Cas. (BNA) 289; 138 Lab. Cas. (CCH) P58,656 (1999).

McGuire v. Elyria, 152 Ohio App.3d 186; 2003 Ohio 1396; 787 N.E.2d 53; 2003 Ohio App. LEXIS 1213 (2003).

Rowe v. Sisters of the Pallottine Missionary Society, 211 W.Va. 16; 560 S.E.2d 491; 2001 W.Va. LEXIS 188 (2001).

Chapter 44

Reporting Illegal, Unethical, or Unsafe Conduct

Susan J. Westrick

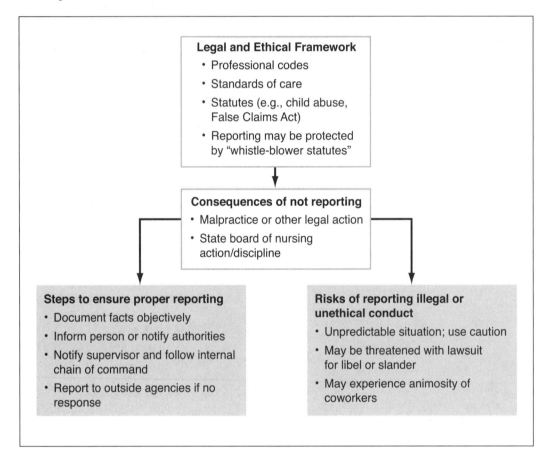

Legal and Ethical Framework
- Professional codes
- Standards of care
- Statutes (e.g., child abuse, False Claims Act)
- Reporting may be protected by "whistle-blower statutes"

Consequences of not reporting
- Malpractice or other legal action
- State board of nursing action/discipline

Steps to ensure proper reporting
- Document facts objectively
- Inform person or notify authorities
- Notify supervisor and follow internal chain of command
- Report to outside agencies if no response

Risks of reporting illegal or unethical conduct
- Unpredictable situation; use caution
- May be threatened with lawsuit for libel or slander
- May experience animosity of coworkers

The nurse is often in a position to recognize conduct of others that is potentially detrimental to the welfare of patients. In such situations, the nurse must seek a satisfactory solution for all parties involved but that ultimately protects the patient's health and safety. In seeking this solution the nurse must weigh the risks and benefits of any action to be taken, as well as the consequences of not taking any action. As in all situations, the nurse is responsible and accountable for such action or inaction (see **Figure 44-1**).

■ LEGAL AND ETHICAL FRAMEWORK FOR DUTY TO REPORT

The following sources provide guidelines for nursing conduct in situations where the nurse questions the actions of others.

1. *Professional codes:* Professional codes provide guidance in many situations that confront the nurse involving the practice of other health professionals. For example, the ANA Code of Ethics for

Nurses (2001) and the International Council of Nurses Code of Ethics for Nurses (2001) mandate that the nurse take appropriate action to safeguard the patient when care is endangered by a coworker or any other person. While these codes identify ethical and not legal duties, they do form standards of care for professional practice that are often used in legal proceedings. It is certainly a part of prudent practice to follow all professional codes for conduct.

2. *Standards of care:* The profession has determined that certain standards of care are required for particular situations. Thus, when a nurse is aware that a standard is not being adhered to by either a person or an agency, an ethical and sometimes a legal duty arises to take corrective action. An example would be if a nurse is aware that OSHA standards are being violated and that patients or staff are likely at risk. This becomes a duty to report the situation to the appropriate authorities, and in some cases the nurse might face serious consequences for not reporting violations.

3. *Statutes:* Most states have mandatory reporting statutes requiring healthcare workers to report child or elder abuse and other kinds of information, such as gunshot or homicide incidents. There are usually fines or other types of sanctions for not reporting. Nurses who work in the school setting or emergency room should be especially mindful of reporting obligations.

■ CASE LAW INVOLVING AN ETHICAL OR LEGAL DUTY TO REPORT

A case involving hospital nurses who made a good faith report to protect an incapacitated and nonverbal adult patient from abuse resulted in the accused filing a lawsuit against the hospital for defamation (*Morganstern v. Mercy Hospital*, 2007). In dismissing the plaintiff's complaint, the court noted that at least five nurses at the hospital stated they observed inappropriate physical conduct by Morganstern, the plaintiff and brother of the patient. In addition there was documentation in the patient's medical record by at least three nurses that they had individually witnessed instances of inappropriate conduct by Morganstern on separate occasions. When this pattern was observed and documented, the nursing staff informed the social worker and ultimately the state Department of Health and Human Services (DHHS). Subsequently, hospital security issued a criminal trespass charge against Morganstern, notified the Portland, Maine police department, and barred him from visiting his sister. Morganstern asserted that hospital staff defamed him through these actions because the staff did not like him, did not conduct an adequate investigation, and accused him in reckless disregard of the truth. However, the court found that nurses are mandatory reporters when "reasonable cause to suspect that an incapacitated or dependent adult … is at substantial risk of abuse, neglect, or exploitation" exists and that those making good faith reports were protected from civil liability. The evidence presented by testimony and affidavits of several nurses and their documentation in the medical record supported the claim of abuse and report to the DHHS.

Other statutes that impact reporting situations involving health and safety are whistle-blowing statutes. These federal or state statutes are designed to protect persons who "blow the whistle" or report employers or others who can retaliate for such action. For example, an employee may be fired for reporting unsafe conditions or inaction of supervisors related to patient safety concerns. In some cases, a whistle-blowing statute could provide protection for the worker in seeking reinstatement after wrongful discharge, or it may prevent the worker from being fired. Some state nurses' associations are actively working to improve whistle-blowing protection for nurses who have been fired for complaining about chronic shortages of staff and other concerns related to patient safety.

The Texas Nurse Practice Act and its whistleblower protection sections that protect against a retaliatory employment decision taken because of an employee's report of a licensed healthcare practitioner was at issue in a case involving nurses who reported a licensed vocational nurse (LVN) to the board of nursing (*Karen Clark, Lavern Worrell, and Jan Woodward v. Texas Home Health Inc.*, 1998). The three plaintiff nurses (the nurses) were serving on a peer review committee for their defendant employer, Home Health. The committee reviewed an LVN, Shaw, whose medical error resulted in a patient's death, and the plaintiffs informed Shaw that the incident must be reported to the Texas Board of Vocational Nurse examiners. They then waited for LVN Shaw's rebuttal and delayed making the actual report. At another meeting of the peer review committee, but before any rebuttal was received from Shaw within the 10-day deadline, the nurses told Home Health that they intended to report the incident. But Home Health's chief executive officer, Sidney Dauphin, expressed concern over the potentially negative consequences if Shaw was reported. He allegedly told the nurses he would personally guarantee their salaries for 10 years if they lost their licenses for failing to report Shaw. At a third meeting the nurses told Home Health they were reporting the incident without any further delay. Without adjourning the meeting, Dauphin immediately removed the nurses from the committee and relieved them of their administrative duties. The nurses then resigned and later sued Home Health, Dauphin, and others under the Nurse Practice Act for retaliatory employment action for reporting a healthcare practitioner, as prohibited by the Texas statute.

The trial court granted summary judgment for the defendants, but the Texas Court of Appeals reversed the decision, in part, and allowed part of the nurses' claim to go forward. The appeals court did not agree with the trial court that just because the actual report was not filed before the adverse employment decision (demotion), the statute did not provide protection for the nurses. The court found that Home Health did have notice that the nurses were making the report to the board and could not hide behind the timing of the actual report when they made the retaliatory acts against these employees. The nurses were demoted after insisting they would report to the proper authorities, and the court found that this is the exact type of retaliatory conduct that the statute is in place to protect. Home Health claimed that it demoted the nurses because they insisted on reporting in their official capacities as administrators for Home Health instead of filing a report in their individual capacities. On the other hand, the nurses claim that they told Home Health that it was critical to report the incident as soon as possible and that they intended to report despite Home Health's disapproval, even if it meant reporting as individuals. The court found Home Health's explanation for the demotion irrelevant because the statute expressly prohibits any adverse employment decision in response to "reporting."

Additionally, Home Health filed a separate lawsuit against the nurses alleging libel and slander based on the nurses' report of Shaw, and the nurses then amended their complaint in this case to include a cause of action for damages and costs incurred as a result of participating in a "peer review." The nurses were not allowed to collect these damages because peer review protection did not apply to review of LVNs. This case illustrates the dilemmas and risks associated with decisions when faced with conflicting expectations of employers and ethical and legal reporting requirements.

A federal statute known as the False Claims Act (FCA) encourages uncovering fraud against the federal government and can be used in medical and agency billing fraud. A civil suit known as *qui tam* lawsuit (where the government is substituted as the plaintiff and brings the lawsuit) can be filed to recover lost money in the government's name. This statute provides whistle-blower protection to the one who makes the claim, and the person may be entitled to a portion of the recovery by the government. While it is sometimes difficult to obtain evidence in these cases, nurses have reported fraud under this statute.

For example, in a lawsuit involving the False Claims Act in the federal district court of Hawaii, the court ruled on a motion by the plaintiffs to compel the defendants to produce certain billing and other records (*United States of America ex rel. Kelly Woodruff, M.D. and Robert Wilkinson, et al. v. Hawaii Pacific Health, et al.*, 2008). In this *qui tam* lawsuit, plaintiffs alleged that the defendants violated the federal False Claims Act, among other charges, by submitting false claims for procedures performed by nurses who were not licensed to perform them. The defendants allegedly submitted false UB-92 forms for the reimbursement of those charges, as well as false cost reports based on these forms. Codes on the forms implied that they were performed by physicians or licensed nurse practitioners with proper physician supervision. These involved procedures that were performed in the newborn intensive care unit (NICU) and also related to other pediatric hematology–oncology procedures. In the motion to compel discovery, plaintiffs sought an additional 255 plus UB-92 forms, access to original microfiche to copy or verify the integrity of the copies produced, electronic evidence related to the cost reports, billing and procedure policies, and documents pertaining to the identified nurses, including call schedules. Some of these records were sought for the years 1997–2001. As part of their request, plaintiffs sought to compel the defendants to

pay for a forensic analysis of their computer systems and files. According to the plaintiffs, the program that defendants used to print the PDF forms that were produced to date is a claims editor program, which can change the content of the claim forms, and the program does not create an audit trail.

The court ruled that most of the documents must be produced by defendants because relevancy, in terms of discovery, is a broad concept that is liberally construed under the Federal Rules of Procedure. They further commented that discovery is designed to define and clarify the issues and is denied only if the information sought has no conceivable bearing on the case. Specifically related to the involved nurses' documentation, requests were also made for their collaborative practice agreements, personnel files for each of the identified nurses, and any personal logs or diaries any identified nurse created or maintained related to the procedures. In this instance the court ruled that the defendant healthcare center had to produce the personnel files of the nurses but only information that indicated whether the nurses performed those procedures in question. The other requested documents related to the nurses did not need to be produced because there was no evidence that these documents were in the defendant's possession.

This litigation is ongoing and underscores the need to have clear and specific documentation of who performed procedures, what their qualifications are, and whether advanced practice nurses or other practitioners are qualified to perform them. Increasingly record keeping is completed in computers and with electronic information systems. One should keep in mind that these records are just as probative as hard copy data and records, and the agency must be able to prove or defend the integrity of these systems.

In another lawsuit, Robbins, a former employee nurse, sued her former employer alleging retaliatory discharge in violation of the False Claims Act (*Pamela Robbins v.*

Provena Hospitals, Inc., 2003). The defendant Medical Center's motion to dismiss was granted in part and denied in part. The plaintiff alleged that she was discharged because of her professional organization activities as chair of the Illinois Nurses Association (INA), the exclusive bargaining agent for the registered nurses at the Medical Center. In this capacity she complained about the adequacy of staffing to the Director of the Illinois Department of Public Health (IDPH), citing inadequate numbers of staff and its effect on patient care. The director advised the nurses to record any delays in patient treatment, and Robbins learned that this type of information could affect the Medical Center's right to participate in and receive reimbursement for Medicare or Medicaid related services. After the meeting, Robbins and other nurses changed the "assignment despite objection" (ADO) forms to expressly notify the Medical Center about delays in patient treatment as a result of inadequate staffing. Robbins also advised the nurses to file the forms with Medical Center supervisors to comply with Illinois regulatory law, which requires nurses to "report unsafe, unethical, or illegal care practice or conditions to the appropriate authorities." The nurses at the Medical Center subsequently filed hundreds of ADOs from 2001–2002, which alleged delays in patient treatment and unsafe staffing levels.

Also in 2002, Robbins and other nurses helped organize public legislative hearings on Illinois House Bill 959, the Patient Safety Act, which proposed to give nurses a role in determining staffing levels and to impose penalties on facilities that refused to do so. Robbins and other nurses attended these televised hearings in March 2002. Before these hearings, Robbins alleges that she was detained and questioned by Medical Center security guards regarding the hearings. She further alleged that a manager confiscated a petition addressed to the IDPH. On May 22, 2002, several nurses were notified that their jobs had

been eliminated. After meeting with human resources and while representing some of these nurses, Medical Center officials placed Robbins on indefinite suspension. She was terminated the next day for allegedly violating an agreement prohibiting nurses from engaging in strikes and work stoppages.

In terms of Robbins's claim that the activities were protected under the FCA, the court found that she did not meet the requisite criteria for such a claim. Specifically while she did put her employer, the Medial Center, on notice that she was complaining to government authorities about the staffing levels, there was no notice that these actions were related to the employer's alleged false claims to the government. However, the court denied the defendant's motion for summary judgment related to two other counts related to retaliatory discharge, so those claims were allowed to go forward for the plaintiff Robbins.

This case illustrates the risks that professional activities, though seemingly valid and important for patient care, can have on one's career. The notion that one is "doing the right thing," even through official channels, does not always protect against negative consequences of the activity. One has to weigh the risks and benefits in such situations and make personal decisions that will uphold one's personal beliefs and professional ethics and integrity.

■ CONSEQUENCES OF NOT REPORTING

Legal or state board of nursing action may be taken against a nurse who does not fulfill a duty to report illegal, unethical, or unsafe conduct of another.

1. Malpractice suits or other legal action can be taken against a nurse for not reporting illegal or unsafe practice by another when the nonreporting results in harm to the patient. In some cases it is the patient who becomes the plaintiff

and alleges that the harm could have been prevented by others who did not report it to proper authorities. The ANA Code of Ethics for Nurses can be used as evidence in malpractice cases to determine the standard of care for nurses' conduct.

Some states have mandatory reporting statutes for healthcare professionals suspected of drug abuse or diversion of drugs. Nurses who do not report these violations risk penalties for nonreporting and could be the subject of actions against them.

2. State board of nursing action imposes penalties for unprofessional conduct by nurses. Unprofessional conduct could include not reporting persons who were harming patients or who were creating issues of health and safety.

■ STEPS TO ENSURE PROPER REPORTING

When a nurse reports illegal, unethical, or unsafe conduct, the following recommended procedures will ensure compliance with standards.

1. Document the facts. The nurse should first document the incident or incidents in a thorough and nonjudgmental manner. The patient's chart should not be used for such comments, but an adverse event or incident report may be used in some circumstances. The nurse needs to record thorough personal notes with specific dates, information, witnesses, and any action taken. This invaluable reference is necessary to validate the person's conduct or the circumstances of concern. In no case should the nurse breach patient confidentiality by copying patient records or data.

2. Inform the person or notify the supervisor or proper authorities. It is recommended that the nurse express appropriate concern to the person whose conduct is in question to clarify the situation and inform the individual of the specific concern for the health or safety of others. Having another person present is recommended because the individual may become defensive or may later misrepresent the information to others. This is especially so if the nurse is confronting a colleague or a physician who may be in a position of power or authority or who is impaired.

3. Notify a supervisor or responsible administrator and follow the internal chain of command and channels. A supervisor should always be notified of the situation, and the nurse should be careful to respect the chain of command. If there is an internal mechanism for reporting such incidents, such as to a committee or union, this should be followed. Many nurses are mistaken in the belief that when they report the situation to supervisors, their responsibility ends. However, it has been confirmed by the courts that the duty does not end there. If there is no response to satisfy the situation and the patient is harmed, the nurse can be responsible for not taking further action. For example, if a physician is still causing harm to a patient and it has been reported to the supervisor with no outcome, the nurse needs to go to a higher authority, such as the medical director.

Using the "chain of command" was at issue in *Whittington v. Episcopal Hospital* (2000) where a high-risk pregnant patient was discharged, readmitted, and died due to delay in dealing with her increasingly dangerous symptoms and delay in treatment. The hospital was held liable for a portion of the damages under a corporate negligence theory, in part because the plaintiff's expert testified that the nurses should have prevented the patient from being discharged the first time as a high-risk patient who had been incompletely evaluated. The expert opined that

> the nurse has an obligation to go to her supervisor and inform the supervisor of this problem that has developed. And the supervisor takes it from there to resolve this conflict of discharging the patient. *It's called the chain of command.* And it has to be used. It should be used. *And the chain of command can go all the way to the chairman of the department or the director of nursing.* (*Whittington v. Episcopal Hospital* at p. 460; emphasis added in case report)

This case underscores the need for nurses to always keep patient safety as the priority, even if it means questioning a medical order and rarely needing to go to someone else (often a nursing supervisor or risk manager) to adequately provide for patient safety. This action is justified when nurses or others know or should know that the patient is in grave danger due to a questionable medical decision. It should not be used for mere disagreement with a medical decision.

4. Report to outside agencies or practice boards. An outside agency may need to be contacted as the next step in seeking a resolution to the problem. The state medical or nursing board should be notified if it involves harmful practice by a health professional. A regulatory agency, such as OSHA, may need to be notified if it is within its area of control.

■ RISKS OF REPORTING ILLEGAL OR UNETHICAL CONDUCT

While the benefits and obligations of reporting questionable conduct that is a threat to health and safety of others outweigh the consequences of not doing so, there are often detrimental effects from reporting. One needs to proceed with care and caution because the risks can be very serious. The accused individual may threaten libel or slander claims against a nurse for reporting his or her conduct. However, the reporting nurse is assured that the truth is an absolute defense to claims that are made in good faith. One may face the animosity of coworkers who consider the reporting nurse to be a traitor or worse. Other forms of retaliation that can occur include job reassignment, demotion, or job loss, as illustrated by the Karen Clark et al. (1998) and Whittington (2000) cases discussed herein.

■ FULFILLING PROFESSIONAL RESPONSIBILITY

In reporting the illegal, unethical, or unsafe practice of others, the nurse is preserving a sense of moral integrity for the profession. The public has a right to expect protection against such harmful conduct by others and to rely on professional nurses to participate fully in its elimination.

■ REFERENCES

American Nurses Association. (2001). *Code of ethics for nurses with interpretive statements.* Washington, DC: Author.

International Council of Nurses. (2000). *Code of ethics for nurses.* ICN, Geneva, Switzerland: Author.

Karen Clark, Lavern Worrell, and Jan Woodward v. Texas Home Health Inc., 971 S.W.2d 435; 1998 Tex. LEXIS 93; 41 Tex. Sup. J. 944; 14 I.E.R. Cas. (BNA) 57 (1998).

Morganstern v. Mercy Hospital, Me. Super. LEXIS 228 (2007).

Pamela Robbins v. Provena Hospitals, Inc., 2003 U.S. Dist. LEXIS 10692 (2003).

United States of America ex rel. Kelly Woodruff, M.D. and Robert Wilkinson, et al. v. Hawaii Pacific Health, et al., 2008 U.S. Dist. LEXIS (2008).

Whittington v. Episcopal Hospital, 2000 Pa. Dist. & Cnty. Dec. LEXIS 361; 44 Pa.D.&C.4th 449 (2000).

Chapter 45

Maternal versus Fetal Rights

Katherine Dempski

A Mother's Rights

- Right to maintain autonomy, bodily integrity, due process, and privacy
- Moral right to determine what will be done with her own person
- Right to be given accurate information, and information necessary to make informed judgments
- Right to be assisted with weighing the benefits and burdens of options in their treatment
- Right to accept, refuse, or terminate treatment without coercion
- Right to be assured that the release of all medical information be prudently restricted

B Situations Where Mother's Rights May Be Diminished

- Requests do-not-resuscitate order
- May not be able to refuse a blood transfusion in some situations (to save the life of the fetus or where she has other children who depend on her)
- Emergency admission during labor or acute illness where mother refuses treatment; questionable whether mother has the capacity to give consent or refuse treatment
- Where the 4 stringent conditions required prior to court intervention have been met

With the development of patients' rights, a pregnant woman presenting in her final trimester creates an inherent conflict to the medical provider. To whom do physicians or nurses owe their first duty—the pregnant woman or the unborn child? Are the rights of the mother subordinated to those of the unborn child? The nurse's role in these situations is a cautious one, but the moral and professional obligation inherent in that role is to treat, regardless of the magnitude of the emotional and moral issues involved. The nurse needs to ensure that the patient's rights are adhered to in the treatment and care plan of each patient.

■ RIGHTS OF THE UNBORN CHILD AND THE MOTHER

The unborn child has a right to be born healthy. *Roe v. Wade* delineated the rights of the fetus and mother based on the degree of viability. The more viable the fetus, the greater degree of rights. When abortion is deemed necessary to save her life, however, the mother's life and health take precedence regardless of the consequence to the fetus.

The rights of the mother are similar to those of any other patient: the right to maintain autonomy and integrity of her body, access to due process, and the right to privacy. The mother's rights according to the *Code of Ethics for Nurses with Interpretative Statements* are listed in **Figure 45-1A**.

The pregnant woman being asked to undergo an extremely invasive procedure to save the baby's life has the right to refuse the treatment and to be free of coercion, even if the fetus is viable. Generally, the more invasive the procedure, the greater degree of maternal rights.

The American Academy of Pediatrics recommends fetal interventions with proven efficacy and low maternal risk. The mother, however, should never be compelled to undergo investigative interventions. In the face of maternal refusal with high probability of fetal harm without intervention and low maternal risk, consultation with the institutional ethics committee should be done, and judicial intervention may become necessary. In contrast, the American College of Obstetrics gives greater weight to the mother's autonomy and advocates maternal counseling and education with judicial review rarely being justified. In its position statement Patient Choice and the Maternal-Fetal Conflict, the American College of Obstetricians and Gynecologists suggest three approaches

to dealing with the competent pregnant woman who refuses treatment: (1) to abide by the patient's decision, allowing her to autonomously determine the course of action, regardless of the consequences; (2) to offer that the woman be cared for by a different provider if the original physician refuses to abide by her request, to give the mother a better chance to be supported; and (3) to petition the court for authorization to proceed against the mother's wishes (the less frequently exercised option).

Courts have been involved in determining the rights of pregnant women in instances of forced monitoring, forced cesarean section, compulsory amniocentesis, and drug testing. Before the decision is made to involve the judicial system, however, the facts of the case must be scrutinized to ascertain the presence of four conditions: (1) a high probability that the fetus will suffer serious harm if the patient's refusal is honored; (2) a high probability that the treatment will prevent or substantially reduce harm to the fetus; (3) no comparable treatment options available; and (4) a high probability that the treatment will also benefit the mother or that the risks to her are minimal. Unless these four conditions are met, the woman's right to autonomy risks being violated with the use of judicial authority.

In these cases, providers need to be cognizant of the fallible nature of testing and the possibility that an ordinarily low-risk procedure, such as cesarean section, could result in serious maternal complications. These unpredictable realities need to be considered when attempting to persuade a pregnant woman to undergo a procedure she has refused.

■ DIMINISHED MATERNAL RIGHTS: CASE LAW ON MATERNAL RIGHT TO REFUSE CESAREAN SECTION

The pregnant woman's right to autonomy is not always absolute (see Figure 45-1B). When the four conditions for judicial review are met, the court will often balance this right with the fetus's chances of survival, the risks of the procedure, and other factors specific to that case. Under this balancing test, some pregnant women have not been required to undergo a medically intricate cesarean, while others have been under court order to receive a life-saving blood transfusion. Besides judicial intervention, some states have diminished maternal autonomy by passing advance directive statutes that remove the DNR option as a healthcare choice for the duration of the pregnancy.

While the Supreme Court has held an unborn fetus is not a person with 14th amendment rights, courts have gone from one extreme (compelling women to undergo surgical intervention) to the other (recognizing maternal right to refuse even if fetal demise is likely). Most courts have held that the fetus may have some protection, but maternal rights weigh more. States have claimed fetuses have no protection under juvenile court, while others have created statutes offering some protectable rights (providing temporary state custody of the unborn fetus).

In *In Re Baby Doe*, the Illinois Appellate Court rejected the state's appeal from the lower court holding that Mrs. Doe could not be compelled into a cesarean section even though the fetus survival rate without the surgical intervention was low and the chance of a maternal death from the procedure was 1:10,000. The state appealed citing the lower court not balancing the rights of the fetus. The appellate court cited to a pregnant woman's right to refuse treatment even when beneficial to the fetus.

A state's right in protecting a fetus was found by the Georgia supreme court in *Jefferson v. Griffin Spalding County Hospital Authority*. A woman had placenta previa. The physicians cited a 50% maternal death rate and 90% fetal death rate without a cesarean section. The woman refused for religious reasons. With a court-appointed attorney for the fetus, a hear-

ing was held at the hospital, and temporary custody of the fetus was granted to a state agency. The woman was compelled to submit to an ultrasound and if the danger persisted would then be compelled to undergo the surgery. The ultrasound showed a shift in the placenta, thereby making the surgery unnecessary, but the court had already laid the groundwork that a mother's right would be diminished in certain circumstances.

Most courts will try to find balance with some fetal protection and the established rights of the mother. In *Pemberton v. Tallahassee Memorial Regional Medical Center*, the state court weighed the "appreciable risk" to the fetus versus the maternal constitutional right to not undergo unconsented surgery. A mother who was compelled to have a cesarean section sued in federal court claiming violation of her constitutional right to procedural due process. The federal court found that when fetal death was almost certain and there was no compelling argument for a vaginal delivery, there was no violation of her constitutional rights to due process.

◼ RESEARCH ON PREGNANT WOMEN

Medical research on pregnant women gives additional duties to an institutional review board. Limitations on including pregnant women in research are limited to where the purpose is to meet the health needs of the mother or fetus, risk to the fetus is minimal, and the activity is the least possible risk for the fetus in achieving the objectives. Informed consent for using research in pregnant women requires informed consent from the competent pregnant woman on behalf of the fetus, as well as the father, unless the research is for the health of the mother or the father is unavailable. The FDA mandates that studies of drugs to treat life-threatening diseases could not exclude women of childbearing age solely based on the perception of fetal risk.

■ DRUG ABUSE

The prevalence of drug abuse has risen among pregnant women. For the most part, the long-term effects of illegal drug use on the fetus are negative. In some states, drug-addicted women are prosecuted for using drugs while pregnant. If arrested and prosecuted prior to the period of viability of the fetus, the mother can be charged with possession, while after viability she is charged with "distribution to a minor." Other states have laws that act to curtail parental rights. Few give pregnant drug users the option of priority access to treatment facilities.

The nurse in this situation is an information provider, discussing options about and assistance with seeking admission into a treatment center. If the mother chooses not to seek treatment and continues to use illegal drugs, she runs the risk of losing her parental rights, and the newborn child may be placed in protective custody. This can cause a backlash. If the mother knows she risks arrest or that her newborn child may be taken from her, she is less likely to seek the treatment required.

Although in many instances drug screening may seem warranted, it is not done routinely. Many institutions believe that if a mother refuses to be tested, the quality of her care will be compromised. Because one cannot be forced to undergo testing, the risk of doing so without consent jeopardizes the patient's right to privacy. Although testing may be done with the best interests of the child in mind, the possible ramification of a positive finding, that of losing her rights as a parent, would be the direct result of the illegally obtained blood sample.

■ AIDS

AIDS is one of the most serious sexually transmitted diseases because it can be life threatening to the newborn. Many states require that medical personnel report all incidences of AIDS to their local health department. The CDC has set forth guidelines both to preserve the patient's privacy and to promote public health through disclosure of the HIV infection. In cases where the reporting of AIDS cases is mandatory, the nurse can breach a patient's confidentiality; the required documentation overrides the patient's privacy.

Mandatory HIV testing has acted to subordinate the usual requirement of obtaining informed consent from the mother for the sake of the fetus. Those who support mandatory HIV testing do so on the grounds that this will enable them to provide the optimum level of care to the newborn. Receiving the HIV drug AZT the last 6 weeks of pregnancy as well as for the first few weeks of the infant's life can reduce an HIV-positive mother from passing on the infection from a 25% chance to about 2–4% if the baby is delivered by a cesarean section (decreases blood exposure from mother to infant). AZT has its own set of side effects, such as anemia and bone marrow toxicity.

At the same time, mandatory testing acts to violate the mother's right to individual liberty and privacy. To ascertain whether mandatory HIV testing of the newborn takes precedent over the rights of the mother, an analysis of the test or procedure is required. If the test or procedure is found to be effective, accurate, and proportionately beneficial to serve its purpose—to protect the health, safety, and welfare of the public—interfering with one's right to privacy and individual liberty will be considered constitutional. With the development of medications that reduce perinatal transmission of HIV and prophylactic regimens that prevent potentially fatal complications, the necessity of mandatory testing is less clear.

States that have enacted HIV testing for pregnant women require counseling of HIV testing as part of routine prenatal care of all women including early treatment benefit to the newborn. The woman may "opt out" with documentation of such in her medical records. At time of delivery the woman would be counseled again as to the benefit of early treatment, and unless she provides specific written refusal, the test will be performed.

■ AMERICAN MEDICAL ASSOCIATION POSITION STATEMENT

Overall, the American Medical Association advocates that the rights of the mother should prevail, except in unusual circumstances. It also adheres to the belief that a decision-making process be in effect to resolve these conflicts. Areas to explore and consider as part of that process include the patient's physical state, the disease process, treatment options, religious beliefs, cultural values, family dynamics, and the legal and financial aspects of the case. In terms of treatment options, technological advances now allow for genetic testing, perinatal diagnosing, fetal surgery, and extensive fetal intensive care facilities. This fact, coupled with the providers' desire and ethical responsibility to do good, further complicates the issue of whose rights prevail.

■ REFERENCES

American College of Obstetricians and Gynecologists Committee on Ethics. (1999). *Patient choice and the maternal-fetal relationship.* Washington, DC: Author.

American Nurses Association. (1976, 2001). *American Nurses Association code for nurses.* Washington, DC: Author.

American Nurses Association. (2001). *Code of ethics for nurses with interpretative statements.* Washington, DC: Author.

Brown, S., Truog, R., Johnson, J., & Ecker, J. (2006, April). Do differences in American Academy of Pediatrics and American College of Obstetricians and Gynecologists positions on ethics of maternal-fetal interventions reflect subtle divergent professional sensitivities to pregnant women and fetuses? *Pediatrics, 117*(4).

Hall, J. (2000). Research with pregnant women and fetuses: Update on ethics and the law. *Journal of Nursing Law, 7*(3).

Honig, J., & Jurgrau, A. (1999). Mandatory newborn HIV testing. *Journal of Nursing Law, 6*(1), 33–37.

In Re A.C., 573 A.2d 1235 (1990).

In Re Baby Doe, 632 N.E.2d 326 (Ill. App. Ct. 1994).

Jefferson v. Griffin Spalding County Hospital Authority, 247 Ga. 86, 274 S.E.2d 457 (Ga. 1981).

Mohaupt, S. M., & Sharma, K. K. (1998). Forensic implications and medical-legal dilemmas of maternal versus fetal rights. *Journal of Forensic Science, 43,* 985–992.

Pemberton v. Tallahassee Memorial Regional Medical Center, 66 F.Supp. 2d 1247 (N.D. Fla. 1999).

Protections for Pregnant Women, Human Fetuses and Neonates Involved in Research, 45 C.F.R. § 46.204–207.

Roe v. Wade, 410 U.S. 113 (1973).

Testing of Pregnant Women and Newborns, Conn. Gen. Stat. Ann. § 19a-593 (2003).

Chapter 46

Futility of Care

Katherine Dempski

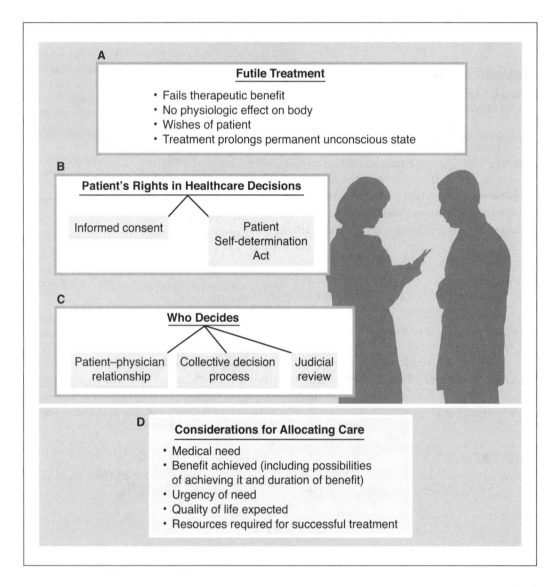

The American Medical Association's code of medical ethics (1997b) states that physicians are not obligated to deliver medical care that in their best judgment will not have a reasonable chance of benefiting the patient. Denial of medical treatment must be based on acceptable standards of care and openly stated ethical principles. Healthcare providers must be aware of the federal statutes and case law that have further complicated the issue of futile care. Recent court decisions look to the futility of medical care when families' wishes to continue and medical recommendations to withdraw collide.

◼ DEFINING FUTILE TREATMENT

Futile treatment is not easy to define (see **Figure 46-1A**). The Hastings Center defines *futility* as care that will not achieve its physiological objective and so offers no physiological benefit to the patient. The term *futility* almost always is used when some treatment is available and may possibly work, but the patient's quality of life is either not worth prolonging or treatment will not improve it. Although futile treatment is often considered "medically unnecessary," that definition alone would encompass such procedures as cosmetic surgery, circumcision, sterilization, in vitro fertilization, etc. Futile care usually is characterized as treatment that does not return the patient to full function or meaningful "quality of life" or life as the patient knew prior to the injury or disease. *Futile* also is used to describe medical treatment that is effective but the patient's quality of life is not perceived as worth prolonging. For example, for an anencephalic infant in acute respiratory distress, intubation is an effective treatment to solve the acute respiratory distress, but it will not cure the anencephaly. In this respect, futile care should not be confused with ineffective treatment. Ineffective treatment does not achieve the desired result.

While there is not clear consensus regarding the definition (local and national medical associations offer various definitions) in general, futile care has these characteristics. The care fails to prolong life or have a physiologic effect or therapeutic benefit for the patient. The patient's wishes will also be weighed. Treatment that prolongs permanent unconsciousness or fails to end dependence on intensive medical care is futile.

◼ SELF-DETERMINATION VERSUS FUTILITY

The doctrine of informed consent ensures that a patient's decision to consent to or refuse medical treatment is an educated one (see Figure 46-1B). The federal law Patient Self-Determination Act (PSDA) of 1991 outlines a patient's right to predetermine his or her own life-and-death decisions regarding medical care. Through advance directives a patient informs the healthcare provider of his or her decision regarding resuscitation, nutrition, hydration, and pain relief when the patient becomes permanently unconscious or terminal (as defined in each state's advance directive statute).

Informed consent and the PSDA preserve the patient's right to refuse medically indicated treatment, but a patient's right to demand medically futile treatment remains uncertain. The President's Commission for the Study of Ethical Problems in Medicine and Biomedical and Behavioral Research found that medical professionals are not obligated to "accede to" the patient's demands when it violates acceptable medical practice. The commission defined informed consent as a "choice among medically acceptable and available options." Informed consent does not translate into a self-determined right to demand what is medically futile. The Hastings Center Guidelines on the Termination of Life-Sustaining Treatment and the Care of the Dying (1987), in accord with the American Medical Association, view physicians as having no ethical obligation to provide futile care.

◼ WHO DECIDES

Medical–legal scholars suggest one of three approaches to the issue of medical futility (see Figure 46-1C). The first avenue is to give deference to the physician–patient relationship. Weight is given to the physician's professional judgment, with the patient's informed consent used as the boundary.

This approach allows the physician and patient the freedom to choose whether the relationship is right for them. The patient has an option to continue care when the physician believes treatment is medically futile. With the physician's help, the patient may transfer to another physician who shares the patient's belief in continuing care. In this approach, the patient's own financial resources or medical insurance may be the limiting factor on receiving care.

The second process involves the collective decisions of the physician, the patient, the family members, the agency, and the judges. An agency's ethics committee is another type of collective decision process. Ethics committees are made up of physicians, nurses, hospital administrators, attorneys, and community members.

When the issue of futile care comes before the courts, it is often because family members wish to continue medical care that the hospitals and physicians determined is futile. In the majority of cases, courts hold that medical care should be continued. Several courts have used federal statutes to determine the issue of medical futility. Congress passed the Emergency Medical Treatment and Active Labor Law (EMTALA) in 1989 to prevent physicians and hospitals from transferring unstable emergency and in-house patients to another facility for insurance purposes. Several courts stated that the EMTALA requires hospitals and physicians to medically treat and stabilize all patients who present to the hospital with an emergency medical condition, even when the treatment may be futile. In *In Re Baby K*, an anencephalic infant continuously presented to the emergency department in acute respiratory distress. The hospital sought a declaratory ruling that future refusal to treat would not violate EMTALA (and other federal statutes) or result in malpractice. The court refused to recognize an exception to EMTALA's requirement that medical emergencies be stabilized and held that the physicians must mechanically ventilate the infant in acute respiratory distress even though the physicians believed it was ultimately futile (*In Re Baby K*, 1994).

Patients have a right to refuse treatment, but do they have a right to demand futile treatment? An adult daughter of a 73-year-old woman with irreversible neurological damage sued the hospital and physicians for making a DNR order over the daughter's wishes. The court looked to the mother's wishes and determined that she would have wanted to be kept alive under these circumstances but held that medical judgment on futility of further treatment outweighed this. Likewise, a probate court ruled continuation of ventilator support and lack of DNR order was "futile invasive measures" and sided with the physicians and guardian ad litem over an adult son who disregarded the physician's and guardian ad litem's recommendation (*Guardianship of Elma Mason*, 1996).

■ USING ETHICS TO ALLOCATE MEDICAL CARE

To safeguard a patient's interest, only medical need may be considered when the allocation of limited medical resources is necessary. Other criteria that are appropriate to consider are listed in Figure 46-1D.

According to the American Medical Association's ethics committee's statements on allocation of medical care (1997a), when medical resources are limited, it may be necessary to prioritize patients so death or poor quality of care is avoided. Nonmedical criteria, such as social standing, financial ability to pay for treatment, patient age, or patient contribution to illness (drug use, smoking, etc.) should not be considered. When there is little difference among the patients with a medical need and the potential for successful outcome, then equal opportunity criteria such as first come, first served is appropriate. The

American Medical Association also recommends that allocation procedures be disclosed to the public and be subjected to the peer review process.

States and hospitals encourage definitions of futile care and policies to guide staff when medical consensus clashes with families' wishes. Policies provide courts with standards of care to follow. State statutes addressing a patient's right to refuse treatment and self-determination of health care often include statements that these acts do not require physicians to give medically inappropriate (futile) care.

Most states provide that a do not resuscitate (DNR) order may not be entered without patient or surrogate consent except under extreme circumstances, such as impossibility.

Policy would guide staff to seek alternatives, such as ethics committee review.

■ REFERENCES

American Medical Association. (1997a). *Code of medical ethics. Allocation of medical care.* Chicago: Author.

American Medical Association. (1997b). *Code of medical ethics. Futile care.* Chicago: Author.

Guardianship of Elma Mason, Mass. App. Ct. No. 96-P-1383 (1996).

Hastings Center. (1987). *Guidelines on the termination of life-sustaining treatment and the care of the dying.*

Herlik, A. (1996). Medicine at the margins: Our national struggle with medically futile treatments. *Journal of Nursing Law, 3*(2), 63–83.

In Re Baby K, 832 F.Supp. 1022 (E.D. Va. 1993), 16 F.3d 590 (4th Cir. 1994).

Chapter 47

Advance Directives and End-of-Life Decisions

Katherine Dempski

Competent individuals can make their wishes known via an advance directive, defined by the PSDA as a written instruction, such as a living will or durable power of attorney, for health care recognized under state law when the individual is incapacitated. Three legal instruments currently meet the act's definition of advance directive (the nurse should refer to each state-specific legislation to ensure the validity of each):

1. *Living will:* A competent adult may prepare a document providing direction as to life-sustaining medical care in the event this individual may become terminal or permanently unconscious. A living will does not appoint a representative to make decisions.
   a. *Terminal:* Incurable or irreversible medical condition that without administration of life support will result in death in a relatively short period of time
   b. *Permanent unconsciousness:* Permanent coma or persistent vegetative state that is irreversible, patient is not aware of self or environment and shows no response to environment
2. *Durable power of attorney/healthcare proxy (DPOAHC):* A durable power of attorney/healthcare proxy enables a competent individual to name someone (usually a spouse, parent, adult child, or other adult) to exercise decision-making authority, under specific circumstances, on the individual's behalf.
3. *Advance directive for health care:* Can be considered a hybrid of the living will and the durable power of attorney/healthcare proxy. Via this tool, an individual will provide precise instructions for the type of care he or she does or does not desire in a number of scenarios. The individual may also appoint a proxy decision maker to help interpret the application of the specific instructions or fill in unanticipated gaps.

As required by the Patient Self-Determination Act (42 U.S.C. 1395), all patients must be advised of their right to make decisions about their health care, including the right to establish written advance directives. Written explanation of these rights must be provided upon admission to the patient or family members of incapacitated patients. CMS Patients' Rights gives patients in facilities accepting Medicare/Medicaid the right to create advance directives for health care, and The Joint Commission is in line with federal regulations that patients be informed about their right to advance directives and the extent the hospital is able to go to honor the directive. A durable power of attorney for health care and a living will and advance directives for health care fit under the umbrella term *advance directives* (see **Figure 47-1**).

■ DURABLE POWER OF ATTORNEY FOR HEALTH CARE

In the durable power of attorney for health-care document, a competent adult appoints a proxy decision maker. This agent, chosen by the patient, has the authority to make decisions about the patient's care and treatment in the event the patient becomes incapable of making such decisions (i.e., the reasoning required to make informed decisions is lacking). Determination of capacity for decision making is done by a primary physician or judicial hearing (see **Figure 47-2**). Ideally, the patient chooses a surrogate with whom a trusted relationship has been established, often a family member or close friend who knows the patient well enough to have had discussions pertaining to end-of-life decisions and treatment choices.

The agent's intent should be to protect the patient's wishes or to act in a manner that fosters the best interests of the patient if the patient's wishes are not known. If the surrogate is not acting in a manner consistent with this or is making what appear to be inappropriate decisions, the nurse needs to protect the patient from the harm that could incur from these acts. These incidents should be reported to the patient's physi-

cian, the nursing supervisor, and the ethics committee.

The application of the durable power of attorney for health care is broad and can range from temporal requests, such as obtaining information about past medical conditions, to those relative to discontinuing life-support systems. In all cases of decision making, if the patient's preference is known, it should take precedence. The agent also should have broad authority to interpret vague statements relative to healthcare choices made by the patient prior to incapacity. If the agent is unaware of such statements, whatever action that advances the best interests of the patient should follow (see **Figure 47-3**).

■ LIVING WILL

Under a written living will, if the patient's condition is deemed "terminal" or if the patient is determined to be "permanently unconscious," life-support systems, including artificial respiration, cardiopulmonary resuscitation, and artificial means of nutrition and hydration may be provided, withheld, or removed. Often a statement from one or two physicians indicating that the patient's condition is not expected to improve is required prior to any action. In drawing a living will, the patient needs to be aware that foregoing life-support measures does not mean that the patient will not be provided measures of pain control or comfort.

Capacity for decision making consists of three basic elements:
1. Ability to evaluate different options
2. The ability to communicate and understand information
3. The ability to reason and to deliberate about one's choices

Figure 47-2   Decision-making capacity.

Durable power of attorney/healthcare proxy (DPOAHC):
• Authority is effective upon determination that the patient lacks capacity
• Ceases effectiveness (revoked) upon recovered capacity of the patient
• Capacity determination is made by primary physician or judicial process
• Decisions are made in accord with patient instruction; absent instruction, decisions are made to the best interest and personal values of the patient
• Usually must be in writing with witness (unless state statute specifies otherwise)
• Some states may recognize oral advance directive under certain conditions, such as statement to healthcare provider or to specified surrogate (such as spouse or adult child)

Living will:
• Forms vary state to state and include state definitions (such as "terminally ill" and "life sustaining treatment")
• Usually applies when patient is terminally ill; not all states include persistent vegetative state
• No designation of agent or surrogate decision maker
• Living will must select or exclude certain provisions of care based on the illness/injury
• Physicians make decisions based on interpretation of the living will

Figure 47-3   Durable power of attorney/healthcare proxy (DPOAHC) and living wills.

■ ADVANCE DIRECTIVES FOR HEALTH CARE

Advance directives for health care may be a hybrid of the living will and durable power of attorney/healthcare proxy (DPOAHC), which combines a proxy with an appointment of a durable power of attorney to make decisions for them but with specific instructions on the type of care desired or not desired.

■ PSYCHIATRIC ADVANCE DIRECTIVES

While the majority of states do not currently have specific state statutes for advance directives of psychiatric care, patients may execute a DPOAHC that applies to mental health treatment preferences. The agent may consent to or refuse treatment for the patient. In the states with statutes, it may be determined

that a properly executed psychiatric advance directive may not be overridden for convenience of providers and may not be automatically overridden when the patient is involuntarily committed. The capacity to execute the DPOAHC is presumed, and the patient may revoke it unless he or she is adjudicated as incapacitated. Physicians may seek adjudication for incapacitation of the patient under state laws.

In *Hargrave v. Vermont*, the plaintiff, who was diagnosed with a serious mental illness, was in "need of treatment" (involuntary commitment). Prior to the admission she properly executed a durable power of attorney and expressly did not authorize her agent to consent to any antipsychotic medications. She was involuntarily medicated against her wishes expressly stated in her durable power of attorney for health care. At issue in the case was whether the state had the right to override a durable power of attorney with involuntary psychiatric medication in a non-emergency situation (patient is not a direct threat to safety of others). The court magistrate held that individuals with mental illnesses should not have to abrogate their statutorily created right to a durable power of attorney for health care when the law does not similarly subject individuals with no mental illness from abrogating their rights. Those with mental illness should execute a durable power of attorney for health care that is afforded the same recognition and enforcement as the advance directives executed by people who do not have mental disability (*Hargrave v. Vermont*, 2001).

■ DO NOT RESUSCITATE ORDERS

Typically, patients are unaware that requests for DNR orders placed in their advance directives are not effective until a physician enters the DNR into the medical record. Implementation of CPR does not require an order, yet withholding CPR does. Standards in practice and state laws presume CPR will be initiated unless a written order precludes it. Furthermore, under various institution's policies on CPR, other measures, such as intubation, may be included and need to be expressly excluded if the patient only desires CPR without intubation. DNR orders need to be reviewed and renewed on a frequent basis as determined by institution policy or state law.

States that do have statutes regarding DNR orders presume the patient's consent to CPR unless there is a written order by a physician responsible for the patient's care and may require it be witnessed. For surrogate decision making to become effective when the patient lacks capacity, the primary physician and a concurring physician will need to document the existence of a terminal condition and that resuscitation is futile.

Perioperative Setting DNR Orders

Terminally ill patients frequently require surgery, whether to repair a broken bone or some other procedure to improve the quality of life. Statistically, a patient suffering a cardiopulmonary arrest while under anesthesia has a better chance of survival than when the arrest is related to the underlying disease. An automatic suspension of DNR orders in the perioperative setting would violate self-determination, but rather DNR orders should be reviewed with the patient and family prior to the surgical procedure (AORN Position Statement, "Perioperative Care of Patients with DNR orders"; concurs with American Society of Anesthesiologists and American College of Surgeons guidelines).

■ NURSE'S ROLE

Nurses' responsibility in advance directives is to educate, document, and communicate. The nurse should document if the patient has signed advance directives or not (and place a copy in the medical record; The Joint Commission, 2008, Standard RI 2.80). The nurse should also communicate the existence of advance directives, including any changes by the patient, to the primary physician. Not communicating the fact that a written living will exists or that the patient made statements regarding end-of-life decisions acts to deny the patient's rights of autonomy and self-determination and sets the stage for a legal cause of action against providers.

In its position statement Nursing and the Patient Self-Determination Act, the ANA suggests that nurses question patients upon admission as to the existence of any advance directives. If none are in place, they should ask if the patient desires to create such a directive. If so, the nurse has the responsibility to see that the patient has the information needed to make an informed decision about treatment and options. The nurse should encourage the patient to ask questions about medical issues as well as the mechanics of advance directives. The nurse also should encourage the patient to be as clear as possible about the choices. If the statements by the patient are of a general nature, such as "no machines to keep me alive," it is the nurse's responsibility to educate the patient.

■ TERMINATION OF LIFE SUPPORT

Terminating life support requires following the patient's written instructions, state statutes, and relevant case law on determining the patient's wishes.

Standards

The Joint Commission addresses compliance with a patient's wishes regarding end-of-life decisions (2008, Standard RI 2.80). The patient receives information on the right to accept or refuse treatment, including resuscitation.

Competent versus Incompetent Patient's Rights

A notable case that has thrust the issue of termination of life support, as well as communicating your wishes regarding life-sustaining measures, to the forefront is *Cruzan v. Director, Missouri Department of Health.* Nancy Beth Cruzan, a 25-year-old woman, lost control of her car in Jaspur County, Missouri. When the paramedics found her, she had no detectable breathing or heart beat, and the paramedics proceeded to resuscitate her. Cruzan lay in a persistent vegetative state—a condition in which a patient exhibits motor reflexes but no significant cognitive function. The family, realizing that there was no chance of Cruzan regaining any of her mental faculties, asked hospital employees to terminate artificial nutrition and hydration procedures. Because that act would cause her death, hospital employees refused to honor the request without court approval. The lower court granted the family's request, finding that Cruzan's

informed conversation with a friend indicated that she would not wish to continue living in her current condition. The Missouri Supreme Court reversed that decision. The higher court recognized a common law doctrine of informed consent but not a broader constitutional right of privacy to refuse medical treatment. The Missouri Supreme Court concluded that the Missouri living will statute embodied a state policy favoring the preservation of life except where the wish to die was established by "clear and convincing evidence." The Missouri Supreme Court also rejected the argument that Cruzan's parents were entitled to order termination of treatment on behalf of their daughter.

Seven years later, the US Supreme Court considered whether life support could be withdrawn from Cruzan's body. The question before the US Supreme Court was whether Cruzan had a right under the US Constitution that would require the hospital to withdraw life-sustaining treatment. The Supreme Court noted that the US Constitution grants a *competent* person the constitutionally protected right to refuse lifesaving hydration and nutrition. Because an *incompetent* patient's rights were in question, the court looked to (and recognized) the Missouri requirement that evidence of the incompetent patient's wishes as to the withdrawal of treatment must be proved by "clear and convincing evidence." As such, the US Supreme Court ruled in June 1990, in a 5–4 decision, that Cruzan's family had not provided clear and convincing evidence to the Missouri court that Cruzan would refuse the life support if she was competent.

After the Supreme Court's decision, a Missouri probate judge ruled that Cruzan's parents had amassed "clear and convincing evidence" that she would not want to persist in her present state of "life." Artificial maintenance procedures were terminated, and Cruzan died 12 days later.

■ SURROGATES

A surrogate may make a decision to withdraw or withhold life sustaining treatment when the patient lacks capacity. Surrogate decisions become effective when a patient has not executed advance directives or appointed an agent by DPOAHC or the agent appointed is not reasonably available. The physician responsible for care determines if the patient is terminal or permanently unconscious (defined by state statutes). The surrogate is responsible to communicate to others that the surrogate has assumed authority. The statute will list the classes in order of priority but in general the order is as follows:

1. Spouse, which may include an adult who shares emotional, physical, and financial relationship of a spouse; revoke if legally separated
2. Adult children
3. Parent
4. Adult siblings
5. Adult grandchildren
6. Adult nieces, nephews, uncles, aunts
7. Adult relative who is familiar with the patient
8. If no members previously listed are available, then an adult who has exhibited concern of the patient and shares values with the patient

Conflicts

When there are numerous members of a class, the majority decision is respected. If the class is split, the providers may refer the case to the ethics committee or other third-party mediator or to a court. If it cannot be resolved, the class may be disqualified and the next priority class consulted.

■ LIABILITY

If medical providers do not follow the instructions of an advance directive, they subject themselves to the same scrutiny and con-

sequences that would occur if they disregarded a refusal to treatment. Some statutes state that healthcare providers must comply with the instructions in a living will. However, in some cases a physician who cannot do so for reasons of conscience can opt to not follow through with the directive. However, there may be a statutory duty to advise the patient and the patient's family of this policy at the time of admission to the facility so that they may be given the option of transferring the patient to a provider who will honor the directive.

Finally, nurses or other medical personnel should not sign as witnesses for any advance directive. The nurse works too closely with the patient, and in certain circumstances, the allegations of undue influence could surface. In most states, the law prevents nurses or other healthcare providers from acting as surrogates for health care for patients. In most states, the advance directive statutes prevent nurses or other healthcare providers from being named as their patients' healthcare agent unless there is a blood relationship.

Not notifying the adult daughter to participate in the decision to withdraw life support resulted in a negligent infliction of emotional distress claim against the hospital. The patient was admitted without advance directives or an appointed agent, and he had not made a statement to his providers regarding his wishes regarding life-sustaining treatment in the end of a terminal illness or permanent unconsciousness. When he suffered an anoxic brain injury, the physicians withdrew life support, and he died 1 week later. The hospital was aware of the daughter's existence, and she was the available next of kin. The court held that the hospital owed a duty to make a reasonable effort to inform known and available next of kin to participate in the decision to remove life support based on what the patient would have wanted. The hospital knew or should have known that without contacting her, she would suffer emotional distress (*Valentin v. St. Francis Hospital and Medical Center*, 2005).

When a consulting neurologist declared that their mother was in a persistent vegetative state, the family requested the primary treating physician to remove the respirator. The patient did not have advance directives, and the son was acting as surrogate, exercising his mother's wishes that she expressed to him. The physician refused stating she would need to be brain dead or the family could seek a court order. During the time the family sought an attorney, the patient was declared brain dead and subsequently expired. The family sued for negligent infliction of emotional distress, and the court held the state probate code had immunity for providers who in good faith did not comply with the family's or patient's request (*Duarte, et al. v. Chino Community Hosp.*, 1999).

■ REFERENCES

American Nurses Association. (1991). *Nursing and the patient self-determination act.* Washington, DC: Author.

AORN. (March 1995, rev. December 2004). *Position statement: Perioperative care of patients with DNR orders.* Denver, CO: Author.

Cruzan v. Director, Missouri Department of Health, 497 U.S. 261 (1990).

Duarte, et al. v. Chino Community Hosp., 72 Cal. App. 4th 849; 85 Cal. Rptr. 2d 521 (Cal. 1999).

Fade, A. E. (1995). Advance directives: An overview of changing right-to-die laws. *Journal of Nursing Law, 2*(3), 27–38.

Hargrave v. Vermont, 2:99 CV 128 (D.Vt. 2001) (upheld 2nd circuit), 2003 WL 21770957 (2nd Cir. 2003).

Patient Self-Determination Act, 42 U.S.C. §§ 1395–1396 (1990).

The Joint Commission. (2008). *Hospital accreditation standards.* Oakbrook Terrace, IL: Author.

Valentin v. St. Francis Hospital and Medical Center, 2005 Conn. Super. LEXIS 2978 (Nov. 2005).

Chapter 48

Assisted Suicide

Katherine Dempski

Assisted suicide: individual provides lethal dose of medication to the patient with intent of ending patient's life

Active euthanasia: provider (not patient) performs drug administration; illegal in the United States

Voluntary euthanasia: patient requests euthanasia

Involuntary euthanasia: patient explicitly opposes

Nonvoluntary euthanasia: patient is incapable of stating wishes

Passive euthanasia:
- Withholding/withdrawing treatment that allows the disease process to take its course
- Patient succumbs to underlying medical condition
- Legally and medically acceptable

Terminal sedation:
- Legally upheld by Supreme Court as distinguished from assisted suicide
- Used in terminal illness with intractable pain, withdrawing life sustaining treatment while intentionally inducing unconsciousness
- Requires consent of patient or surrogate

The terms *assisted suicide* and *euthanasia* generally mean aiding or assisting another person to kill himself or herself, or killing another person at his or her request, often called "active voluntary euthanasia." The US Supreme Court has determined there is no constitutional right to physician-assisted suicide whether by liberty right (*Washington v. Glucksberg*, 1997) or equal protection (*Vacco v. Quill*, 1997). The Supreme Court clearly distinguished the withdrawal of life support to passively allow the disease to kill the patient versus intentionally administering a medication that will kill the patient. In both *Washington* and *Vacco*, the Court upheld two state statutes that prohibited assisted suicide in all instances, including patients with a terminal illness. Providing palliative treatment for those in intractable pain and near death or terminating life support per the patient's wishes are generally not considered to be assisted suicide. Nurses should be aware of these differences (see **Figure 48-1**).

■ STATE INTEREST IN PRESERVING LIFE

Assisted suicide involves a decision concerning one's own body; as such it falls within the realm of personal liberty that government may not enter. However, the state has an obligation to protect life simply because of its existence. This conflict between personal autonomy (which includes the right to refuse medical treatment) and the state's interest in preserving life leaves the nurse in the middle of a legal and ethical entanglement.

■ DISTINGUISHING ASSISTED SUICIDE FROM PERSONAL AUTONOMY

Nurses providing patient care are concerned with defining assisted suicide versus honoring the patient's wishes regarding palliative care and termination of life support. Two notable cases involving terminating life support provide some guidelines. The first began with Karen Quinlan, a young adult hospital patient who had been in a coma for approximately 1 year and was being kept alive by a respirator (*In Re Karen Quinlan*, 1976). The New Jersey Supreme Court, in a unanimous decision based on the patient's right to privacy, permitted the father to seek physicians and hospital officials who would agree to remove the respirator. The court said that if the responsible attending physician concluded that there was no reasonable possibility of Karen Quinlan's return to cognitive and sapient life and that the life-support apparatus be discontinued, they should consult the hospital ethics committee or similar group at the institution where she was hospitalized. If the ethics committee agrees, the life-support system may be withdrawn, and the action will be without any civil or criminal liability on the part of any participant, whether guardian, hospital, physician, or others.

In its ruling, the New Jersey Supreme Court laid down a procedure insulating the physician from liability. Ethics committees were formed to free healthcare providers from using their own self-interest and fear of legal ramifications to make decisions on the well-being of their dying patients.

In the second case, *Cruzan v. Director, Missouri Department of Health* (1990), a 25-year-old woman sustained life-disabling injuries after a car accident. The family asked to have any and all life-sustaining measures removed.

Both the hospital and the courts of Missouri denied this family request. The US Supreme Court upheld the state court decision, citing the state's right to legislate the type of evidence it will accept to prove an incompetent person's desires for life-support termination. The court emphasized that preservation of life was paramount unless there was clear and convincing evidence that the patient wished otherwise under those circumstances (such as a persistent vegetative state).

The difference between assisted suicide and permissive termination of life support is the question of intent. For the latter, a patient's *informed* refusal of treatment is recognized as legal and even a constitutionally mandated right, the patient's right to personal autonomy. Assisted suicide, even in the face of intractable pain or terminal illness, is not legal because the *intent* is to kill and usually involves the deliberate act of providing a means to cause death.

■ PROTECTION AGAINST CLAIMS

In 1974 and 1980 the American Medical Association proposed that decisions not to resuscitate be formally entered in the patient's progress notes and communicated to all staff. When applied and followed correctly, it provides evidence that the healthcare providers followed the patient's wish (and right) to refuse unwanted medical treatment. Many hospitals have published policies about withdrawal or nonapplication of life-prolonging measures. It is paramount that healthcare providers be very aware of these standards, protocols, and procedures.

While the Supreme Court noted in *Vacco v. Quill* (1997) that there is no constitutional right to physician-assisted suicide, the question was left to the states to legalize. Oregon became the first state to enact a physician-assisted suicide statute, The Oregon Death with Dignity Act (ODWDA, 1997) permitting competent, terminally ill adults to obtain a prescription for a lethal dose of medication intended for self-administration. The act contains strict guidelines to ensure safeguards in implementing the act in an effort to improve end-of-life care for citizens of Oregon. Data related to the "success" of the act are mixed, but advocates point to the positive outcomes for patients in terms of self-determination.

The ODWDA was challenged in *Gonzales v. Oregon* (2006). Under the ODWDA, a physician who prescribes or dispenses lethal doses of drugs to terminally ill patients within certain safeguards will be protected from criminal or civil liability. The Court held that the Attorney General could not use the federal Controlled Substance Act to prohibit physicians from prescribing the regulated medications used in assisted suicide under the ODWDA. Specifically, the Court held the Controlled Substance Act does not allow the federal government to control state-assisted suicide laws.

■ NURSE'S ROLE

The ANA Position Statement on Assisted Suicide (1994b) concludes that nurse participation in assisted suicide violates the Code of Ethics for Nurses. The role of the nurse in end-of-life decisions includes promoting comfort, pain relief, and permissive withdrawal or withholding of life support. The ANA acknowledges that administering pain medication with the intent of alleviating pain may risk hastening death but that this does not constitute assisted suicide. The underlying cause of death is the natural disease process. A nurse may not deliberately aid in the termination of another's life.

The ANA further acknowledges that the withdrawal of nutrition and hydration should be decided by the patient or surrogate with the nurse continuing expert nursing care.

The ANA Position Statement on Active Euthanasia (1994a) states that the nurse should not participate in active euthanasia

because it would be a violation of the Code of Ethics for Nurses.

■ CONFLICTING PROFESSIONAL VIEWS

It has been long cultivated for healthcare professionals to respect the patient's wishes to refuse or to discontinue life-prolonging treatment. Physicians and nurses may hold some views that make it difficult to act in ways that would be consistent with their own express support for patient autonomy. Most clinicians are uncertain about what the laws, ethics, and the respected professional standards state. In addition to this uncertainty, clinicians are less likely to withdraw treatments than to withhold them for a variety of other reasons, including psychological discomfort with actively stopping a life-sustaining intervention; discomfort with the public nature of the act, which might occasion a lawsuit from disapproving witnesses even if the decision were legally correct; and fear of sanction by peer review boards.

■ ARGUMENTS AGAINST ASSISTED SUICIDE

Legalization of physician-assisted suicide creates fear of abuses resulting from undue influence and coercion, financial incentives, inadequate determinations of mental competence, mistaken diagnosis of illness as terminal, inadequate diagnosis of depression, inadequate treatment for pain, ineffective communication, and impatience of medical personnel. However, not recognizing and setting forth some sort of framework in which to operate in the realm of assisted suicide may exacerbate the risk of abuse of decision-making power.

■ REFERENCES

American Nurses Association. (1992, April 2). *ANA position statement: Foregoing nutrition and hydration.* Washington, DC: Author.

American Nurses Association. (1994a). *ANA position statement: Active euthanasia.* Washington, DC: Author.

American Nurses Association. (1994b). *ANA position statement: Assisted suicide.* Washington, DC: Author.

Chopko, M. E., & Moses, M. F. (1995). Assisted suicide: Still a wonderful life? *Notre Dame Law Review, 70,* 519.

Cruzan v. Director, Missouri Department of Health, 497 U.S. 261 (1990).

Gonzales v. Oregon, 546 U.S. 243 (2006).

In Re Karen Quinlan, 355 A.2d 644 (N.J. S. Ct. 1976) reversing, 348 A.2d 80 (N.J. S. Ct. 1976).

Rose, T. (2007). Physician-assisted suicide: Development, status, and nursing perspectives. *Journal of Nursing Law, 11*(3), 141–151.

Scofield, G. R. (1997). Natural causes, unnatural results, and the least restrictive alternative. *Western New England Law Review, 9*(2), 351.

Vacco v. Quill, 117 S. Ct. 2293 (1997).

Volker, D. (2007). The Oregon experience with assisted suicide. *Journal of Nursing Law 11*(3), 152–162.

Volker, D. L. (1995). Assisted suicide and the terminally ill: Is there a right to self-determination? *Journal of Nursing Law, 2*(4), 37–47.

Washington v. Glucksberg, 521 U.S. 702 (1997).

Part V Review Questions

1. A 44-year-old obese woman is admitted to the hospital for an evaluation of numerous vague complaints. She has seen several physicians and undergone several tests over the years, but her symptoms have not been diagnosed. She has been taking narcotics for her pain, as prescribed by her private physician. When the nurse is in her presence, she moves in a painful manner, making frequent references to her discomfort and inability "to do anything." However, when the nurse is observing her without her knowledge, she has no difficulty moving and does not reveal any signs of pain on movement. The admitting physician writes an order for the narcotics as requested by the patient. What should the nurse do first?

   (A) Follow the order and give her a dose upon her first request
   (B) Talk to the physician about the observation
   (C) Refuse to give her the medication when she requests it and tell her why
   (D) Spend some time talking with the patient before she requests a pill to try to get an understanding of her needs, both physical and emotional

2. The nurse is treating two patients with the same condition. The nurse believes that all patients should be fully informed as to their conditions and prognoses. One of these patients is very interested in learning more about the condition, while the other could care less. In fact, he stated, "I don't want to know. This whole thing scares me to death. I just want to get it over with and get out of here." The nurse should:

   (A) Walk away in frustration, complaining to colleagues about the incident
   (B) Talk to the physician about the patient's denial, suggesting that a psychiatric evaluation is in order
   (C) Tell the patient that the nurse understands and start talking about the condition
   (D) Speak to the patient privately about his concerns to ascertain what, in fact, he does know about the condition and prognosis

3. Which of the following steps should the nurse take *first* in fulfilling a professional duty to report a colleague who is not completing nursing tasks in a safe manner for patients?

   (A) Report the conduct to the nurse's supervisor
   (B) File a complaint with the state board of nursing
   (C) Check to see if others have noticed this by seeking validation from other coworkers
   (D) Inform the individual and state specific concerns

4. A nurse has witnessed a physician diverting drugs for his own use and signing

them as given to patients. The physician told the nurse to "keep quiet" about it. If the nurse does not report this potentially harmful conduct for patients, the nurse:

(A) Should be safe from consequences because the physician has the authority to prescribe drugs
(B) May be subject to disciplinary action by the state board of nursing
(C) Will only be at risk if actual harm does come to a patient because of this
(D) Will fulfill professional responsibility if the nurse confronts the physician (if safe to do so) and documents in personal notes what was seen

5. A pregnant woman comes into the emergency room. She is talking incoherently and acting paranoid. Her labor is processing rapidly, and the nurse has difficulty hearing a fetal heart tone. The physician examines her and makes the decision to perform a cesarean section. When the patient hears this, she reacts violently, shouting that she "will not be cut!" What should the nurse do first?

(A) Get an immediate order for diazepam
(B) Tell the physician that in spite of the patient's drugged state, she has refused to undergo a cesarean section
(C) Question the patient about her fears, if able to, and try to determine if it is feasible to educate her as to the risks and benefits of cesarean section
(D) Leave her to attend to other patients who are more cooperative and less combative

6. A woman comes into the emergency department and is 8 months pregnant. She is experiencing contractions. She tells the nurse she has had no prenatal care. She also tells the nurse she has had multiple sexual partners and in fact does not know which one is the father of her unborn baby. The nurse should:

(A) Listen, take the patient's vital signs, and make a note of it in the chart
(B) Tell the patient that she will need to undergo AIDS testing and remind the physician to order it as part of regular blood work
(C) Advise the patient that she should have an AIDS test and that if the result is positive, this finding will have to be reported to the local health agency
(D) Do nothing

7. When allocating medical care in an equality situation, it is necessary that:

(A) The patient's physician assist in the decision
(B) The patient's age and quality of life be considered
(C) The allocation be based on first come, first served basis
(D) The patient's contribution to the illness be considered because a smoker who refuses to quit smoking should not be given a lung transplant prior to someone who never smoked

8. In a community hospital emergency department, an 80-year-old man presents with chronic obstructive pulmonary disease complicated by a 65-year history of smoking two packs of cigarettes per day. He arrives in the department with his family at least once a month in acute respiratory distress requiring intubation and respiratory support. After a few days in the intensive care unit, he is discharged back to a hospice program. There is no indication that he is incompetent, but his condition is terminal. The medical and nursing staff agree that he is wasting hospital resources because there is no cure and he continues to smoke even as he is hooked up to his oxygen tank. The appropriate action to take the next time he comes to the emergency department is to:

(A) Refuse to intubate him and get a court order to declare him incompetent (no one who continues to smoke while on oxygen is competent)

(B) Continue to intubate him as needed for the acute respiratory arrest

(C) Refuse to intubate and get a physician to order DNR

(D) Do none of the above

9. A 24-year-old victim of a serious motor vehicle accident told the nurse that he does not want heroic measures to save his life. The nurse first should:

(A) Ignore the statement and attend to other patients

(B) Tell him he is not thinking clearly and walk away

(C) Ask him to be more specific and report the results of this conversation to the charge nurse and attending physician

(D) Talk to family members about how they feel about his decision

10. An 84-year-old mother of six has been hospitalized after fracturing her hip. The incident caused a major setback in her independence, and she will no longer be able to manage her affairs. One of her sons has approached her about signing a durable power of attorney for health care, which would name him as having that authority. The nurse notices that he speaks to her rudely and in a manner that is a little threatening. The nurse first should:

(A) Encourage the mother to sign the document, assuring her everything will work out

(B) Speak to the mother privately about her concerns, if any, and preferences, and report the findings to the charge nurse and social worker in charge of her case

(C) Speak to the family members about the options available and leave it to them to decide

(D) Report the observations about the son to the charge nurse only

11. The Patient Self-Determination Act (PSDA) requires that:

(A) Patients make living wills when admitted to hospitals

(B) Healthcare providers receiving Medicare or Medicaid funds apprise patients of their right to make advance directives

(C) All inpatient facilities must provide special counselors to help patients fill out advance directives

(D) Nurses discuss living wills or healthcare proxies with any patient who is terminal

12. A landmark case in the area of life-ending treatment is the Cruzan case. This case involved the family's desire to end life-sustaining treatment for Nancy Cruzan, who was in a persistent vegetative state. The outcome of this US Supreme Court case was that the court:

(A) Would not allow the termination of life support because the patient was not competent and could not express her wishes

(B) Required that states have statutes in place before decisions like this could be made

(C) Stated that the US Constitution would grant a competent person a constitutionally protected right to terminate life-sustaining treatment and extended this to incompetent patients when consistent with the state statute's requirements

(D) Struck down the provision of the state statute that required "clear and convincing" evidence of the incompetent patient's wishes in such situations

13. Arguments that have been advanced against legalizing assisted suicide include all *except*:

    (A) Patients may be influenced by financial concerns to select this option
    (B) Medical personnel may make a mistaken diagnosis of a terminal condition
    (C) Disabled persons may be urged to die as a form of conserving resources
    (D) There has been no Supreme Court decision about the issues surrounding assisted suicide

14. A nurse is administering large doses of morphine to a terminally ill patient. The nurse is concerned that these actions may be considered assisted suicide. The law permits this intervention if:

    (A) The nurse has a physician's order that allows the nurse to set the patient's dosage of the morphine without any dosage parameters
    (B) The patient's family has requested this action
    (C) The nurse is implementing pain relief as a therapeutic intervention with no intent to harm the patient or cause his death
    (D) There is a statute permitting assisted suicide by physicians in the state

Part V Answers

1. *The answer is D.*

   Although talking to the physician may be in order, to give the patient the respect she deserves, a conversation with her is the first action. This recognizes the patient's autonomy and gives the nurse a chance to obtain information about the patient. Ultimately, the nurse will be able to draw upon that information when making ethical decisions. Giving her the medication in spite of the nurse's beliefs would be contrary to beneficence. Refusing to give the medication denies the patient's rights to autonomy and acts to create an adversarial, authoritarian relationship.

2. *The answer is D.*

   The nurse needs to comprehend this patient's level of understanding and can only do that by speaking with him. He may have unfounded fears about his health and prognosis that the nurse could help to correct and alleviate. Although the nurse's duty is to provide truthful information to all patients, to do so in this case could cause harm and therefore violate the principle of non-malfeasance. A specialized approach to each patient is necessary to give patients the respect they deserve.

3. *The answer is D.*

   The person whose conduct is questioned should be informed before other actions are taken. Specific facts and circum-

stances should be addressed, and the nurse should document these facts in personal notes. Answer C is a step that can be taken but with caution; the nurse does not want to appear to be influencing the opinion of others, and it is safest to inform the person first. Answer A would occur after the person is on notice but could occur shortly after this. Answer B may be necessary in some instances but would not be the first step.

4. *The answer is B.*

   The nurse risks disciplinary action by not reporting, based on the idea that the nurse is not protecting patients from potential harm. This is a serious unethical and illegal act that needs to follow all the steps for proper reporting of such incidents. Answer A is incorrect because these acts are not permitted even with prescriptive authority. Answer C is incorrect because actual harm does not have to be shown; placing patients at risk is enough. Answer D does not go far enough in taking definitive action to prevent harm.

5. *The answer is B.*

   This is the first response in this situation. One should also consider C, however. In spite of her drugged state, the patient has a right to be informed and educated about what is at stake. By ascertaining the comprehensive ability of the patient and relaying the risks and benefits to both herself and her baby, the nurse may provide her with enough information to at least make an informed refusal. Assuaging her fears regarding the surgery should be part of the information process as well. This should all be done in a noncoercive manner.

6. *The answer is C.*

The nurse needs to advise the patient, without emotion or coercion, of the effect of HIV on her unborn baby, with the hope that the information will encourage the mother to undergo the test for the sake of her child's health. The nurse should also inform the patient that most states mandate the reporting of positive AIDS test results. A and D fall below the standard of care, and B is incorrect because HIV testing of pregnant women is voluntary in a majority of states.

7. *The answer is C.*

A is incorrect because usually the ethics committees make the allocation determinations. Although it may be necessary for the treating physician to add medical input and answer quality-of-life questions, ethicists advise that the treating physician not be in the forefront of the decision because it may damage the physician–patient relationship, which is based on trust. B is incorrect because ethicists advise that patient's age not be considered. D is incorrect because ethically the patient's contribution to the disease should not be considered.

8. *The answer is B.*

Unless there is a court order to the contrary, the staff must continue to intubate the patient. The nurse could request a team meeting with the patient and family and an ethics committee review. A is incorrect because there is no indication

(even smoking) to declare incompetence, and even if he was incompetent, his guardian could seek medical care on his behalf, so the issue of futile care is not solved solely by this action. C is incorrect because the sequence is wrong (DNR status must be determined first). Furthermore, physicians must have a competent patient's agreement for DNR status (DNR status is a collaborative decision and not unilaterally done by a physician).

9. *The answer is C.*

If a patient makes a clear statement about an end-of-life decision, it needs to be taken seriously. Reporting his statement to the charge nurse and attending physician is required. Document the statement in the chart. Unless the patient has a history of suicidal tendencies or his prognosis is not deemed to be poor, discussion with the family is not the first action to take. He needs to be educated as to the mechanics of life-support systems and needs to be made aware of his options to withhold or discontinue one or all systems.

10. *The answer is B.*

The nurse's first obligation is to the patient. Assuming the patient is capable, the nurse must inform the patient of the options available (durable power of attorney for health care and living wills) and what signing these documents means to her care and ability to make decisions. The nurse needs to encourage the patient to be honest about her concerns, with assurances that anything said will be held in confidence from those whose interests may be affected. Reporting the incident to the charge nurse is necessary, but the nurse's responsibility does not stop there. An assessment of the patient's capacity is also necessary. This should be pointed out to the physician as well.

11. *The answer is B.*

    Any healthcare provider who receives these federal funds must provide information to individuals about the laws that govern advance directives (living wills or healthcare proxies or agents) in their state. The PSDA does not create these rights but refers to patients and others being informed of the rights under these state statutes. Answer A is incorrect because there is no requirement that a patient complete an advance directive. Answer C is incorrect because it is often healthcare personnel (nurses, social workers, etc.) who implement the PSDA. Answer D is incorrect because there is no requirement that nurses do this, although often it is the nurse who provides this information. Also it applies to all patients, not just those who are terminally ill.

12. *The answer is C.*

    The court upheld the state statute that required "clear and convincing" evidence of the incompetent's wishes while finding a constitutional right to terminate life-sustaining nutrition and hydration. Answer A is incorrect because the right was extended to incompetent patients while upholding states' rights to implement standards for determining the incompetent's wishes. Answer B is incorrect because statutes are not required by states.

Answer D is incorrect because the "clear and convincing" standard required by the state statute was upheld by the Court.

13. *The answer is D.*

    This is not one of the arguments against assisted suicide because the Supreme Court has decided that there is no constitutional right to assisted suicide. However, the door was left open to let states deal with the issue with the possibility that a statute could be upheld in the future. Answers A, B, and C contain reasons that have been advanced for possible abuse of any legalized assisted suicide law.

14. *The answer is C.*

    The nurse is clearly within legal and ethical boundaries if there is no intent to cause the patient's death and the medication is being administered to provide for pain relief. Answer A is incorrect because the order would not be valid if it permitted the nurse to adjust the dosage without dosage parameters. Answer D is incorrect because even if there is a statute, the nurse would not be allowed to implement this because the statement says this is permitted for physicians. B is incorrect because this must be done with a physician order to relieve pain, not hasten death. Dosage should be set at the minimum to relieve pain.

Basic Legal Research

Susan J. Clerc

Nurses are increasingly exposed to information about the law and legal processes in professional literature and within the healthcare environment. Guidelines presented in this section will help you find, read, use, and cite authoritative legal references.

■ HOW TO READ A LEGAL CITATION

Citations that are frequently encountered in legal research refer to case law, statutes, or regulations. These citations are part of a uniform system of citation for legal references.

Case Law

Cases are published in book sets called *reporters*. Each set has an abbreviation, and you can find dictionaries of the abbreviations online by typing words like "law citation abbreviations" into a search engine. Your local library might have a copy of *The Standard System of American Legal Citation*, usually referred to as the "Blue Book," the standard source for legal citation.

Cases are often published in several places simultaneously. One, some, or all of these might be included in a citation. The official

reporter is listed first, and that's really the only one you need. If a case is very recent, it might not have an official citation yet and will have a docket number instead.

The citation of a case tells you the case name, whether it's a federal or state case, and the date it was decided. Some citation styles put the decision date at the end and others put it after the name of the case.

Figure A-1 illustrates the citation for a Supreme Court case showing the parallel citations.

The case *Cruzan v. Director, Missouri Dept. of Health* is a US Supreme Court case decided in 1990. The case is published in volume 497 of *U.S. Reports,* beginning on page 261. The case is also published in volume 110 of *Supreme Court Reporter* beginning on page 2841 and in volume 111 of *Lawyer's Edition 2nd Series* beginning on page 224.

Federal Court of Appeals, also referred to as Circuit Court, cases are published in *Federal Reporter* (F., F.2d, F.3d). Federal District Court cases are published in *Federal Supplement* (F. Supp.).

People v. Kevorkian was a Michigan Supreme Court case decided in 1994 and is published in volume 447 of *Michigan Reports*, beginning

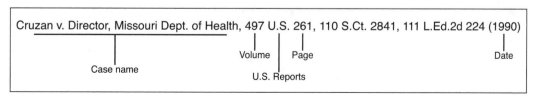

Figure A-1

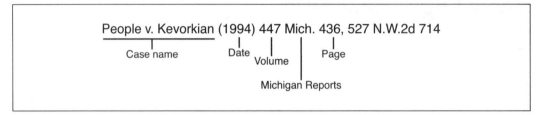

Figure A-2

on page 436 (see **Figure A-2**). It also appears in volume 527 of West's *Northwest Reporter 2nd Series*, beginning on page 714.

Statutes and Regulations

The examples in **Figure A-3** tell you where to find the Americans with Disabilities Act (ADA), a federal statute, in three different sources.

The first example is a Public Law. The first number is the Congress, the second is the order in which the law was passed; 101-336 is the 336th law passed by the 101st Congress.

The second example is a *Statutes at Large* citation. At the end of each Congress, Public Laws are published in *Statutes at Large* in the order they were passed. The ADA begins on page 327 of *Statutes at Large* volume 104.

The third example is for the *U.S. Code* (U.S.C.), the subject arrangement of all the current laws of the United States. Each subject area is called a title (e.g., Public Welfare is Title 42, Labor is Title 29, etc.), and one title can comprise several physical volumes. Be aware that public laws are often divided and distrib-

uted among titles depending on the content. For example, most of the ADA is in Title 42, but some sections are in Title 47 and Title 29.

If you want to see the text of a law as it was passed, look for the Public Law or the *Statutes at Large* citation. The *U.S. Code* is the law as it currently exists, including amendments since it first passed into law.

State statutes follow the same pattern of publication: public law or act, session laws similar to *Statutes at Large*, then subject codification in the state code.

States vary on how statute citations are written, but many use an abbreviation for the state code followed by a section number, while others include a chapter or title number (see **Figure A-4**).

Regulations are the rules formulated by agencies to implement the broader statutes. Federal regulations are published in the *Code of Federal Regulations* (C.F.R.), which is organized by titles and sections, like the U.S.C. Citations for state regulations vary; some look like state statute citations while others look like the C.F.R. and U.S.C. model (see **Figure A-5**).

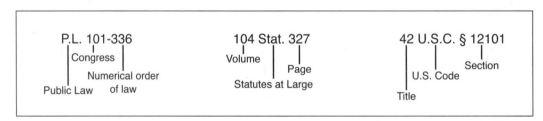

Figure A-3

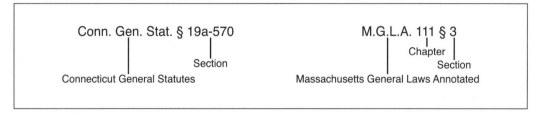

Figure A-4

■ HOW TO SEARCH

Searches are most often done using computer-based methods. This yields the most current and readily available information. As you begin, the more you know about a topic or issue before you search, the easier it will be to find what you're looking for.

Try looking for newspaper or magazine articles before you look for the text of an opinion, statute, or regulation. Not only will the information you find help you in your search, but articles often provide analysis and context that explain the significance of the law.

The most valuable information you can have before starting a search is the citation because it is unique. If you don't have a citation, get as many of the following pieces of information as you can before searching a database or Web site:

- Is it a case, a statute, or a regulation?
- Is it federal or state?
- If it's a state case or law, which state?
- What is the name of the case, or the name of at least one party to the case? If it's a statute, was there a popular name

like PATRIOT Act or No Child Left Behind Act?
- What year was the case decided or statute passed?
- What was the legal issue?

Regardless of what electronic database or search engine you decide to use, read the directions. Every database has unique features. For example, sometimes you need to put quotation marks around a phrase to search it as a phrase instead of individual words (e.g., "penal code" versus penal and code).

You will always receive multiple hits of cited references in your result list. Cases go through several courts, parties may join or leave the case, etc. Every time an event impacts the case, a new document is generated. There is no perfect way to determine which item in your result list is the one you are searching for; you will need to look at each of them. A general guideline, especially for Supreme Court cases: If it's long, it's the one you're looking for.

Remember that there are unpublished cases, and those are ones you won't find. For example, if the initial case was a jury trial,

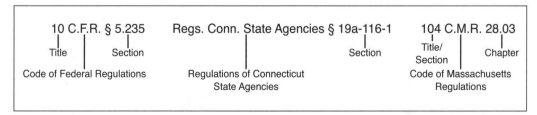

Figure A-5

you're better off looking for newspaper reports that tell you the verdict than wasting your time in a database. If the verdict was appealed, you can probably find the appellate case.

For explanations of legal concepts, landmark cases, and other law-related matters, use an encyclopedia or other reference book. *West's Guide to American Law* is written in plain English, meant for laypeople, and can be found in most public libraries. You should also be able to find several reference books about landmark cases—ask the reference librarian. If you're reasonably conversant in legalese, *American Jurisprudence (AmJur)* and *American Law Reports (ALR)* are options. Both are available online in *Westlaw Campus Research*. Law libraries will have the print versions. *AmJur* has briefer entries, while *ALR* aims to be comprehensive.

■ WHERE TO SEARCH

Find a public library, community college, or state university near you that has *LexisNexis Academic Research* or *Westlaw Campus Research*. These are college versions of the databases that law firms and law schools use and are only available in libraries. State colleges are open to the community, although they usually place some limits on access. Don't be afraid to ask. Both of these databases provide a depth and breadth of material not available on public access Web sites, and they also provide a lot of cross-linking—if you're reading a case and want to see the statutory authority, you click on the link and the statute appears. Both of them also include

indicators of whether the material is still good law. Finally, and most importantly, if you go to a library, a librarian will help you.

There are several publicly accessible Web sites you can use, too, including FindLaw (http://lp.findlaw.com), Justia (http://www.justia.com), and Public Library of Law (http://www.plol.org). Both FindLaw and Public Library of Law require registration (it's free) before displaying results. You can also use individual state pages to locate statutes and regulations, and individual Courts' Web pages for recent opinions. For example, the Connecticut General Assembly Web site is found at http://www.cga.ct.gov; the US Supreme Court's Web site is at http://www.supremecourtus.gov.

Table A-1 is a chart that indicates what material the two commercial publishers and three of the public Web sites have.

■ READING A CASE FOUND ONLINE

All of the Web sites or databases in Table A-1 display results differently, but the official language of the opinion, statute, or regulation remains the same regardless of where you find it.

Figures A-6 through A-9 (found on pages 306–309) are examples of the same Supreme Court case—*Scheidler v. National Organization for Women*, 537 U.S. 393 (2003)—as it appears on the Supreme Court's Web site and in *Westlaw Campus Research*.

Other federal and state cases look slightly different, but they will always include the official language of the opinion, the concurring opinion(s), and the dissent(s), as well as the date and holding.

Table A–1   Comparison of Legal Reference Sources

US Supreme Court	All	All	1893+	All	1892+
US Court of Appeals	Yes. Coverage may vary by Circuit	1891+	1995/6 for most Courts with some older, and links to other sites	1950+	Yes. Dates may vary by Circuit
US District Courts	Yes. Coverage may vary by District	1789+	Links to District Court Web sites	2004+	No
US Code	Subject search	Subject search	Subject search	Title links	Link to House of Representatives U.S.C. page
C.F.R.	Subject search	Subject search	Subject search	Title links	Link to GPOAccess C.F.R. page
State Supreme Courts	Yes	Yes	Yes. Dates vary	No	1997+
State Appeals Courts	Yes	Yes	Yes. Dates vary	No	Yes
State Trial Courts	Yes	Yes	No	No	No
State Codes	Yes	Yes	Links to outside sources	Yes	Links to outside sources
State Regulations	Yes	Yes	Links to outside sources	No	Links to state pages

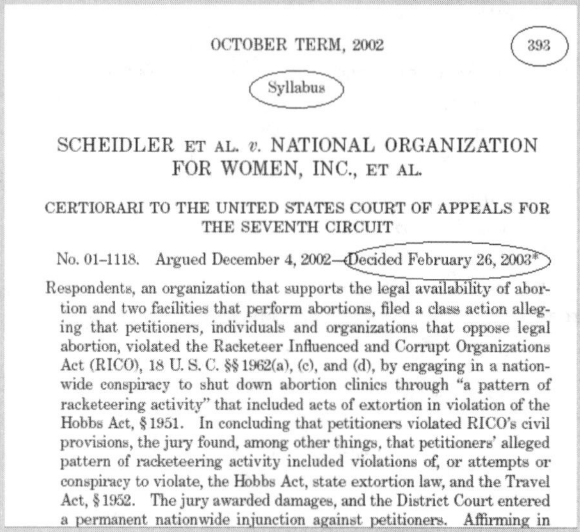

OCTOBER TERM, 2002

393

Syllabus

SCHEIDLER ET AL. *v.* NATIONAL ORGANIZATION FOR WOMEN, INC., ET AL.

CERTIORARI TO THE UNITED STATES COURT OF APPEALS FOR THE SEVENTH CIRCUIT

No. 01–1118.   Argued December 4, 2002—Decided February 26, 2003*

Respondents, an organization that supports the legal availability of abortion and two facilities that perform abortions, filed a class action alleging that petitioners, individuals and organizations that oppose legal abortion, violated the Racketeer Influenced and Corrupt Organizations Act (RICO), 18 U. S. C. §§ 1962(a), (c), and (d), by engaging in a nationwide conspiracy to shut down abortion clinics through "a pattern of racketeering activity" that included acts of extortion in violation of the Hobbs Act, § 1951.   In concluding that petitioners violated RICO's civil provisions, the jury found, among other things, that petitioners' alleged pattern of racketeering activity included violations of, or attempts or conspiracy to violate, the Hobbs Act, state extortion law, and the Travel Act, § 1952.   The jury awarded damages, and the District Court entered a permanent nationwide injunction against petitioners.   Affirming in

This is the page from *U.S. Reports* as displayed on the Supreme Court's Web site. Some public access Web sites (like FindLaw) use a similar display. Notice the page number in the upper right hand corner. This case is 537 U.S. 393.

The Syllabus is a summary provided in the Reporter. It's repeated wherever you find the case, but is not part of the official opinion.

After the name of the case, you'll see the date it was argued and the date it was decided.

Figure A-6

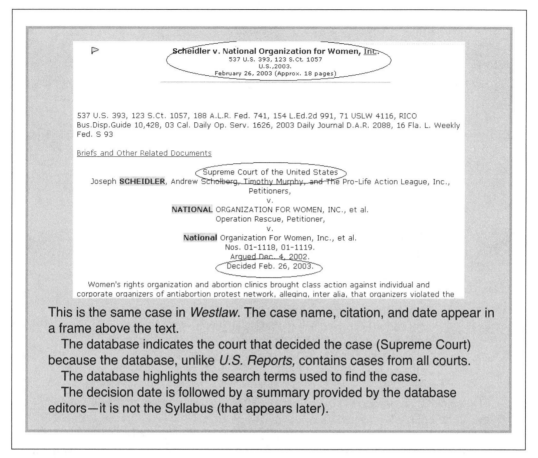

This is the same case in *Westlaw.* The case name, citation, and date appear in a frame above the text.

The database indicates the court that decided the case (Supreme Court) because the database, unlike *U.S. Reports,* contains cases from all courts.

The database highlights the search terms used to find the case.

The decision date is followed by a summary provided by the database editors—it is not the Syllabus (that appears later).

Figure A-7

Cite as: 537 U. S. 393 (2003)   397

Opinion of the Court

CHIEF JUSTICE REHNQUIST delivered the opinion of the Court.

We granted certiorari in these cases to answer two questions. First, whether petitioners committed extortion within the meaning of the Hobbs Act, 18 U. S. C. § 1951. Second, whether respondents, as private litigants, may obtain injunctive relief in a civil action pursuant to 18 U. S. C. § 1964 of the Racketeer Influenced and Corrupt Organizations Act (RICO). We hold that petitioners did not commit extortion because they did not "obtain" property from respondents as required by the Hobbs Act. We further hold that our determination with respect to extortion under the Hobbs Act renders insufficient the other bases or predicate acts of racketeering supporting the jury's conclusion that petitioners violated RICO. Therefore, we reverse without reaching the question of the availability of private injunctive relief under § 1964(c) of RICO.

The official opinion doesn't begin until p. 397. Preceding it are the Syllabus and the list of counsel.

Notice that the official citation is provided at the top of every page.

Before the opinion, you would also see the list of concurring and dissenting opinions. Opinions always appear in this order: majority opinion, concurring opinion(s), dissenting opinion(s). Some cases only have a majority opinion.

Figure A-8

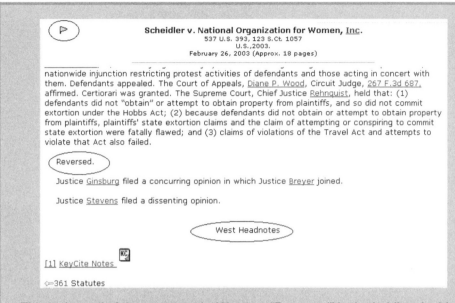

This is the end of the summary in *Westlaw*. "Reversed" is the holding. In this case, the Supreme Court reversed the decision of the Court of Appeals. You might also see Affirmed, or Reversed and remanded (sent back to the lower court for further action).

Westlaw and *Lexis Nexis* both insert Headnotes between the summary and the beginning of the Syllabus. Both databases use the notes as a way of linking cases on similar points of law.

The yellow flag in the upper left hand corner is a link to the case history—other cases that have cited Scheidler and how they treated it.

This is the beginning of the opinion in *Westlaw*. Notice that the language is exactly the same as in the example above.

Westlaw and *Lexis Nexis* both provide the pagination of the printed case. The opinion begins on p. 397 in *U.S. Reports.* The other number, 1062, refers to *Supreme Court Reporter,* the print equivalent of *Westlaw.*

Figure A-9

Index

U

unconsciousness, permanent, 282
undue hardship, definition of, 218
unions, 191–192, 204–205
United American Nurses (UAN), 204–205
United Network for Organ Sharing (UNOS), 132, 135–136
unlicensed assistive personnel (UAP)
  definition of, 45*f*
  delegation to, 25, 45–51
  failure to supervise, 49–50

V

Vacco v. Quill, 289, 290–291
veracity, ethical decision making and, 258*f*
verdicts, 5
violence. *See also* abuse
  community, 240
  documentation of, 241
  family, definition of, 114
  against nurses, 238*f*, 239–240

against patients, 238–239, 238*f*
  risk management and, 241
vulnerable adults
  abuse of, 115–116
  definition of, 115

W

Washington v. Glucksberg, 289
whistle-blowing statutes, 204, 263–265, 267–268
Williams v. West Virginia Board of Examiners, 49–50
Winkelman v. Beloit Memorial Hospital, 214–215
witnesses. *See also* expert witnesses, nurses as; testimony
  nurses as, 28–31
workers' compensation, 187
  civil actions and, 12
workplace(s)
  hostile, 234
  safety, 192–193
  sexual harassment in, 233–237
  violence, 238–241